Malarial Subjects

Malaria was considered one of the most widespread disease-causing entities in the nineteenth century. It was associated with a variety of frailties far beyond fevers, ranging from idiocy to impotence. And yet, it was not a self-contained category. The reconsolidation of malaria as a diagnostic category during this period happened within a wider context in which cinchona plants and their most valuable extract, quinine, were reinforced as objects of natural knowledge and social control. In India, the exigencies and apparatuses of British imperial rule occasioned the close interactions between these histories. In the process, British imperial rule became entangled with a network of nonhumans that included, apart from cinchona plants and the drug quinine, a range of objects described as malarial, as well as mosquitoes. *Malarial Subjects* explores this history of the co-constitution of a cure and disease, of British colonial rule and nonhumans, and of science, medicine and empire. This title is also available as Open Access.

ROHAN DEB ROY is Lecturer in South Asian History at the University of Reading. He received his PhD from University College London, and has held postdoctoral fellowships at the Centre for Studies in Social Sciences Calcutta, at the University of Cambridge, and at the Max Planck Institute for the History of Science in Berlin. He has been a Barnard-Columbia Weiss International Visiting Scholar in the History of Science.

SCIENCE IN HISTORY

Series Editors

Simon J. Schaffer, University of Cambridge

James A. Secord, University of Cambridge

Science in History is a major series of ambitious books on the history of the sciences from the mid-eighteenth century through the mid-twentieth century, highlighting work that interprets the sciences from perspectives drawn from across the discipline of history. The focus on the major epoch of global economic, industrial and social transformations is intended to encourage the use of sophisticated historical models to make sense of the ways in which the sciences have developed and changed. The series encourages the exploration of a wide range of scientific traditions and the interrelations between them. It particularly welcomes work that takes seriously the material practices of the sciences and is broad in geographical scope.

Malarial Subjects

Empire, Medicine and Nonhumans in British India, 1820–1909

Rohan Deb Roy

University of Reading

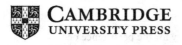

CAMBRIDGE
UNIVERSITY PRESS

CAMBRIDGE
UNIVERSITY PRESS

University Printing House, Cambridge CB2 8BS, United Kingdom

One Liberty Plaza, 20th Floor, New York, NY 10006, USA

477 Williamstown Road, Port Melbourne, VIC 3207, Australia

314-321, 3rd Floor, Plot 3, Splendor Forum, Jasola District Centre, New Delhi - 110025, India

79 Anson Road, #06-04/06, Singapore 079906

Cambridge University Press is part of the University of Cambridge.

It furthers the University's mission by disseminating knowledge in the pursuit of education, learning and research at the highest international levels of excellence.

www.cambridge.org
Information on this title: www.cambridge.org/9781316623619

DOI: 10.1017/9781316771617

First published 2017
First paperback edition 2019

A catalogue record for this publication is available from the British Library

ISBN 978-1-107-17236-4 Hardback
ISBN 978-1-316-62361-9 Paperback

Cambridge University Press has no responsibility for the persistence or accuracy of URLs for external or third-party internet websites referred to in this publication, and does not guarantee that any content on such websites is, or will remain, accurate or appropriate.

For Joyasree and Amitabha Deb Roy

Contents

Illustrations

Acknowledgements

This book was conceived in Calcutta, developed in London, reconceptualised and rewritten in Cambridge and Berlin, and ultimately completed in Reading. It has taken me more than ten years. I am deeply indebted to many institutions and individuals. The Wellcome Trust Centre for the History of Medicine at University College London awarded me a three-year doctoral studentship (2005) as well as the Roy Porter Prize (2006), which enabled me to put together my doctoral dissertation. I have since then held postdoctoral fellowships at the Centre for Studies in Social Sciences Calcutta (2009–2010), at the Department of History and Philosophy of Science at the University of Cambridge (2011–2013), and at the Max Planck Institute for the History of Science in Berlin (2013–2015). A generous Medical History and Humanities grant from the Wellcome Trust (ref. 091630/Z/10/Z) supported my time in Cambridge. I am also grateful to the Governing Body of Christ's College, Cambridge, for including me as a postdoctoral affiliate. I spent a part of the fall of 2012 in New York as the Barnard-Columbia Weiss International Visiting Scholar in the History of Science. I thank colleagues in these different institutions for their support while I was working on this book.

My teachers in Calcutta have inspired me, ever since I was an undergraduate, to pursue professional research. Subhas Ranjan Chakraborty and Rajat Kanta Ray at Presidency College, and Bhaskar Chakrabarty, Shireen Maswood, Madhumita Majumdar and Samita Sen at the University of Calcutta exposed me to the various predicaments of South Asian history. I was introduced to interdisciplinary research when I was a student at the Research and Training Programme at the Centre for Studies in Social Sciences Calcutta. The courses offered by Sibaji Bandyopadhyay, Gautam Bhadra, Pradip Bose, Partha Chatterjee, Rosinka Chaudhari, Tapati Guha-Thakurta, Janaki Nair, Manas Ray and Lakshmi Subramanian continue to inform my work. The last ten years have witnessed my own transition from a student to a faculty member. I thank my colleagues at the Department of History at the University of Reading for setting exemplary standards of collegiality.

I am grateful to Lucy Rhymer, Commissioning Editor at the Cambridge University Press, as well as the two anonymous readers for their insights and incisive suggestions. Simon Schaffer and Jim Secord included this book as part of the Science in History series, and along with Lucy, oversaw the transition of the draft manuscript into a book. I can never thank them enough. Sanjoy Bhattacharya (my supportive PhD supervisor) and David Arnold, Partha Chatterjee, Anne Hardy, Mark Harrison and Peter Robb commented extensively on a full draft of my doctoral dissertation, and in so doing, inspired its substantial recasting. Deborah Coen, Angela Creager, James Delbourgo, Cathy Gere, Philipp Lehmann and Sujit Sivasundaram offered crucial suggestions on the introductory chapter. Bodhisattva Kar, Chitra Ramalingam and Pratik Chakrabarti devoted their precious time in commenting on a chapter each. Megan Barford, James Hall and James Poskett read multiple drafts of different parts of the manuscript, and I am especially grateful to them. I thank the generous staff at the Asiatic Society, the National Library, and the West Bengal State Archives in Calcutta, the National Archives of India in New Delhi, the British Library, London Metropolitan Archives and the Wellcome Library in London, and the Whipple Library, the Centre for South Asian Studies library and the University Library in Cambridge for all their help. Without the support of Ashim Mukhopadhyay and Kashshaf Ghani, my research at the Asiatic Society and at the National Library would have remained incomplete. Kamalika Mukherjee and Abhijit Bhattacharya shared with me their unique knowledge of the archives at the Centre for Studies in Social Sciences in Calcutta. Apurba Podder and Will Acquino helped this technologically challenged historian with the preliminary formatting of the manuscript.

Parts of Chapter 3 were published in Saurabh Dube (ed.) *Modern Makeovers: The Oxford Handbook of Modernity in South Asia,* (New Delhi: Oxford University Press, 2011). An earlier version of Chapter 5 was published as 'Quinine, Mosquitoes and Empire: Reassembling Malaria in British India, 1890–1910' in *South Asian History and Culture,* 4.1 (January 2013). I thank the editors and anonymous readers for their critical feedback.

I am particularly grateful to Deborah Coen and Sujit Sivasundaram for their intellectual generosity. I thank Ishita Banerjee-Dube, Chris Bayly, Dipesh Chakrabarty, Supriya Chaudhuri, Hal Cook, Roger Cooter, Joya Chatterji, Lorraine Daston, Faisal Devji, Saurabh Dube, Sven Dupre, Shruti Kapila, Joan Landes, Veronika Lipphardt, Hugh Raffles, Anupama Rao, Biswajit Ray, Anne Secord, David Sepkoski, Sonu

Shamdasani, Emma Spary and John Harley Warner for their encouraging comments and incisive suggestions.

My fellow-travellers Siraj Ahmed, Guy Attewell, Jenny Bangham, Sharmadip Basu, Varuni Bhatia, Moinak Biswas, Prasanta Chakravarty, Teri Chettiar, Anirban Das, Rajarshi Dasgupta, Rohit De, Rajarshi Ghose, Bodhisattva Kar, Nayanika Mathur, Durba Mitra, Hannah Newton, Surabhi Ranganathan, Utsa Ray, Shrimoy Roy Chaudhury, Jonathan Saha, Uditi Sen, Michael Stanley-Baker and Sanjukta Sunderason set inspiring standards of scholarly integrity and imagination. While pursuing their own exciting works, Atig Ghosh, Sukanya Sarbadhikary, Anandaroop Sen, Kaustubhmani Sengupta and especially Upal Chakrabarti welcomed me during my visits to New Delhi. I am always indebted to them for their warmth and affection.

Urmimala Ghosh and Sreecheta Das, and Rekha and Amal Bhowmick provided me a home in Calcutta on innumerable occasions when the manuscript was being researched, written and revised. I hoped to write an engaging book that Samar Das would have appreciated! My grandfather, M. L. Deb, almost reached a hundred years hoping to see my book in print, before giving up all too suddenly. I thank Rinki Deb Ray and Pradip Bhowmick for being there for me.

Joyasree and Amitabha Deb Roy are amongst my very best friends. I am privileged to have them as my parents: A cliché has never been truer! I am following in their footsteps by pursuing academic research and teaching. All along, they have quietly and wholeheartedly supported me. This book is dedicated to them. Shinjini Das has endured a quinine-bitter-half over the past decade, while developing her own research and career in South Asian history. For her companionship, patience and invaluable perspectives that have enriched me, and this project, I say: Thank you!

Abbreviations

BL	British Library, London
BMJ	British Medical Journal
CSSSC	Centre for Studies in Social Sciences, Calcutta Archives
Economic-Products	Economic Products Branch
Finance, Miscellaneous	Financial Department, Miscellaneous Branch
General, General	General Department, General Branch
General, Industry-Science	General Department, Industry and Science Branch
General, Medical	General Department, Medical Branch
General, Miscellaneous	General Department, Miscellaneous Branch
General, Sanitation	General Department, Sanitation Branch
Home, Jails	Home Department, Jails Branch
Home, Medical	Home Department, Medical Branch
Home, Patents	Home Department, Patents Branch
Home, Port Blair	Home Department, Port Blair Branch
Home, Public	Home Department, Public Branch
Home, Sanitary	Home Department, Sanitary Branch
IMG	Indian Medical Gazette
LMA	London Metropolitan Archives
Municipal, Medical	Municipal Department, Medical Branch
Municipal, Sanitation	Municipal Department, Sanitation Branch
NAI	National Archives of India
NL	National Library, Calcutta
Political, Medical	Political Department, Medical Branch
Prog.	Proceedings
Rev-agriculture	Revenue and Agriculture Department

Rev-agriculture, Agriculture	Revenue and Agriculture Department, Agriculture Branch
Rev-agriculture, Famine	Revenue and Agriculture Department, Famine Branch
Rev-agriculture, Forests	Revenue and Agriculture Department, Forests Branch
WBSA	West Bengal State Archives, Calcutta
WL	Wellcome Library, London

Introduction
Side Effects of Empire

Malaria remains one of the indelible hallmarks of the postcolonial world. It is also a trope through which various communities identify themselves. Today, malaria continues to dominate agendas of the World Health Organization, multinational philanthropy, research in tropical medicine, electoral politics, medical journalism and governance. In recent decades, novelists have appropriated malaria as a central problematic of anti-realist fiction[1] or have mentioned the presence of anti-malarial drugs in the traveller's kit as an indicator of persisting western psychoses about erstwhile British colonies.[2] Malaria is also considered to be a signifier of the limits of postcolonial modernity, development and democracy. This is most evident in contemporary India, where reports have described malaria as an endemic agent, shaping the encounters between Maoist insurgents and state-endorsed paramilitary forces in the interiors.[3]

In recent years, malaria has been acknowledged to be a globally relevant disease, which shaped the patterns of a variety of world historical processes: human settlements in Ancient Rome, the European colonisation of the 'New World', the demography of agrarian England, nationalist reconstructions and ethnic conflicts in the twentieth century, and the Cold War. Many historians have engaged with contemporary medical science to explain malarial outbreaks in the wider non-European world in the nineteenth and twentieth centuries in terms of social inequalities, racial degenerations, poverty, hunger, water stagnation and ill-conceived

---

[1] A. Ghosh, *The Calcutta Chromosome: A Novel of Fevers, Delirium and Discovery* (New Delhi: Ravi Dayal Publishers, 1996).

[2] A. Roy, *The God of Small Things* (London: Flamingo, 1997), 266.

[3] Special Correspondent, 'Maoist Link to Malaria', *The Telegraph* (Thursday, October 29, 2009), www.telegraphindia.com/1091029/jsp/frontpage/story_11672759.jsp [retrieved on 24 March 2014]; S. Ravi, 'Indian Police fighting Maoists "dying of malaria"', BBC (Tuesday, 23 February 2010), http://news.bbc.co.uk/1/hi/world/south_asia/8529615.stm [retrieved on 24 March 2014].

and carelessly implemented government projects.[4] Twentieth-century (or even more recent) scientific understandings of malaria have been invoked to diagnose mortalities and to analyse events in earlier centuries.[5] Other kinds of scholarship have situated efforts to eradicate malaria within the social histories of newly consolidated nation-states, as well as global geopolitics.[6]

Rather than taking scientific medicine as an explanatory frame, this book aims to explain the processes through which scientific medical knowledge about malaria itself was put together. It extends the premise that medical or scientific knowledge has been a product of contingent historical processes.[7] To understand the widespread significance of malaria in the contemporary world, many recent books have examined the history of malaria in the twentieth century.[8] Instead, I focus on the long nineteenth century, and explore the intellectual, cultural and political histories of the ways in which the category was reconsolidated and sustained as an object of natural knowledge and social control. The nineteenth century deserves more scholarly attention, in its own right, as a

[4] See, for example, A. Samanta, *Malarial Fever in Colonial Bengal, 1820–1939: Social History of an Epidemic* (Kolkata: Firma KLM, 2002); M. Humphreys, *Malaria: Poverty, Race and Public Health in the United States* (Baltimore: Johns Hopkins University Press, 2001), 3, 8, 68; R. M. Packard, *The Making of a Tropical Disease: A Short History of Malaria* (Baltimore: Johns Hopkins University Press, 2007), 13, 19–35, 249–250; K. Yip (ed), *Disease, Colonialism and the State: Malaria in Modern East Asian History* (Hong Kong: Hong Kong University Press, 2009).

[5] R. Sallares, *Malaria and Rome: A History of Malaria in Ancient Italy* (Oxford: Oxford University Press, 2002); Packard, *The Making of a Tropical Disease*, 17–35; J. L. A. Webb Jr, *Humanity's Burden: A Global History of Malaria* (Cambridge: Cambridge University Press, 2008), 32–49; J. R. McNeill, *Mosquito Empires: Ecology and War in the Greater Caribbean* (Cambridge: Cambridge University Press, 2010).

[6] F. M. Snowden, *The Conquest of Malaria, Italy 1900–1962* (New Haven: Yale University Press, 2006); M. Cueto, *Cold War, Deadly Fevers: Malaria Eradication in Mexico, 1955–1975* (Baltimore: Johns Hopkins University Press, 2007).

[7] I particularly draw upon research which has hinted at how historical insights about malaria since the early twentieth century were shaped by colonial discourses about race and civilisation, questions of nationalism and ethnicity, and the liaisons between warfare and industry. See for example, S. M. Sufian, *Healing the Land and the Nation: Malaria and the Zionist Project in Palestine, 1920–1947*, (Chicago and London: University of Chicago Press, 2007); L. B. Slater, *War and Disease: Biomedical Research on Malaria on the Twentieth Century* (New Brunswick: Rutgers University Press, 2009); W. Anderson, *Colonial Pathologies: American Tropical Medicine, Race and Hygiene in the Philippines*, (Durham: Duke University Press, 2006), 207–225; D. Arnold, '"An ancient race outworn": Malaria and Race in Colonial India, 1860–1930', in W. Ernst and B. Harris (eds), *Race, Science, Medicine, 1700–1960* (London and New York: Routledge, 1999), 122–143; M. Harrison, '"Hot beds of disease": Malaria and Civilisation in Nineteenth-Century British India', *Parassitologia*, 40 (1998), 11–18.

[8] For example, Snowden, *The Conquest of Malaria*; Sufian, *Healing the Land and the Nation*; Slater, *War and Disease*; Cueto, *Cold War, Deadly Fevers*; J. L. A. Webb Jr, *The Long Struggle Against Malaria in Tropical Africa* (Cambridge: Cambridge University Press, 2014).

significant phase in the history of malaria, rather than being treated as a period characterised by flawed archaic understandings about the disease, which would be rectified eventually in course of the next century.[9] Embarking on this project, I soon realised that malaria was perceived as amongst the most active and commodious disease-causing entities during much of the century. It was associated with a variety of debilities far beyond fevers, ranging from idiocy to impotence. Malaria was not a self-contained category. Rather, malaria was co-constituted with political discourses and practices relating to a network of plants, events, places, drugs and insects. Nor were narratives about malaria confined within nationally bounded geographies or the territorial units reified by area studies. British India, the focus of this book, was an integral part of an interconnected world in which malaria, cinchona plants, the drug quinine (extracted from cinchona barks) and subsequently mosquitoes were co-constituted.

In exploring the makings and persistence of malaria as an enduring diagnostic category, I have drawn upon particular strands within constructivist histories of science and medicine, and historical epistemology, more generally.[10] Invoking the vocabulary common to these overlapping genres of scholarship, this book analyses how malaria, cinchonas, quinine and mosquitoes were co-produced, maintained and repaired as prepackaged, self-evident, ready-made and black-boxed categories in British India.[11] But such an analysis needs to be combined with a

---

[9] Existing books on the history of malaria in the nineteenth century include the 1940s classic E. H. Ackerknecht, *Malaria in the Upper Mississippi Valley, 1760–1900* (Baltimore: The Johns Hopkins Press, 1945). Paul Winther's *Anglo-European Science and the Rhetoric of Empire: Malaria, Opium and British Rule in India, 1756–1895* (Oxford: Lexington Books, 2005) provides a close reading of the various findings of the Royal Commission on Opium of 1894 on the status of opium as an anti-malarial. Chapter 3 of this book adopts an alternative approach while building on Arabinda Samanta's important work *Malarial Fever in Colonial Bengal.*

[10] These different approaches have in common their shared critique of scientific determinism. For an engaging commentary on constructivism see J. Golinsky, *Making Natural Knowledge: Constructivism and the History of Science* (Chicago and London: University of Chicago Press, 2005). For historical epistemology see L. Daston, 'Historical Epistemology', in J. Chandler, A. I. Davidson and H. Harootunian (eds.), *Questions of Evidence: Proof, Practice and Persuasion Across the Disciplines,* (Chicago and London: University of Chicago Press, 1994), 282–289.

[11] For knowledge as an object of maintenance and repair see B. Latour, 'Whose Cosmos, Which Cosmopolitics? Comments on the Peace Terms of Ulrich Beck', *Common Knowledge* 10, 3 (2004), 459; for 'prepackaged' see, L. Daston, 'Science Studies and the History of Science', *Critical Inquiry* 35, 4 (Summer 2009),807, 811; for a critique of the 'self-evident method' in the histories of science, see S. Shapin and S. Schaffer, *Leviathan and Air Pump: Hobbes, Boyle and the Experimental Life* (New Jersey: Princeton University Press, 1985), 4–13. For a broader conceptualisation on self-evidence see S. Schaffer, 'Self Evidence', in Chandler, Davidson and Harootunian (eds), *Questions*

historiography that has exposed the overlapping trajectories of modernity and empire.[12] Indeed, the entrenchment of integrated regimes of modernity and empire since the late eighteenth century necessitated the proliferation of categories of rule and knowledge. Such categories have over time appeared legitimate, commonsense, credible, foundational and even universal across the expanses of the colonial world and beyond. The stories explaining the making and naturalisation of these categories, it has been suggested, might reveal 'the ambivalences, the contradictions, the use of force, and the tragedies and the ironies' that have attended the histories of modern empires.[13] An eclectic range of such categories, from the economic[14] to the primitives,[15] or indeed population,[16] were historically produced or remade in a variety of conjunctures engendered by modern empires and their legacies both within Europe and its colonies. Like many of these categories and processes, the circulation of words like malaria, quinine and cinchona was augmented in post-Enlightenment Europe and Victorian and Edwardian England. In the course of the nineteenth century, these were reconfigured as natural, inevitable and relevant in distant corners of the British Empire. The predicaments of the wider colonial world in turn reshaped and sustained them, while also redefining the ways in which these were understood in Europe itself.

Malaria established itself as a recurrent category amongst government officials in British India and other parts of the colonial world by the third quarter of the century. Its status as a valid and credible category was seldom in doubt within the bureaucracy even as its meanings and physical characteristics were upheld as imprecise, fluid and contentious. Various commentators considered malaria simultaneously as familiar and

---

of Evidence, 56–91. For 'black box' and 'readymade science' see B. Latour, *Science in Action: How to Follow Scientists and Engineers through Society* (Cambridge, Mass.: Harvard University Press, 1987), 2–4.

[12] For an elaboration of the overlaps between modernity and empire, see for example S. Dube, 'Terms that Bind: Colony, Nation, Modernity', in S. Dube (ed), *Postcolonial Passages: Contemporary History-writing on India* (New Delhi: Oxford University Press, 2004), 1–37. See also, P. Chatterjee, *Black Hole of Empire: History of a Global Practice of Power* (New Jersey: Princeton University Press, 2012), xi–xii.

[13] D. Chakrabarty, 'Postcoloniality and the Artifice of History: Who Speaks for "Indian" Pasts?', in Ranajit Guha (ed), *A Subaltern Studies Reader:1986–1995* (New Delhi: Oxford University Press, 1997),288.

[14] T. Mitchell, *Rule of Experts: Egypt, Techno-politics, Modernity* (Los Angeles: University of California Press, 2002),4; see also M. Goswami, *Producing India: From Colonial Economy to National Space* (Chicago and London: University of Chicago Press, 2004).

[15] P. Banerjee, *The Politics of Time: 'Primitives' and History Writing in a Colonial Society* (New Delhi: Oxford University Press, 2006).

[16] A. Bashford, *Global Population: History, Geopolitics, and Life on Earth* (New York: Columbia University Press, 2014); S. Hodges, 'Governmentality, Population and the Reproductive Family in Modern India', *Economic and Political Weekly*, 39, 11 (March 13–19, 2004), 1157–1163.

enchanting, hackneyed and enigmatic, quotidian and dreadful.[17] Despite or perhaps because of this, malaria continued to be imagined as the most flexible, elusive and yet ubiquitous disease-causing entity through much of the century. The effects of malaria were reported to have been encountered in diverse and disparate geographical terrains across the colonial world and beyond: from inhospitable military trenches to long-distance sea voyages, from monotonous plains to eventful frontiers, from sunbaked deserts to impenetrable ravines and jungles. Both as a material and a metaphor, it was invoked consistently in narratives about travels and settlements. Malaria found itself entangled with the diagnoses of an exhaustive range of everyday and spectacular illnesses; the management of individual and collective bodies; the prejudices of smell, colour and class; efforts to make sense of lands, landscapes and objects; and debates about agricultural improvement, land revenue as well as urban and sanitary governance. A few decades later in 1923 when Rabindranath Tagore, by then a Nobel laureate and later apotheosised as the national poet of India, called for a 'war with malaria', the category had already acquired newer connotations, often in consonance with shifting patterns in late-imperial politics.[18] At the same time, it continued to occupy the centre stage in vernacular imagination as a crucial node of anti-colonial resistance and nationalist reconstruction, percolating into the arena of provincial print cultures.

In situating the different understandings and practices relating to malaria within various layers of imperial history, this book provides an occasion for extending the conversations between the histories of science and medicine on the one hand and scholarship on empire and postcolonial studies on the other. It speaks to the concerns opened up by an interrelated field of scholarship, which over the past two decades has been described variously as histories of colonial medicine, histories of science and empire, global and postcolonial histories of science.[19]

---

[17] See for instance, R. Deb Roy, 'Mal-areas of Health: Dispersed Histories of a Diagnostic Category', *Economic and Political Weekly*, 42, 2 (January 13–19, 2007),123. See also, M. Worboys, 'From Miasmas to Germs: Malaria 1850–1879', *Parassitologia*, 36 (1994), 61–68.

[18] R. Thakur, 'Samavaye Malaria Nibaran' ('Malaria Eradication Through Cooperatives: Text of lecture delivered on 29th August 1923'), in *Rabindra Rachanabali*, Volume 13 (Calcutta: West Bengal Government, November 1990), 795–798.

[19] These have emerged to be extremely rich fields of scholarship. For an overview on the field of colonial medicine, see P. Chakrabarti, *Medicine and Empire, 1600–1960* (Basingstoke: Palgrave Macmillan, 2014). See also R. Deb Roy, 'Science, Medicine and New Imperial Histories', *British Journal for the History of Science*, 45, 3 (September 2012): 443–450. Critical commentaries on the historiography of imperial, global and postcolonial science include R. Macleod (ed), *Nature and Empire: Science and the Colonial Enterprise, Osiris, 15* (Chicago: University of Chicago Press, 2000);

These multi-sited histories have revised in many ways the received imperial and nationalist geographies of scientific and medical knowledge formation.[20] Apart from exposing patterns of connections and correspondence between colonies held by various European imperial states, these histories have discarded narcissistic and Eurocentric narratives of triumphalism, progress and unilateral diffusion of scientific knowledge from Europe to the rest of the world. The increasing emphasis on a variety of non-European actors and sources have not only added multiple accents to the histories of early-modern and modern sciences but have also diversified our insights into their textures, vocabularies and dictions.[21] Themes such as translation, exchange, circulation, racism and violence have now emerged as crucial in understanding the making of modern science and medicine.

Despite methodological admonishments implicit in these works, various existing histories have continued to focus exclusively on colonial administrative policies, and have often tended to reify at face value the official categories of scientific and medical governance. Similarly, single-minded emphases on vernacular processes of translation and cultural difference have not done enough to question the façade of an originally unbiased domain of colonial-state-endorsed metropolitan scientific knowledge. There has been a growing awareness of the need then to go beyond scholarly models that either internalise the epistemological foundations of the colonial state or continue to romanticise an autonomous, exotic and incommensurable indigenous sphere.[22] The case of malaria

S. Sivasundaram, 'Sciences and the Global: On Methods, Questions and Theory', *Isis*, 101, (2010), 146–158; S. Hodges, "The Global Menace", *Social History of Medicine*, 25, 3 (2012), 719–728; W. Anderson, 'From Subjugated Knowledge to Conjugated Subjects: Science and Globalisation, or Postcolonial Studies of Science', *Postcolonial Studies*, 12, 4 (2009), 389–400; E. Kowal, J. Radin and J. Reardon, 'Indigenous Body Parts, Mutating Temporalities, and the Half-lives of Postcolonial Technoscience', *Social Studies of Science*, 43, 4 (2013), 465–483.

[20] For the expression 'multi-sited histories', see W. Anderson, 'Postcolonial Histories of Medicine', in F. Huisman and J. H. Warner (eds), *Locating Medical History: The Stories and Their Meanings* (Baltimore and London: Johns Hopkins University Press, 2004),287.

[21] For example P. B. Mukharji, *Nationalizing the Body: The Medical Market, Print and Daktari Medicine* (London and New York: Anthem Press, 2009); K. Sivaramakrishnan, *Old Potions, New Bottles: Recasting Indigenous Medicine in Colonial Punjab* (New Delhi: Orient Longman, 2006); R. Berger, *Making Ayurveda Modern: Political Histories of Indigenous Medicine in North India, 1900–1955* (Basingstoke: Palgrave Macmillan, 2013); G. Attewell, *Refiguring Yunani Tibb: Plural Healing in Late Colonial India* (Hyderabad: Orient Blackswan, 2007); S. Alavi, *Islam and Healing: Loss and Recovery of an Indo-Muslim Medical Tradition, 1600–1900* (Basingstoke: Palgrave Macmillan, 2008).

[22] A recent wave in the histories of medicine in South Asia has succinctly critiqued the category 'indigenous'. These include Attewell, *Refiguring*; Alavi, *Islam and Healing*; Sivaramakrishnan, *Old Potions*; Berger, *Making Ayurveda Modern*; Mukharji, *Nationalizing the*

inspires historians to contest long-held distinctions between an objective as well as sacrosanct world where knowledge is produced and a messy outside world where knowledge is consumed, resisted and displaced.[23] Thus here I return to the mainstream category of public health and to factories, laboratories, plantations and government files to interrogate the surviving myths of stability and autonomy prevalent about some of the most celebrated and apparently insulated sites of modern science and medicine.

Rather than focusing only on official policy makers, I propose to locate (wherever feasible) the European, colonial and vernacular sources in a single analytic field[24] to examine not only predictable differences, but also revealing overlaps between them. As the story of how the histories of cinchonas, malaria, quinine and eventually mosquitoes and the intimacies between them were shaped unfolds, in the following chapters, it will be clear that the concerns of a range of institutions, groups and individuals were enmeshed. I explore the interplay between a variety of sources: bureaucratic records relating to the medical and sanitary departments of the colonial state; correspondence involving the office of the Secretary of State for India; private papers of London-based drug-manufacturing families; annual reports of dispersed cinchona plantations and quinine factories; widely circulating medical journals and military manuals; Bengali vernacular literature and advertisements; and reports and memoirs written by peripatetic physicians, phyto-chemists, geographical explorers, entomologists, botanists, geologists and chemical examiners within British India and beyond. Bengal, from where most of my non-English examples are drawn, was home to one of the earliest cinchona plantations and quinine factories to have been established in the colonial world, even as it continued being recounted in various sources as amongst the more intensely malarial provinces of the British Empire. Witness to one of the most enduring encounters with colonial rule in modern history,

---

Body. For a critical overview of this literature, see P. B. Mukharji, 'Symptoms of Dis-Ease: New Trends in Histories of "Indigenous" South Asian Medicines', *History Compass*, 9, 12 (2011), 887–99.

[23] Even Michel de Certeau frames the 'devious...dispersed', 'innumerable and infinitesimal' 'tactics of consumption' in opposition to 'the centralised and spectacular...dominant cultural economy' of production. See, M. de Certeau, *The Practice of Everyday Life* (Los Angeles and London: University of California Press, 1984), xi–xxi. For the overlaps between the worlds of science and its public, institutional research and spectacular performance, see for instance S. Qureshi, *Peoples on Parade: Exhibitions, Empire and Anthropology in Nineteenth-Century Britain* (Chicago and London: University of Chicago Press, 2011).

[24] A. Stoler and F. Cooper, 'Between Metropole and Colony: Rethinking a Research Agenda', in A. Stoler and F. Cooper (eds), *Tensions of Empire: Colonial Cultures in a Bourgeois World* (London and Los Angeles: University of California Press, 1997), 4, 15.

Bengal provides various examples not only of how practices and knowledge relating to malaria were circulated, translated, appropriated and contested across linguistic contexts, but also of the ways in which colonial modernity, medical conceptions about the body and provincial print markets interacted to shape vernacular public culture.

Malarial Subjects covers the period 1820 to 1909: from the discovery of quinine in Paris to the organisation of the Imperial Malaria Conference in the British Indian summer capital at Simla. As I have hinted already, this period witnessed gradual shifts in the ways malaria was perceived: from being an elusive and generic cause of many diseases to its reconfiguration as the name of a mosquito-borne parasitic fever disease; from being an essential theme in asserting colonial difference and governance to emerging as an agenda in nationalist reconstruction and development. Over this period, various plants including eucalyptus, sunflower and opium[25] were attributed with properties to cure diseases associated with malaria. However, despite changes in the epistemological and political meanings of malaria, quinine (extracted from cinchona barks) continued to figure throughout the period, as its most enduring and quintessential remedy. These two categories were projected as invariably connected.

The structure of this book reflects how, during the period of around ninety years covered here, the figure of quinine informed understandings about the disease/disease-causing entity it was supposed to remedy. Taken together, Chapters 1 and 2 show that the establishment of cinchona plantations in colonial Dutch Java, French Algeria and British India in the 1850s coincided with considerable redefinition of malaria as a colonial disease. Besides, while the word malaria was certainly not absent in sources available in English in the eighteenth century, an unprecedented circulation of the category across the British Empire followed the discovery of quinine in 1820. John MacCulloch's treatise published in 1827, seven years after quinine was discovered, was widely recognised as the first book-length English work on malaria. Moreover, while examining the making of Burdwan fever, an epidemic attributed to malaria in the Bengal presidency in British India in the 1860s and 1870s, Chapter 3 indicates that quinine often functioned as a quick-fix diagnostic agent to determine the malarial identity of enigmatic maladies. A patient could be retrospectively diagnosed as malarial if s/he had recuperated after consuming quinine. Chapter 4 argues that quinine itself was not a homogenous, stable or inflexible entity. But rather, as hinted in the final chapter, quinine was adaptive instead to the shifts within

---

[25] For example, see Winther, *Anglo-European Science*.

imperial rule and to the changing meanings of malaria. The Imperial
Malaria Conference of 1909, an important event towards the end of the
period covered by the book, was organised in Simla in the wider context in which the therapeutic properties attributed to quinine were questioned, and reasserted in the wake of significant readjustments in the
aetiology of malaria.

Malarial Subjects therefore questions the predictable teleological
sequences of scientific knowledge production, which various histories
of colonial science and medicine often take for granted. In such a
schema, problems inevitably precede the solutions they tend to necessitate; an answer is possible only after a question has been posed; cures
are responses to well-defined maladies, which have already revealed
themselves. This book, in contrast, presents an overlapping history of
quinine and malaria to expose various ways in which cures and their
diseases, solutions and their problems could sustain and shape one
another.[26]

At the same time, each chapter focuses on individual scientific and
medical categories to examine how British imperial rule in India reconsolidated or engendered them: a plant (cinchonas), a diagnostic category
(malaria), an epidemic (Burdwan fever) and a drug (quinine). The final
chapter reveals the imperial networks through which the histories of a
group of insects (mosquitoes) and malaria were entangled in the 1900s,
and how these entanglements in turn affected the social and political
meanings of quinine. This book joins existing efforts to critique colonial rule by exposing how certain aspects of the 'taken for granted intellectual framework' of British colonialism were consolidated.[27] Such an
exercise also enables me to extend the prevailing insights into the links
between Empire and the production of natural knowledge.[28] Indeed,
the production of social and scientific perceptions about the constellation of *natural artifacts* explored here, as well as the establishment of

---

[26] While commenting on Ludwick Fleck's work on syphilis, David Bloor hints at a
closely similar idea in *Wittgenstein: A Social Theory of Knowledge* (New York: Columbia
University Press, 1983), 34–36.

[27] Shapin and Schaffer, *Leviathan and Air Pump*, 6.

[28] For example, R. Drayton, *Nature's Government: Science, Imperial Britain and the
'Improvement' of the World* (New Haven: Yale University Press, 2000); S. Sivasundaram,
Nature and the Godly Empire: Science and the Evangelical Mission in the Pacific (Cambridge and New York: Cambridge University Press, 2005); Macleod, *Nature and Empire*;
D. Arnold, *The Tropics and the Travelling Gaze: India, Landscape and Science, 1800–1856*
(Seattle: University of Washington Press, 2006); P. Anker, *Imperial Ecology: Environmental Order in the British Empire, 1895–1945* (Cambridge, Mass.: Harvard University Press,
2001); R. H. Grove, *Green Imperialism: Colonial Expansion, Tropical Island Edens and
the Origins of Environmentalism, 1600–1860* (Cambridge: Cambridge University Press,
1996).

interrelationships between them were enabled considerably by various kinds of connections held together by the British Empire. This history reconfirms how Empire occasioned not only the imbrications of the apparently unconnected worlds of colonial governance, vernacular cultures, medical knowledge and pharmaceutical commerce, but also structured the ways in which British India was linked to events, sites and processes in South America, Dutch Java, Ceylon, Burma, Mauritius, German and British Africa, and Trinidad.

The arrival of cinchonas to be planted in British India in the late 1850s coincided with the end of the Sepoy mutiny, and the transfer of the political authority to govern significant parts of the subcontinent from the East India Company to the British Crown. This book ends around 1909; the year when the first Imperial Malaria Conference was organised as well as the Morley Minto Reforms were enacted, a few years before the onset of the World War I. The decades in between witnessed a particular phase of imperial rule, which was marked by an unprecedented convergence of regimes of knowledge, biopolitics and political economy in British India.[29] This was reflected in the interconnected network of conversations about agricultural improvement, class, colours, credibility, diseases, distance, drugs, expertise, factories, field-works, governance, insects, labour recruitments, laboratories, legitimacies, markets, places, plants, plantations, purities and races about to be explored in this book. This phase, which Stoler and Cooper have described as the 'embourgeoisement of imperialism', was also characterised by the emergence of a newer commitment to govern the moralities, productivities and individual conducts of imperial subjects on either side of the colonial divide.[30] Unsurprisingly, these concerns fed into ensuing conceptions about colonial bodies, health, diseases and their cures. During these decades,

---

[29] A. Appadurai, 'Number in the Colonial Imagination', in C. Breckenridge and P. Van der Veer, (eds), *Orientalism and the Postcolonial Predicament: Perspectives from South Asia* (Philadelphia: University of Pennsylvania Press, 1993), 314–39; D. Arnold, *Colonizing the Body: State Medicine and Epidemic Disease in Nineteenth-Century India* (Los Angeles and London: University of California Press, 1993); M. Harrison, *Climates and Constitutions: Health, Race, Environment and British Imperialism in India, 1600–1850* (New Delhi: Oxford University Press, 1999); K. Raj, *Relocating Modern Science: Circulation and the Construction of Scientific Knowledge in South Asia and Europe, 1650–1900* (Palgrave Macmillan: Houndmills and New York, 2007), 181–222; P. Chatterjee, 'The Disciplines in Colonial Bengal', in P. Chatterjee (ed), *Texts of Power: Emerging Disciplines in Colonial Bengal* (Minneapolis and London: University of Minnesota Press, 1995), 1–29. Incidentally, this phase also reveals the overlapping foundations of imperial and nationalist discourses in British India. See particularly, P. Chatterjee, 'The Constitution of Indian Nationalist Discourse', in P. Chatterjee, *Empire and Nation: Selected Essays* (New York: Columbia University Press, 2010/1987), 37–58; M. Goswami, 'From Swadeshi to Swaraj: Nation, Economy, Territory in Colonial South Asia', *Comparative Studies in Society and History*, 40, 4 (October, 1998), 609–636.

[30] Stoler and Cooper, 31.

exigencies and apparatuses of Empire reshaped not only the meanings and contours of individual categories, such as cinchonas, quinine, malaria and mosquitoes, but also engendered the terms of intimate interactions between them.

However, imperial constructs such as cinchonas, quinine, malarial objects or mosquitoes were enabling artifacts rather than passive, inert or vacuous (non)entities. The predominant anthropocentrism in conventional political histories of empire has begun to be contested by historians who have commented variously on the multiple careers of animals, materials and plants in British imperial history.[31] I build upon and extend further the possibilities inherent in these works to argue that Empire itself was reconsolidated while shaping the histories of nonhumans such as cinchona plants, objects considered as malarial, the drug quinine, mosquitoes and even parasites. Therefore, the word nonhumans used in this book does not refer to animals alone. But rather, it explores the symbiotic dynamics between the British Empire, on the one hand, and a spectrum of other-than-humans (including materials and organisms), on the other.

The British Empire was clearly not a monolithic, unchanging, omnipotent agent or a 'totalising efficacy'.[32] Rather than homogenizing it as a coherent point of origin or a preordained institutional framework, or a distant overarching entity, Empire can be interpreted more incisively as a constellation of processes, which was coming into being along with the script that it was putting together.[33] There has been an increasing awareness of the ways in which the dominant themes in

---

[31] For cultural histories of animals in colonial India, see for example J. E. Hughes, *Animal Kingdoms: Hunting, the Environment and Power in the Indian Princely States* (Cambridge, Mass.: Harvard University Press: 2013). For plants, see for instance Drayton, *Nature's Government*; for veterinary turn in the histories of medicine see S. Mishra, 'Beasts, Murrains and the British Raj: Reassessing Colonial Medicine in India from the Veterinary Perspective, 1860–1900', *Bulletin of the History of Medicine*, 85, 2 (2011), 587–619. For materials and science in the wider imperial world, see, P. Chakrabarti, *Materials and Medicine: Trade, Conquest and Therapeutics in the Eighteenth Century* (Manchester and New York: Manchester University Press, 2010); H. J. Cook, *Matters of Exchange: Commerce, Medicine and Science in the Dutch Golden Age* (New Haven: Yale University Press, 2007).

[32] Kowal, Radin and Reardon, 'Indigenous Body Parts', 470.

[33] Here I draw upon reassessments about modern states in general and colonial and postcolonial states in particular. See, T. Mitchell, 'Society, Economy and the State Effect', in G. Steinmetz (ed), *State/Culture: State Formation After the Cultural Turn* (Ithaca: Cornell University Press, 1999), 76–97. Mitchell argues elsewhere that 'the issue of power and agency' should be seen as a 'question instead of an answer known in advance'. See T. Mitchell, 'Can the Mosquito Speak?', in *Rule of Experts: Egypt, Techno-politics, Modernity* (Berkeley and Los Angeles: University of California Press, 2002), 53. For the ways in which the state is experienced and reconfigured in the everyday, see for example, J. Saha, 'A Mockery of Justice: Colonial Law, the Everyday State and Village Politics in the Burma Delta, c. 1890–1910', *Past and Present*, 217, 1 (2012), 187–212;

mainstream political and cultural history – capital, democracy, enlightenment, the everyday, modernity, romanticism – did not only engender but were in turn permeated and delimited by nonhumans such as animals, oil, automata, technology, metals, machines and alike.[34] Similarly, I uncover how imperial artifacts such as cinchonas, malarial objects, quinine and mosquitoes, in turn, deepened the structural, ideological, prejudicial, biopolitical, as well as physical foundations of Empire itself. Nonhuman objects and organisms (like cinchonas, quinine, mosquitoes, malarial objects), medical knowledge about them and Empire were not only entangled, but to quote Donna Haraway, were also 'becoming with' one another.[35] The history of malaria therefore provides an occasion to probe the constitutive intersections amongst the nineteenth-century worlds of medicine, nonhumans and empire.

Recent histories on a diverse range of topics have shown renewed interest in undertaking the bold challenge to narrate the materiality of nonhuman objects and organisms by transgressing the conventional confines of discourse analysis and the history of ideas.[36] In the process, significant histories of medicine and the environment have

---

J. Wilson, *The Domination of Strangers: Modern Governance in Eastern India, 1780–1835* (Basingstoke: Palgrave Macmillan, 2008), 4, 9–18, 183–185.

[34] N. Shukin, *Animal Capital: Rendering Life in Biopolitical Times* (Minneapolis and London: University of Minnesota Press, 2009); T. Mitchell, *Carbon Democracy: Political Power in the Age of Oil* (London and New York: Verso, 2011); S. Schaffer, 'Enlightened Automata', in W. Clark, J. Golinski and S. Schaffer (eds), *The Sciences in Enlightened Europe* (Chicago and London: University of Chicago Press, 1999), 126–165; D. Arnold, *Everyday Technology: Machines and the Making of India's Modernity* (Chicago and London: University of Chicago Press, 2013); N. Wickramasinghe, *Metallic Modern: Everyday Machines in Colonial Sri Lanka* (New York and Oxford: Berghahn Press, 2014); J. Tresch, *The Romantic Machine: Utopian Science and Technology after Napoleon* (Chicago and London: University of Chicago Press, 2012).

[35] D. Haraway, *When Species Meet* (Minneapolis and London: University of Minnesota Press, 2008), 2, 23–27. Other theoretical formulations, which indicate co-constitution of authors, objects and knowledge, include D. E. Pearse, 'Author', in F. Lentricchia and T. McLaughlin (eds), *Critical Terms for Literary Study* (Chicago and London: University of Chicago Press, 1990), 113. See also, F. Trentmann, 'Materiality in the Future of History: Things, Practices and Politics', *The Journal of British Studies*, 48, 2 (April 2009), 297, 300; S. Kirsch and D. Mitchell, 'The Nature of Things: Dead Labor, Nonhuman Actors, and the Persistence of Marxism', *Antipode*, 36 (2004), 688.

[36] For a critical engagement with conventional social constructivism and on the methodological challenges of talking about materials and objects, see Golinsky, *Making Natural Knowledge*, 1–45. See also, P. Joyce, 'What is the Social in Social History?', *Past and Present*, 205 (November, 2009), 175–210; B. Braun and S. J. Whatmore (eds), *Political Matter: Technoscience, Democracy and Public Life* (Minneapolis and London: University of Minnesota Press, 2010); T. Bennett and P. Joyce (eds), *Material Powers: Cultural Studies, History and the Material Turn* (London and New York: Routledge, 2010); J. Bennett, *Vibrant Matter: A Political Ecology of Things* (Durham and London: Duke University Press, 2010); R. Drayton, 'Maritime Networks and the Making of Knowledge', in

drawn upon the sciences almost immediately.[37] There is a need to go beyond descriptions of straightforward materiality or uncontaminated nonhuman agency often revealed in scientifically informed histories. Therefore I am inspired by Timothy Mitchell's pioneering first chapter in *Rule of Experts*, which evokes the figure of mosquitoes in mid-twentieth-century Egyptian history, to interrogate straightforward notions of agency prevalent in social theory. Yet, Mitchell does not open up for analysis the contingent histories of medical entomology through which mosquitoes were labeled as vectors of malaria earlier in the century.[38] In this book I explore ways to trace the inscriptions of materials and objects while examining the links between the production of scientific knowledge and Empire.[39] Therefore I examine the empowering properties acquired by cinchona plants, malarial objects, mosquitoes and different forms of quinine, while social perceptions and scientific knowledge about them was being produced by imperial assemblages and associations.[40] These categories and entities under construction were not passive, impotent, inflexible, unresponsive or insignificant. I analyse the

D. Cannadine (ed), *Empire, the Sea and Global History* (Basingstoke: Palgrave Macmillan, 2007), 74–78; P. Chatterjee, T. Guha-Thakurta, B. Kar, 'Introduction', in P. Chatterjee, T. Guha-Thakurta and B. Kar (eds), *New Cultural Histories of India: Materiality and Practices* (New Delhi: Oxford University Press, 2014), 12–17.

[37] Gregg Mitman points out in a stimulating article how 'environmental history appropriates scientific knowledge to grant agency to nature', citing the works of William McNeill, Alfred Crosby and Jared Diamond. G. Mitman, 'In Search of Health: Landscape and Disease in American Environmental History', *Environmental History*, 10, 2 (April 2005),192. Other scholars have drawn upon medical entomology to recognise mosquitoes as historical agents. For example, McNeill, *Mosquito Empires*; Webb, *Humanity's Burden*, 32–49.

[38] Mitchell, 'Can the mosquito speak?' 19–53.

[39] A similar plea to combine narratives of 'historical contingency with the matter-of-fact hard materialism of science studies' has been evident in P. B. Mukharji, 'The "Cholera Cloud" in the Nineteenth-Century "British World": History of an Object-without-an-essence', *Bulletin of the History of Medicine*, 86 (Fall, 2012), 303–332. See also, R. Deb Roy, 'Quinine, Mosquitoes and Empire: Reassembling Malaria in British India, 1890–1910', *South Asian History and Culture*, 4,1 (January 2013), 65–86.

[40] Works that have been particularly instructive for me include Mitchell, 'Can the mosquito speak?', 38–40, 50; L. White, 'Tsetse Visions: Narratives of Blood and Bugs in Colonial Northern Rhodesia, 1931–39', *Journal of African History*, 36 (1995), 219–245; S. Jansen, 'An American Insect in Imperial Germany: Visibility and Control in the Making of the Phylloxera in Germany, 1870–1914', *Science in Context*, 13, 1 (2000), 31–70. For historical sociologies of commodification see for example, A. Appadurai, 'Introduction: Commodities and the Politics of Value', in A. Appadurai (ed), *The Social Life of Things: Commodities in Cultural Perspective* (Cambridge: Cambridge University Press, 1986), 3–60; W. van Binsbergen, 'Commodification: Things, Agency, and Identities', in W. van Binsbergen and P. Geschiere (eds), *Commodification: Things, Agency and Identities: The Social Life of things Revisited* (Berlin/Muenster/Vienna/London: LIT, December 2005), 9–51. For the ways in which objects impacted variously while being commoditised and culturally constituted in the colonial world see S. Mintz, *Sweetness and Power: The Place of Sugar in Modern History* (New York: Penguin Group, 1985);

extent to which these, whether as categories undergoing constitution or as deployed metaphors, or as objects of knowledge, governance and production were, as Bruno Latour suggests, 'modifying a state of affairs by making a difference'.[41] Quinine, mosquitoes, cinchonas and other nonhumans could make variously their presence felt while being constituted by discourses and practices enabled by Empire. Thus it might be simplistic to conceive of them as willful, full-fledged, autonomous, preordained and straightforward actors wholly independent of the political circumstances they found themselves in.

Therefore, this book reasserts the need for political histories of British Empire to be more attentive to the lessons of science studies, an interdisciplinary field that takes the agency and existence of nonhuman objects and creatures as a central point of inquiry.[42] Science studies scholars have suggested that the imbrication of nonhumans in various actions can be shown to be both simultaneously constructed and real.[43] They have undertaken the challenge to narrate the capabilities of nonhuman objects and organisms while resisting the temptations of scientific reductionism and biological determinism. In their theoretically more ambitious moments, science studies scholars have contested essentialist and straightforward notions of agency itself. They have argued that agency (and even existence) should be considered the exclusive monopoly of neither autonomous humans nor nonhumans. Instead, they point out that these are properties of collectives or assemblages of humans and nonhumans, subjects and objects.[44]

T. Burke, *Lifebuoy Men, Lux Women: Commodification, Consumption and Cleanliness in Modern Zimbabwe* (Durham: Duke University Press, 1996).

[41] B. Latour, *Reassembling the Social: An Introduction to Actor-Network Theory* (Oxford: Oxford University Press, 2005), 72 and 52.

[42] Golinsky, *Making Natural Knowledge*, 1–45; Daston, 'Science Studies and the History of Science'.

[43] See Latour, *Reassembling the Social*, 88–93, 44–73; B. Latour, 'The Promises of Constructivism' in D. Ihde and E. Selinger (eds), *Chasing Technoscience: Matrix of Materiality* (Bloomington: Indiana University Press, 2003), 27–46. I. Hacking, *Social Construction of What?*, (Cambridge, Mass. and London: Harvard University Press, 1999), 1–34; D. Haraway, 'Situated Knowledges: The Science Question in Feminism and the Privilege of Partial Perspective', in M. Biagioli (ed), *Science Studies Reader* (New Delhi and London: Routledge, 1999), 175–76, 183–85; S. Sismondo, 'Some Social Constructions,' *Social Studies of Science*, 23, 3 (August 1993), 516, 519–22; and Kirsch and Mitchell, 'The Nature of Things,' 697–702. Also see Nicole Shukin on 'rendering' in *Animal Capital*, 20–27.

[44] Latour, 'A Collective of Humans and Nonhumans,' in *Pandora's Hope: Essays in the Reality of Science Studies* (Cambridge, Mass.: Harvard University Press, 1999), 174–193; Haraway, 'Situated Knowledges', 179, 185; B. Latour, *We Have Never Been Modern* (Cambridge Mass.: Harvard University Press, 1993), 136–138; Latour, *Reassembling the Social*, 72; B. Latour, 'On the Partial Existence of Existing and Nonexisting Objects,' in

While drawing upon some of these insights, this book also hopes to demonstrate how scholarship about empire might, in turn, situate these lessons of science studies within enduring historical contexts, by revealing the ways in which nonhumans (or indeed collectives of humans and nonhumans) were implicated within histories of violence, expansion and intercultural exchange. Attention to the history of British Empire in South Asia will uncover not just how cinchonas, malarial objects, quinine and mosquitoes were reshaped in the long nineteenth century. Focus on colonial South Asia will further show that these plants, materials and insects did not constitute a self-sufficient and autonomous world of nonhumans. But rather, specific socio-material assemblages that proliferated in the British imperial context sustained them. I also suggest that imperial biopolitics in British India were founded on the simultaneous processes of anthropomorphism, animalisation and dehumanisation, which, on occasions, blurred the distinctions between humans and nonhumans/subjects and objects.[45] Attribution of lifelike properties (if not human characteristics) to cinchonas, quinine, malarial objects and mosquitoes converged with and stoked exclusionary narratives about race, place, colour, purity, primitives, class and labour.

The title of this book *Malarial Subjects* simultaneously draws on different uses of the word subjects. In a public lecture delivered in London in March 1882, the British Indian bureaucrat Joseph Fayrer deployed the expression 'malarial subjects' to refer to patients suffering from 'various symptoms of the malarial poison' ranging from remittent fever to 'a variety of indefinite complaints'.[46] Going beyond the overt medical connotation of the original expression, the title of this book signals at the imperial context in which the lecture was delivered. Malaria had emerged by then as an extensively deployed trope to describe colonial

L. Daston (ed), *Biographies of Scientific Objects*, (Chicago: University of Chicago Press, 1999), 253, 256, 258.

[45] On dehumanisation, see the historiography on 'primitives', for example, K. Ghosh, 'A Market for Aboriginality: Primitivism and Race Classification in the Indentured Labour Market of Colonial India', in G. Bhadra, G. Prakash and S. Tharu (eds), *Subaltern Studies X: Writings on South Asian History and Society* (New Delhi: Oxford University Press, 1999), 8–48; J. Fabian, *Time and the Other: How Anthropology Makes its Object* (New York: Columbia University Press, 1983); Banerjee, *Politics of Time*. See also S. Muthu, *Enlightenment Against Empire* (New Jersey: Princeton University Press, 2003), 11–71. On anthropomorphism see L. Daston and G. Mitman, *Thinking with Animals: New Perspectives on Anthropomorphism* (New York: Columbia University Press, 2005). This point about the dual move of anthropomorphizing and dehumanizing in relation to enlightenment Europe has been made most eloquently by Simon Schaffer in 'Enlightened Automata'. Also see H. Raffles, 'Jews, Lice and History.' *Public Culture*, 19, 3 (Fall, 2007), 521–566; Jansen, 'An American Insect in Imperial Germany'.

[46] J. Fayrer, 'First Troonian Lecture on Climate and the Fevers of India', *Lancet*, 119, 3055 (March 18, 1882), 423–426; 467–470.

lands, landscapes and people. Besides, Fayrer's status as an authority on malaria was connected to his long career as a bureaucrat in British India. His examples of native people, who figured in his narrative as either vulnerable to or immune from malaria, were drawn from various parts of the colonial world including Algeria, Burma, India, Guinea or the West Indies.[47] *Malarial Subjects* therefore indicates that various medical and colonial identities were bound by nineteenth-century histories of the category malaria. The title of the book also acknowledges that malaria attracted the attention of a variety of intellectual persuasions. The medical history of malaria was shaped by contributions from geologists, geographers, meteorologists, chemists, economic-botanists, engineers, natural historians and entomologists. In a more methodological sense malaria provides opportunity for deeper conversation between the apparently disparate historiographies of empire, medicine and nonhumans. Finally, the history of malaria can also provide the occasion to complicate the received distinctions between the subject and the object. In history writing, the word subject is variously understood to mean the subjugated, or an acting agent, or a product of relationships of power. I ask in this book if these different conceptualisations of the subject can be extended to incorporate the nonhuman. In the process, I also urge that the binary of human and nonhuman itself needs to be historicised.

[47] Ibid.

1 'Fairest of Peruvian Maids'

Planting Cinchonas in British India

The real Eldorado of India is Cinchona.[1]

Where Andes hides his cloud-wreathed crest in snow
And roots his base on burning sands below;
Cinchona, fairest of Peruvian maids,
To health's bright goddess, in the breezy glades
Of Quito's temperate plains, an altar reared,
Trilled the loud hymn, the solemn prayer preferred.[2]

Europeans owed their initial encounters with cinchona plants to the consolidation of Spanish imperial rule in the interiors of South America. As objects of commerce and knowledge, cinchonas had been made to travel from South America to various corners of Europe and beyond since the mid-seventeenth century.[3] However the mid-nineteenth century was particularly significant in the history of the cinchonas as the Dutch, British and French colonial governments began to express a new interest in these plants. The 1850s, as many historians have shown, witnessed the beginnings of organised attempts to collect and transport cinchona seeds and plants from 'natural' South American forests towards the sites of 'experimental plantations' in colonial Africa and the East and

---

[1] F. C. Daukes to Secretary, Government of Bengal, Medical and Municipal Department, 27 June 1881, Simla. *Home, Medical,* June 1881 47–49 A (NAI).

[2] Cited in the title page of W. D. Hooker, *Inaugural Dissertation upon the Cinchonas, their History, Uses and Effects* (Glasgow: Edward Khull, Dunlop Street, 1839).

[3] S. Jarcho, *Quinine's Predecessor: Francesco Torti and the Early History of Cinchona* (Baltimore and London: Johns Hopkins University Press, 1993); M. J. Crawford, *Empires Experts: The Politics of Knowledge in Spain's Royal Monopoly of Quina, 1751–1808* (unpublished doctoral dissertation, University of California, San Diego, 2009); A. Holger Maehle, *Drugs on Trial: Experimental Pharmacology and Therapeutic Innovation in the Eighteenth Century* (Amsterdam: Rodopi, 1999), 223–309; D. Bleichmar, 'Atlantic Competitions: Botanical Trajectories in the Eighteenth-Century Spanish Empire', in J. Delbourgo and N. Dew (eds), *Science and Empire in the Atlantic World* (New York and Abingdon: Routledge, 2007), 242–244.

West Indies, particularly, Dutch Java, British India, Ceylon and Jamaica and French Algiers.[4]

In the wider histories of colonialism, plants have figured variously as objects of collection, classification, profit, intrigues and collaboration,[5] as sources of military prowess,[6] as nodes of resistance,[7] as markers of geographical distinction and cultural difference,[8] as emblematic of rural social life, livelihoods, adaptations and reinventions,[9] and even as signifiers of memory amongst postcolonial refugees.[10] Plants have often been situated at the interstices of the histories of imperial science, evangelism, commerce and politics.[11] Drawing on these broader concerns, historians like Richard Drayton and Kavita Philip, who have commented on the establishment of colonial cinchona plantations, have shown how the globalised networks of economic botany, plantation capital and imperial ideology informed one another.[12]

---

[4] R. Drayton, *Nature's Government: Science, Imperial Britain, and the 'Improvement' of the World*, (New Haven: Yale University Press, 2000), 207–211; K. Philip, *Civilising Natures: Race, Resources and Modernity in South Asia* (Hyderabad: Orient Longman, 2004), 240; A. Mukherjee, 'The Peruvian Bark Revisited: A Critique of British Cinchona Policy in Colonial India', *Bengal Past and Present*, 117 (1998), 81–102; L. H. Brockway, *Science and Colonial Expansion: The Role of the British Royal Botanic Gardens* (New Haven: Yale University Press, 2002), 104, 117–125. See also, M. Honigsbaum, *The Fever Trail: The Hunt for the Cure for Malaria* (London: Macmillan, 2001); F. Rocco, *Quinine: Malaria and the Quest for a Cure that Changed the World* (London: Harper Collins, 2003).

[5] Bleichmar, 'Atlantic Competitions', 225–252; D. P. Miller and P. H. Reill (eds), *Visions of Empire: Voyages, Botany and Representations of Nature* (Cambridge and New York: Cambridge University Press, 1996); J. Endersby, *Imperial Nature: Joseph Hooker and the Practices of Victorian Science* (Chicago: University of Chicago Press, 2008), 1–30.

[6] D. Headrick, *The Tools of Empire: Technology and European Imperialism in the Nineteenth Century* (Oxford: Oxford University Press, 1981), 58–79.

[7] L. Schiebinger, *Plants and Empire: Colonial Bioprospecting in the Atlantic World* (Cambridge Mass.: Harvard University Press, 2004), 142–149.

[8] D. Arnold, 'Envisioning the Tropics: Joseph Hooker in India and the Himalayas, 1848–1850', in F. Driver and L. Martins (eds), *Tropical Visions in an Age of Empire* (Chicago and London: University of Chicago Press, 2005), 142–143.

[9] W. Beinart and L. Worshela, *Prickly Pear: Social History of a Plant in the Eastern Cape* (Johannesburg: Wits University Press, 2013), 8–10.

[10] R. Dasgupta, 'Justice in a Landscape of Trees', http://humanitiesunderground.wordpress.com/2012/08/05/justice-in-a-landscape-of-trees/ [retrieved on 29 April 2013].

[11] S. Sivasundaram, *Nature and the Godly Empire: Science and Evangelical Mission in the Pacific, 1795–1850* (Cambridge: Cambridge University Press, 2005), 175; M. T. Bravo, 'Mission Gardens: Natural History and Global Expansion, 1720–1820', in L. Schiebinger and C. Swan (eds), *Colonial Botany: Science, Commerce and Politics in the Early Modern World* (Philadelphia: University of Pennsylvania Press, 2005), 49–65.

[12] Drayton, *Nature's Government*, 207–210, 230, 231; Philip, *Civilising Natures*, 240–267. See also L. Veale, *A Historical Geography of the Nilgiri Cinchona Plantations, 1860–1900* (unpublished doctoral dissertation, University of Nottingham, 2010); A. R. Hoogte and T. Pieters, 'Science in the Service of Colonial Agro-Industralism: The Case of Cinchona

This chapter builds upon these existing histories to examine the ways in which the image of cinchonas as valuable plants were historically produced and maintained.[13] It follows the historical efforts to circulate and plant cinchonas in British India in the 1850s and 1860s to reveal how and why a set of material properties was ascribed to these plants. These decades marked, I argue, an occasion for the reconstitution of cinchonas as a political symbol, as a valuable commodity and as an object of botanical knowledge. The commodity status of cinchonas was reinforced through various 'localised negotiations'.[14]

Colonial geographers, planters, botanists and bureaucrats reaffirmed, shared and sustained amongst themselves the impression that the cinchonas were valuable plants through certain recurrent vocabulary, strategies and practices. The discourses, techniques and predicaments associated with circulating and planting cinchonas in British India during this time suggests the production of a colonial bureaucratic consensus about these plants. Further, this consensus was internalised beyond the confidential files of the imperial state. Interest in cinchonas was reflected not only in widely cited memoirs, unpublished travel narratives and routine bureaucratic correspondence, but also in the aspirations of private planters, local Rajas, distant newspaper reporters, contending vernacular advertisements, photographers and illustrators amongst others.

The commodification of cinchonas in British India of the 1850s and 1860s was achieved through the official detailing of the intense physicality of these plants. Cinchonas were projected not as vacuous, unresponsive objects but as variously living, surviving, changing, decaying, dying, corporeal entities. Cinchonas figured as rare, distant, alien, brittle, sensitive, delicate, feminine beings which were difficult to tame in British Indian plantations. Yet, the construction of cinchonas as invaluable rarities coalesced with programmatic visions about the plausibility of managing and naturalising cinchonas in British India, and these plants appeared suitably malleable. Thus in various plantation records in the 1860s, cinchonas could appear as both enchanting and profane, both exotic and accessible, as a symbol of the distant and also of the everyday.

Cultivation in the Dutch and British East Indies, 1852–1900', *Studies in the History and Philosophy of Biological and Biomedical Sciences*, 47, PA (September 2014), 12–22.

[13] Philip mentions the word 'commodification' in pages 240, 268, 270, but does not elaborate. For maintenance and repair, see B. Latour, 'Whose Cosmos, Which Cosmopolitics? Comments on the Peace Terms of Ulrich Beck', *Common Knowledge* 10, 3 (2004), 459.

[14] For 'localised negotiations' see E. C. Spary, 'Of Nutmegs and Botanists: The Colonial Cultivation of Botanical Identity', in L. Schiebinger and C. Swan (eds), *Colonial Botany: Science, Commerce and Politics in the Early Modern World* (Philadelphia: University of Pennsylvania Press, 2005), 203.

The history of the imperial production of such a liminal plant can be variously meaningful. First, it makes possible an engagement of approaches in the cultural histories of (particularly botanical) knowledge production with insights available in the existing histories of commoditisation.[15] It also enables a deeper conversation with newer works, which have begun to analyse the historical ascriptions of lifelike properties to politically significant plants.[16] Efforts to commodify cinchonas were intimately linked to the assertions about their lively properties. Secondly, human and nonhuman assemblages enabled the making and sustenance of the cinchonas in British India. Cinchonas were as much shaped by some of the necessary constituents of the 'material culture of colonial botany' in the mid-nineteenth century like Wardian cases, steamers, small pots, herbariums, plantations, royal gardens and so on, as they were by the priorities of human actors like planters, bureaucrats, botanists and geographers.[17] Thirdly, circulation from one part of the world to another appears to have been a transformative experience for these plants. Cinchonas not only adapted to newer habitats, but also acquired newer experts, identities and functions. In what follows, cinchonas are revealed as a mutating entity rather than stable and unchanging. Finally, in various ways, cinchona plants and Empire shared a symbiotic relationship. The apparatuses and exigencies of imperial rule predominantly occasioned the status of cinchonas as valuable objects of plantation in the 1850s and 1860s. Efforts to plant cinchonas in British India, in turn, reinforced and sustained an imperial network of ideologies, protocols, travels, connections, botanical rivalries, correspondence, exclusions and prejudices.

Discovery of an Event

In 1820, French chemists Pierre Joseph Pelletier (1788–1842) and Jean Bienaime Caventou (1795–1887) claimed to have detected the presence of two distinctly different alkaloids in the grey, yellow and red varieties of cinchona barks. They named these two different 'salifiable bases', cinchonine and quinine. In 1820 it was uncertain whether this constituted a

---

[15] Ibid; Spary, 'Of Nutmegs', 187–203; P. Anker, *Imperial Ecology: Environmental Order in the British Empire, 1895–1945* (Cambridge, Mass.: Harvard University Press, 2001).

[16] L. Totelin, 'Botanizing Rulers and their Herbal Subjects: Plants and Political Power in Greek and Roman Literature', *Phoenix*, 66, 1–2 (2012), 122–144; S. Gibson, *Animal, Vegetable, Mineral? How Eighteenth-Century Science Disrupted the Natural Order* (Oxford: Oxford University Press, 2015), 149–178.

[17] L. Schiebinger and C. Swan, 'Introduction' in Schiebinger and Swan (eds), *Colonial Botany*, 13–15.

momentous achievement. Immediate responses from the scientific community in Paris were lukewarm. Pelletier had to wait for another five years before he was promoted. He became a professor at the School of Pharmacy in Paris in 1825. Formal recognition in the form of an award reached them after seven years in the form of the Montyon Prize, which they shared in 1827, the first and perhaps only award they ever received. Pelletier was made a member of the Academy of Sciences in Paris twenty years later in 1840. That was two years before he died at the age of fifty-four. Caventou was promoted to professorship fifteen years later in 1835.[18]

Amongst contemporary studies on the chemistry of cinchona barks their accomplishment appeared significant but unexceptional. From the mid-eighteenth century cinchona barks had attracted the attention of many reputed continental phytochemists. Histories of these studies tend to be teleological success stories, dotted with big names.[19] Knowledge about the chemistry of cinchona barks has been shown in these narratives to proceed from one significant milestone to another, with each breakthrough tending to verify, build upon, refine or correct previous understandings. For instance, it has been shown how Pelletier derived hints from studies about morphine and opium by the Hanoverian apothecary F. W. Serturner (1783–1841) between 1806 and 1818.[20] It has been pointed out that in 1820 Pelletier and Caventou's success lay in 'reinvestigating'[21] and correcting 'a mistake'[22] in the chemical characterisation of cinchonine by Bernardino Antonio Gomes. Gomes, a Portuguese naval surgeon, had apparently treated a cinchona extract with caustic potash and obtained an alkaloid product, which he named cinchonino in 1810.[23] Gomes, in turn, was trying to 'purify'[24] an almost similar vegetable substance detected in the bark of the cinchona trees by Andrew Duncan Junior (1773–1832) of Edinburgh. At the beginning of the nineteenth century, Duncan Junior called that vegetable substance cinchonin. Similar studies concerning the alkaloid-chemistry of different varieties of cinchona barks did not end in 1820. In 1829, Pelletier himself claimed to refine his earlier findings and suggested the presence of a third alkaloid aricine in the cinchona barks. In 1852, Louis Pasteur named two newer alkaloids as quinidine and cinchonidine. Pasteur

---

[18] L. F. Haas, 'Pierre Joseph Pelletier (1788–1842) and Jean Bienaime Caventou (1795–1887)', *Journal of Neurology, Neurosurgery and Psychiatry*, 57 (1997), 1333; G. E. Trease, 'Pierre-Joseph Pelletier (1788–1842): The Discoverer of Quinine', *British Journal of Pharmaceutical Practice*, 2, 7 (1980), 32–33; Maehle, *Drugs on Trial*, 282–283.

[19] LaWall, 'The History of Quinine', *Medical Life*, 38, 4 (April 1931), 195–216.

[20] Maehle, *Drugs on Trial*, 282–283. [21] Trease, 'Pierre-Joseph Pelletier'.

[22] Maehle, *Drugs on Trial*, 282–283. [23] Trease, 'Pierre-Joseph Pelletier'.

[24] Maehle, *Drugs on Trial*, 282–283.

suggested that quinidine had earlier been located in the cinchona barks by L. Henry and Auguste Delondre in 1833, while F. L. Winckler had 'isolated' cinchonidine in 1844.[25] By 1871, phytochemists had already traced the presence of around eleven such alkaloids in the barks of different varieties of cinchonas.[26] Besides, from the early 1840s considerable attention had been devoted towards analysing the constituents of the roots of the cinchonas.[27]

In retrospect, amongst innumerable such analyses into the chemistry of cinchona barks since the late eighteenth century, the accomplishment of Pelletier and Caventou in 1820 stands out. Such recognition results from the extensive market response to quinine in particular. Commercial considerations had from the late-seventeenth century necessitated studies of cinchonas. A wide range of healing qualities was attributed to the barks of the cinchona trees in Europe since then. Physicians and pharmacologists had around this time begun analysing whether certain species of cinchona barks were more medically efficacious than others. It was hoped that by identifying particular cinchona species which were best endowed with therapeutic properties, these analyses would provide a rationale for the traders in making profitable choices. European traders dealing in cinchona barks, it was believed, could then invest in the most valuable trees.[28]

The historian Andreas Holger Maehle has shown how the therapeutic properties of the barks were examined through *in vitro* and animal experimentations, chemical tests and microscopic observations, and clinical case histories in the hospitals, army, navy and private practices.[29] By the early eighteenth century some general criteria for the assessment of barks became known: considerable emphases were, for instance, laid on 'colour, consistency and taste' of the barks.[30]

The belief that the curative potentials attributed to cinchona barks could most reliably be explained in terms of 'an active principle' emerged in the late eighteenth century. This was made possible by the gradual entrenchment of a new language of science, evident in the sustained confidence expressed by commercial interests in the emerging discipline of organic chemistry. It was suggested that the curative agent inherent in cinchona barks could be a chemical, an alkaloid or a salifiable base.

---

[25] LaWall, 'The History of Quinine', 210.
[26] J. Broughton, 'Chemical and Physiological Experiments on living Cinchonae', *Philosophical Transactions of the Royal Society of London*, 161 (1871), 1–15.
[27] T. Anderson, to W. Grey, No. 333, 11th February 1862. *Home, Public*, 22nd February 1862, 54–58 A. (NAI).
[28] S. Tomic, 'Chemical Analysis of Plants: The Case of Cinchona', *Annals of Science*, 58, 3 (2001), 287–309. Also Bleichmar, 'Atlantic Competitions', 243.
[29] Maehle, *Drugs on Trial*, 268–273.   [30] Ibid., 275.

In its 'pure form', it was hoped, it could be 'chemically analysed', 'isolated', 'discovered' by the phytochemists. Fifty years between 1779 and 1829 witnessed the publication of more than three hundred monographs about the chemistry of the cinchona barks.[31] These studies were published from various parts of Europe – including present-day France, England, Germany, Scotland, Russia, Sweden and Holland.[32] These appeared inseparably bound up with the necessities of commerce, especially in providing advice to investors in selecting more valuable species of cinchonas.[33] To ascertain the pharmaceutical properties inherent in different varieties of cinchona barks, the Harveian Society of Edinburgh 'laudably decreed two prize medals'.[34]

Late eighteenth century onwards, alkaloid chemistry had a symbiotic relation with the market. Traders in the cinchonas depended on phytochemists for ratification of their business decisions. At the same time, alkaloid chemistry established its legitimacy by deriving patronage from commercial interests. It is unsurprising then that some of the early breakthroughs in the field of alkaloid chemistry were attained in relation to articles which would eventually be considered commercially viable. The first alkaloid was claimed to be isolated in Paris in 1803. It was later named as narcotine. Morphine was isolated from opium in 1806; strychnine was isolated from Nux Vomica in 1818; caffeine was 'found' in 1821.[35]

The disparate roles of alkaloid-chemist and trader often overlapped. It has been pointed out that most of the early researchers of alkaloids were pharmacists and many discoveries were made in their shops. Charles Deronse, who is attributed with the glory of isolating narcotine, was a French pharmacist. F. W. Serturner, a Hanoverian apothecary, isolated morphine. Pelletier followed the footsteps of his father in directing the Pelletier Pharmacy. K. E. W. Meissner (1792–1855), who 'found'

---

[31] H. Hobhouse, *Seeds of Change: Five Plants that Transformed Mankind* (New York: Harper Collins, 1987), 14.

[32] Ibid.

[33] For instance, R. Kentish, *Experiments and Observations on a New Species of Bark, Showing its Great Efficacy in Very Small Doses, also a Comparative View of the Powers of the Red and Quilled Bark; Being an Attempt Towards a General Analysis and Compendious History of the Valuable Genus of Cinchona, or the Peruvian Bark* (London: J. Johnson, 1784); W. Sanders, *Observations on the Superior Efficacy of the Red Peruvian Bark, in the Cure of Fevers* (London: J. Johnson, 1782); J. M. H. Moll, 'William Saunders, 1743–1817', *Journal of Medical Biography*, 1 (November 1993), 235.

[34] J. Relph, *An Inquiry into the Medical Efficacy of a New Species of Peruvian Bark, Lately Imported into this Country Under the Name of Yellow Bark Including Practical Observations Respecting the Choice of Bark in General* (London: James Phillips, 1794).

[35] Trease, 'Pierre-Joseph Pelletier'.

sabadilline in the Cevadilla seeds, was a Prussian apothecary; F. F. Runge, who 'found' caffeine, was a German pharmacist.[36]

The first and the most sustained effort towards propagating the virtues of quinine came from an experimental physiologist based in Paris, Francois Magendie, in the 1820s. It is hardly surprising that in successive texts he overtly addressed the market. In his *Formulary*, published first in 1821, he was inspiring druggists to initiate extensive manufactures of quinine. He however did not confine himself into advertising the virtues of quinine alone, and was equally emphatic in asserting the medicinal attributes of almost every other 'newly isolated alkaloids', such as iodine, bromine, morphine, strychnine, veratrine and emetine besides quinine.[37] This text went into several editions and was translated into several languages.

Even before the first North American edition of this book, which was translated by Dr Robley Dunglinson, was published in 1824, businessmen Farr and Kunzi had started selling quinine to customers at 16 dollars per ounce. In 1823, a company based in Philadelphia named Rosengarten and Sons claimed to manufacture quinine from cinchona barks on a commercial scale.[38] A physician, Dr John Sappington (1776–1856), who practiced medicine on a farm near Arrock Rock in central Missouri, claimed to sell pills of quinine sulphate as John Sappington's anti-fever pills. He is reported to have made a fortune out of such business.[39] In London, Luke Howard, a retail pharmacist since 1795, set up a quinine factory in 1823.[40] In the same year, a pharmacist named Pietro Peretti (1781–1864) set up a quinine factory in Rome.[41] In 1826, Riedel, a Swiss apothecary, began selling quinine at eight dollars an ounce in Berlin.[42] Thus, by the mid-1820s, drug manufacturers of varying statures, backgrounds and pedigrees in Europe and North America had started investing in quinine production.

---

[36] Ibid.

[37] F. Magendie, *Formulary for the Preparation and Mode of Employing Several New Remedies: Namely, Morphine, Iodine, Quinine* (London: Thomas and George Underwood, 1824). Translated from the French of the third edition of Magendie's 'Formulaire' by C. T. Haden.

[38] LaWall, 'The History of Quinine', 206–209.

[39] W. A. Strickland, 'Quinine Pills: Manufactured on the Missouri Frontier (1832–1862)', *Pharmacy in History*, 25, 2 (1983), 61–68.

[40] J. H. Kirkwood and C. H. Lloyd, *John Eliot Howard: A Budget of Papers on His Life and Work*, (Oxford: Lloyd, 1995), 13–14.

[41] *A Ledger of Peretti's Pharmacy, Rome dated 1823, in Which Are Entries of the Method of Preparation of Quinine Salt, the Purchase of Quinine, Pulverization, Price etc...* 1823 (WL).

[42] LaWall, 'The History of Quinine', 195–216.

In 1839, William Dawson Hooker, eldest son of the influential botanist William Jackson Hooker and brother of Joseph Dalton Hooker, the future director of the Royal Botanic Gardens at Kew, had applied for induction into the faculty of physicians and surgeons at the University of Glasgow. He wrote his inaugural dissertation on 'Cinchonas, their history, uses and effects'. This dissertation explained the extensive currency of quinine in pharmaceutical businesses in the 1830s.[43] Hooker attributed 'knowledge of the virtues of the Peruvian barks' solely to 'modern chemistry'. He suggested that modern chemistry brought precision and clarity of knowledge about the therapeutic properties of cinchona barks. Quinine, he argued, removed the uncertainties that characterised cinchona trade. By projecting quinine into the fore, it appears, 'modern chemistry' provided a definite indicator for measuring the values of each individual cinchona tree. Hooker suggested that quinine could be clearly measured, identified and distinguished from less valuable alkaloids by certain precise features.[44] He provided details of chemical tests to detect adulterated versions of quinine. He suggested separate tests (with sugar, sulphate of lime, boracic acid, margaric acid, stearine, starch etc) for detecting adulterations of quinine.[45]

However, such promising laboratory manifestoes should be read with caution, as they do not necessarily indicate quotidian commercial practice. Existing histories have shown that different alkaloids inherent in cinchona barks were 'in all practical possibilities' indiscriminately referred to as quinine.[46] Many medics continued to believe that the combined effects of all the constituents of the cinchona barks made it an effective remedy.[47] Hooker himself suggested that quinine, cinchonine and aricine were closely similar alkaloids in their chemical composition. They seemed to minutely vary only in their content of oxygen.[48]

It appears then that quinine, most generally, circulated in the market as well as in clinical practice as a convenient point of reference. Since the 1820s, quinine was projected to signify the collective virtues of cinchona plants. Quinine figured as a symbol, which defined enduring pursuits of a myriad of individuals, interests and institutions relating to the cinchonas. It emerged as an acceptable category around which different correspondences, negotiations, comparisons and competitions could revolve.

---

[43] Hooker, *Inaugural Dissertation*, 18–19.   [44] Ibid., 19.   [45] Ibid., 24.
[46] Hobhouse, *Seeds of Change*, 14–15.   [47] Maehle, *Drugs on Trial*, 283.
[48] Hooker, *Inaugural Dissertation*, 19–20.

Quinine, since the mid-1820s, revealed considerable overlap between men of knowledge and men of commerce. The physician John Sappington, who made enormous money from selling pills of quinine in the early 1820s, eventually turned his medical business over to his sons in 1838 and began to devote more time in dealing in livestock, finance and land speculation. In 1844, he wrote a book called *The Theory and Treatments of Fevers*.[49] By 1826, Pelletier himself started manufacturing quinine on a commercial scale.[50]

Botanical knowledge and commercial aspirations, however, converged most emphatically in the careers of different members of the Howard family in London. Throughout the nineteenth century the Howards were arguably the most influential business interests in quinine.[51] Luke Howard had been a retail pharmacist since 1795. However his main interest lay in meteorology and his work on cloud formations over London earned him a Fellowship of the Royal Society in 1821. In 1823, however, he claimed to have dissociated pure form of quinine from other less valuable alkaloids present in the cinchona barks.

It was left to his son, John Eliot Howard, who initiated large-scale profitable manufacture of quinine on a commercial sense in the late 1850s (see Figure 1.1). By then, the Howards had advertised themselves as leading experts in England of knowledge about cinchona and its various extracts. Howard was in immediate correspondence with an elaborate network of travelling botanists from Europe who had ventured into the South American forests of Bolivia and Peru. He participated in an epistolary world of botanical knowledge production, and regularly exchanged letters and ideas with Hugh Algernon Weddell in Paris, Clements Markham in London and Hermann Karsten in Berlin.[52] In such an exclusive world the correspondents endorsed themselves as experts by referring to or citing from the works of one another.[53] In 1857, in recognition of his status as an expert on quinine he was inducted into the Linnean Society. In 1858 he purchased an entire collection of cinchona barks from Professor Pavon of Madrid. In 1862 Howard translated the professor's manuscript into English and edited a pictorial representation of his collections. He called it *Illustrations of Neuva Quinologia*

---

[49] Strickland, 'Quinine Pills'.   [50] Trease, 'Pierre-Joseph Pelletier'.

[51] Kirkwood and Llyod, *John Eliot Howard*, 13–14.

[52] Weddell, Markham and Karsten were French, British and German botanical explorers in the 'Cinchona forests' of South America from the early to mid-nineteenth century.

[53] J. E. Howard, *Illustrations of Neuva Quinologia of Pavon* (London: Lovell Reeve and Co, 1862). See also C. R. Markham, 'Preface', *Travels in Peru and India* (London: John Murray, 1862), v–x.

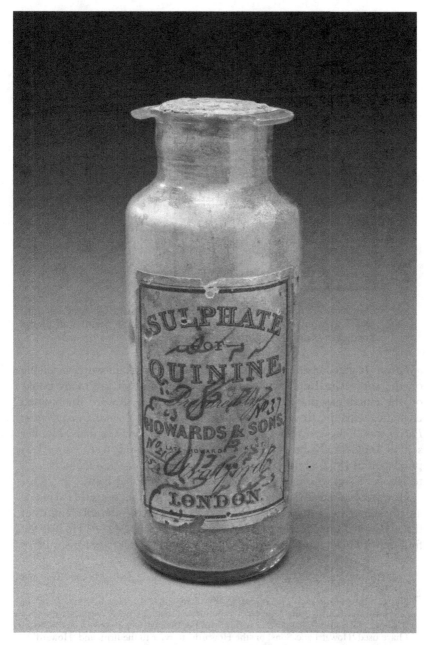

Figure 1.1 Photograph of a bottle of quinine bearing the label Howards and Sons, c.1860–1910, Credit: Wellcome Library, London.

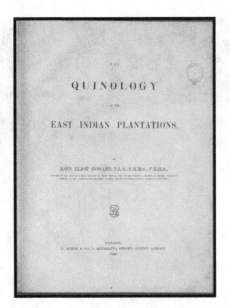

Figure 1.2 Title page of John Eliot Howard's *The Quinology of East Indian Plantations*, 1869. Reproduced by the kind permission of the Syndics of Cambridge University Library.

of Pavon. It was considered amongst the most important works available on the subject in English, and this was one amongst the many books on the cinchonas that he would eventually write. Howard maintained close ties with the Royal Botanic Gardens at Kew. *Neuva Quinologia of Pavon* was dedicated to the then-director of the Kew Gardens, Hooker senior. Incidentally, he dedicated his subsequent work (see Figure 1.2) published in 1867, entitled *The Quinology of the East Indian Plantations*,[54] to Hooker's son who had by then become influential at Kew.

Howard could also boast of thriving political connections. He acted as an advisor to the British Government in India for considerable lengths of time. Howard's nephew joined Howard and Sons in 1871.[55] He was the founder of Society of Chemical Industry as well as the Royal Institute of

---

[54] J. E. Howard, *The Quinology of the East Indian Plantations* (London: Lovell Reeve and Co, 1869).

[55] Nineteenth-century sources referred to this firm either as 'Howards and Sons' or 'Howard and Sons'. India Office correspondence that this book engages with used 'Howard and Sons' while referring to this firm. For the sake of consistency, in this book, I have used 'Howard and Sons' or 'the Howards' to refer to the firm, and 'Howard' to refer to the individual, John Eliot Howard.

Chemistry. His son David Lloyd Howard joined the family business in 1888. He followed the footsteps of his predecessors and set up the Association of British Chemical Manufacturers, Drug and Fine Chemical Manufacturer's Association and Wholesale Drug Trade Association.[56] The successes of the family in the field of quinine manufacture and circulation can only be studied in reference to such interconnected networks amongst the worlds of chemistry, commerce and politics. Over much of the nineteenth century the Howards were recognised as amongst the leading authorities in the science of quinine manufacture in the British Empire. They were also predominant players in most of the commercial ventures involving that commodity. I will explore in Chapter 4 the ways in which this explicit nexus between pharmaceutical capital and botanical knowledge played itself out.

In the late 1850s and early 1860s, quinine began to attract the attention of colonial governments in French Algeria, Dutch Java and British India. Medical commerce and colonial rule had long shared an intimate relationship.[57] The establishment of experimental cinchona plantations at various locations in these colonies converged with attempts to write credible histories of cinchona trees. Such histories formed parts of memoirs written by officials who were associated with the transfer of cinchona seeds and plants from South America to these British, Dutch and French colonies. Clements Robert Markham's *Travels in Peru and India* and Gustav Planchon's *Peruvian Barks* are amongst the most detailed texts in this genre of writing.[58] These narratives revealed themselves as long hagiographies of quinine. Different episodes involving two centuries of European association with forests in South America were repackaged variously as stories, legends, facts, rumours and incidents associated with quinine. The 'history' of the Peruvian forests that emerged from such narratives effectively conveyed the impression of indispensability of cinchona barks in curing various maladies. Quinine emerged retrospectively in these narratives as the precise cause that made cinchona trees valuable. Existing anecdotes from the annals of Spanish colonisation of Latin America were retold in the mid-nineteenth century as necessary components of broader pre-histories of quinine. Even when medical science was unaware of its existence, it was suggested, patients had benefited from quinine.

---

[56] Kirkwood and Lloyd, *John Eliot Howard*, 14.

[57] For instance P. Chakrabarti, *Materials and Medicine: Trade, Conquest and Therapeutics in the Eighteenth Century* (Manchester and New York: Manchester University Press, 2010).

[58] Markham, *Travels in Peru and India*, v–x. See also, G. Planchon, *Peruvian Barks* (London: George E. Eyre and William Spottsiwoode 1866).

'An interval of only forty years intervened between the pacification of Peru and the discovery of its most valuable product', Markham wrote.[59] A Jesuit priest's recovery in 1600 mentioned by J. de Jussieu at Malacotas was now attributed to the curative powers of quinine. Similarly, quinine was retrospectively recognised in the writings of Clements Markham or Gustave Planchon as the unknown agent which famously cured Don Juan Lopez de Canizares, the Spanish Corregidor of Loxa in 1630 and the wife of the Fourth Count of Chinchon at Lima in 1638. Nineteenth-century narratives rewrote the penetration of Jesuit Acuna's fraternity into the forests bordering on the upper waters of the Amazon and subsequent formation of settlements as disinterested explorations in search of quinine.[60] Different varieties of drugs attributed to the cinchona barks (i.e. salutary powder, Countess's Powder, Jesuit's Powder,[61] cinchona red, *'sel essentiel febrifuge'*)[62] were now appropriated within the expansive history of quinine. These were now recognised as imperfect and lesser versions of 'pure, raw quinine'.[63]

Quinine was also invoked to explain various contemporary political developments. Quinine was described as that medical wonder which could explain British military successes in expeditions in the Walcheren and along the river Niger, and the sustenance of troops from Peshawar to Pegu.[64] The use of quinine in earlier centuries, it was conjectured, could have '[change(d)] the history of the world'. Markham lamented that the 'greatest and most patriotic of England's rulers' could have lived longer had the use of quinine been current: 'Oliver Cromwell was carried off by ague'.[65] Even the death of Alexander the Great was explained in terms of the 'want of a few doses of quinine'.[66] Such overemphasis on the glory of quinine often led to the renaming of the tree and the landscape with which it was associated. In the mid-nineteenth century cinchona trees were often referred to as 'quinine trees'.[67] South American forests that were considered the natural home of cinchonas were designated as 'quinine forests'.[68] The cinchona-growing provinces of South America began being mentioned as the 'quinine region'.[69]

At the same time, quinine was advertised as the cure for not only an extensive range of fevers, but also dysentery,[70] sore throat,[71] alarming

---

[59] Markham, *Travels*, 3.   [60] Ibid., 6.   [61] Planchon, *Peruvian*, 1.
[62] Markham, *Travels*, 17.   [63] Planchon, *Peruvian*, 34.   [64] Markham, *Travels*, 519.
[65] Ibid.   [66] Ibid.   [67] Planchon, *Peruvian*, 4–6.
[68] Anderson to Grey. *Home, Public*, 22 February 1862, 54–58 A., (NAI).
[69] Planchon, *Peruvian*, 6.
[70] J. Macpherson, *On Bengal Dysentery and Its Statistics* (Calcutta: Thacker, 1850).
[71] D. J. Brackenridge, 'On the Use of Quinine as a Gargle in Diphtheritic, Scarlatinal, and Other Forms of Sore Throat', *Practitioner*, 15, 86 (August 1875), 110–114.

head symptoms,[72] impotence,[73] and toothache[74], amongst other conditions. In view of such prestige subsequently endowed on quinine, the
accomplishments of Pelletier and his colleagues in 1820 began to be
considered a moment of great discovery in the standard histories of
medicine. Markham wrote, 'This medicine, the most precious of all
those known in the art of healing, is one of the greatest conquests made
by man over the vegetable kingdom'.[75] The memory of the discovery of
quinine in 1820 was carefully restored and magnified. To commemorate
eighty years of the discovery a bronze statue of Pelletier and Caventou in
their academic robes was erected in Paris in the Boulevard Saint Michel
in 1900.[76] Figure 1.3 shows that Ernest Board celebrated the discovery
again in the 1910s in an oil painting. Soon thereafter original samples of
quinine and cinchonine attributed to Pelletier and Caventou began being
displayed as a museum relic in exhibitions across London.[77] Further in
1970, a stamp was released to commemorate the 150th anniversary of
the discovery of quinine.[78]

'Pleasantest Episode of British Rule in India'[79]

In the early 1860s, the event of discovery was invoked in many imperial
narratives, which sought to justify the transfer of cinchona plants and
seeds from various corners of South America towards possible destinations of colonial plantations in British India, French Algeria and Dutch
Java. Published in 1862, Clements Robert Markham's *Travels in Peru
and India* is one of the earliest and most widely cited amongst these
accounts.[80] As a professional geographer, Markham was credited with
having explored the forests of Peru and the frontiers of Bolivia much
before the project had been conceived. In 1859, he was entrusted by the
British government to lead an exploration into the interiors of the South
American forests. The purpose of the expedition was to identify different

---

[72] R. L. Bowles, 'Alarming Head Symptoms After Violent Exercise in Hot Weather,
Relieved by Quinine', *BMJ*, 1, 34 (22 August 1857), 711.
[73] L. J. Jordan, *Specification of Lewis Jacob Jordan: Tonic* (London: Great Seal Printing
Office, 1861) (WL).
[74] M. A. F. Mannons, *Specification of Marc Antoine Francois Mannons: Elixir* (London:
Great Seal Patent Office 1862) (WL).
[75] Markham, *Travels*, 20.   [76] Trease, 'Pierre-Joseph Pelletier'.
[77] 'Original Preparations by Pelletier', (Credit: Wellcome Library, London. M0011461).
[78] Haas, 'Pierre Joseph Pelletier'.
[79] D. Hanbury, 'Review of a Memoir of the Lady Ana de Osorio, Countess of Chinchon
and Vice-Queen of Peru with a Plea for the Correct Spelling of the Chinchona Gneus
by Clements R. Markham' in D. Hanbury, *Science Papers: Chiefly Pharmacological and
Botanical* (London: Macmillan and Co, 1876), 475.
[80] Markham, *Travels*, v–x.

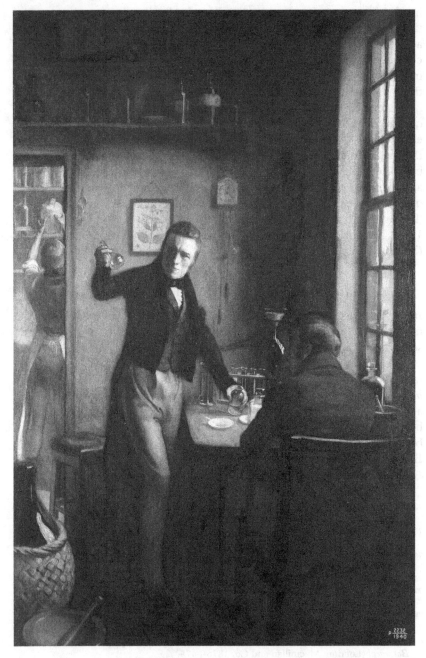

Figure 1.3 Oil painting of Pelletier and Caventou discovering quinine by Ernest Board, c. 1910–20. Credit: Wellcome Library, London.

species of cinchonas in their natural habitats. Seeds and plants belonging to these different varieties were then to be shipped towards the British ports in India. Markham spent most of his time exploring the forests of the Peruvian province of Caravaya. Botanists claiming almost equal experience in the region assisted Markham. Richard Spruce engaged himself in Chimborazo, Robert Cross explored New Grenada while G. J. Pritchett traversed the forests of Huanuco and Huamalies.[81] Existing works have already explored in great detail the challenges faced by them during this expedition.[82] This section closely reads from *Travels in Peru and India* to reveal the ways in which Markham was justifying efforts to establish cinchona plantations in British India. It argues that travel accounts like this reinforced the image of cinchonas as valuable items.

In Markham or Planchon's accounts these plants figured not only as objects of enduring botanical interest, but also as commodities which were in great demand in the 1850s. Cinchonas were described as sources of enormous revenue. For instance, Markham mentioned that from the four Bolivian ports of Arica, Islay, Payta and Guayaquil, the export of cinchona barks in 1859 amounted to around 912,900 lbs, which was valued at £59,076.[83] Such obvious commercial significance was further underscored by predictions that the world's only natural cinchona reserves (in South America) were on the verge of extinction. Markham blamed the Spanish governments in South America and the republics that succeeded them for their mismanagement of the only natural cinchona reserves in the world. These governments had allegedly failed to control an unbridled trade in cinchona barks.[84] This, he argued, had set the stage for the exhaustion of the cinchona trees. He projected the fear of the depletion of the cinchona trees altogether in view of enormous yearly exports of cinchona barks. Markham suggested that the British were not alone in their concern about the possibility of imminent extinction of the cinchona trees in their natural homeland. French, Dutch and Spanish explorers in the South American forests since the mid-eighteenth century (beginning with La Condamine, Humboldt and Ruiz) had supposedly predicted the exhaustion of cinchona trees.

Markham argued that many French, Dutch and British botanists and explorers, amongst his contemporaries, had proposed the cultivation of cinchonas in colonial plantations elsewhere as a means to protect these

[81] Planchon, *Peruvian*, 45–46.

[82] Philip, *Civilising Natures*, 238–272; Brockway, *Science and Colonial Expansion*, 112–117.

[83] Markham, *Travels*, 571–572.

[84] C. Perez, *Quinine and Caudillos: Manual Isidoro Belzu and the Cinchona Bark Trade in Bolivia, 1848–1855* (unpublished doctoral dissertation, University of California at Los Angeles, 1998); Brockway, *Science and Colonial Expansion*, 111.

plants from extinction. Dr Forbes Royle, reporter on Indian Products to the East India Company, as early as 1839 in his *Illustrations of Himalayan Botany*, recommended the introduction of cinchona plants from South America to different parts in India.[85] Markham pointed out that similar experiments were recommended by botanists and explorers Dr Weddell, M. Delondre and M. Fee in the French colonies, particularly in Algeria in the 1840s, and that earlier amongst a host of Dutch botanists, Blume had insisted on the introduction of cinchona plants into Dutch Java.[86] Thus, Markham described the transplantation of cinchonas in the Dutch, French and British colonies as a response to a shared imperial anxiety.

The arrival of these valuable sources of quinine within a few years after the Sepoy mutiny of 1857, it was claimed, would initiate the 'pleasantest episode of British rule in India'.[87] Cinchonas were upheld as objects which symbolised the benevolent transition of imperial power in British India from the East India Company to the Crown.[88] By being a part of the process of bringing cinchonas to India, Markham imagined himself as engaged in an everlasting service to the colonial poor in India:

Thus England will leave behind her by far the most durable monument of the benefits conferred by her rule. The canals and other works of the Moguls were in ruins before the English occupied the country; but the melons which the Emperor Baber, the founder of the Mogul dynasty, introduced into India, and which caused him to shed tears while thinking of his far-off mountain home, still flourish around Delhi and Agra. Centuries after the Ganges canal has become a ruin, and the great Vehar reservoir a dry valley, the people of India will probably have cause to bless the healing effects of the fever dispelling chinchona-trees, which will still be found on their southern mountains.[89]

He suggested that the British imperial project of extracting cinchonas from the interiors of South American forests was not only justified, but also legitimate. Markham refused to view the introduction of cinchona plants from South America to South India as a radical break from the past. It appeared to be part of a longer history of continuous travel of commodities from South America and their subsequent domestication in India:

India owes to South America the aloes which line the roads in Mysore, the delicious anonas, the arnotto-tree, the sumach, the capsicums so extensively used in

---

[85] D. Williams, 'Clements Roberts Markham and the Introduction of the Cinchona Trees into British India, 1861,' *The Geographical Journal*, 128, 4 (December 1962), 432.

[86] Markham, *Travels*, 46.   [87] Hanbury, 'Review of a Memoir', 475.

[88] Philip, *Civilising Natures*, 240, 256–267; Drayton, *Nature's Government*, 231.

[89] Markham, *Travels*, 61.

native curries, the pimento, the papaw, the cassava which now forms the staple food of the people of Travancore, the potato, tobacco, Indian corn, pine-apples, American cotton, and *lastly, the chinchona*: while the slopes of the Himalayas are enriched by tea-plantations, and the hills of Southern India are covered with rows of coffee trees.[90]

At the same time, he dispelled apprehensions that the establishment of cinchona plantations in British, Dutch or French colonies would injure the cinchona trade controlled by Peru and Ecuador.[91] On the contrary, Markham argued that the setting up of the colonial plantations in distant parts of the imperial world was conceived as pedagogical measures, which would eventually benefit the South Americans themselves. Competitions with the barks produced in the Indian and Javanese plantations, he hoped, would teach them to appreciate the value of the cinchona trees more than ever before. This in turn would inspire them to carefully preserve and protect these trees in their immediate locales. Once the cinchona plantations in Java and South India bloomed, Markham envisioned, the South Americans would benefit from such experiences. Beyond the enclaves of naturally sprouted forests, Markham thought, the South Americans would then learn to grow and rear cinchonas within enclosed and manicured spaces of plantations. Therefore in the abstruse logic of colonial exchange, he eventually situated the South Americans as beneficiaries:

Hitherto they have destroyed the chinchona trees in a spirit of reckless short sightedness, and thus done more injury to their own interests than could have possibly arisen from any commercial competition; but it may be that the influence of peace and education will inaugurate a new system in time to come, that more enlightened views will prevail, and that they themselves may undertake the cultivation of a plant which is indigenous to their forests, but which up to this time they have most foolishly neglected. It will then be a pleasure to supply them with the information which will have been gained by the experience of cultivators in India, and thus *to assist them in the establishment of plantations on the slopes of the eastern Andes*.[92] (Emphasis mine.)

Moreover, cinchonas were situated by Markham at the heart of an unwritten contract. He argued that the British government in India exercised a legitimate right over the cinchonas that grew in South America:

Under any circumstances the South Americans, who owe to India the staple food of millions of their people, and to the Old World most of their valuable products – wheat, barley, apples, peaches, sugar cane, the vine, rice, the olive, sheep, cattle,

---

[90] Ibid., 60.   [91] Ibid., 338.   [92] Ibid.

and horses- have *no right to desire to withhold* from India a product which is so essentially necessary to her welfare.[93] (Emphasis mine.)

Representing the British Empire in South America, Markham could hardly afford to be sympathetic to the memory of Spanish colonialism. He dedicated three chapters in his *Travels in Peru and India* towards detailing the exploitative aspects of Spanish rule.[94] Markham claimed to read the minds of the Peruvian Indians better than their immediate or erstwhile rulers. He suggested that the Peruvians had communicated to him their will 'to promote a friendly interchange of the products of the New and Old worlds'.[95] He explained that the many acts of resistance to these British, French and Dutch ventures were results of shrewd instigations engineered by short-sighted, local officials:

The foolish decree issued in Ecuador on the 1st of May, 1861, as well as the numerous obstructions thrown in my way in southern Peru, may be imputed either to the narrow minded selfishness of half educated officials; or to the ignorant patriotism of backwoodsmen. These are feelings that are not shared by either the educated few, or by the Indian population.[96]

As an object of circulation, cinchona plants performed considerable commercial, epistemological and ideological functions for the British Empire in India in the late 1850s and early 1860s. In the memoirs of imperial handlers like Markham, these plants figured as what Harold Cook calls a 'matter of exchange', which South Americans could share with the wider imperial world in return for necessities, knowledge and goodwill.[97]

Distant and Delicate

Travel memoirs, bureaucratic reports, sketches and paintings were amongst the sites where the journey of the cinchonas from South America to various parts of British India was narrated. These narratives entwined intimate descriptions of the fragile physicality of these plants with ceaseless suggestions about their exalted status as valuable commodities in British India. Detailed accounts of the hardships involved in transporting a delicate plant from a distant part of the world tended to underscore the exotic value of the cinchonas. To that extent, cinchonas were hardly exceptional amongst attention-seeking commodities

[93] Ibid., 338–339.   [94] Ibid., vi.   [95] Ibid., 339.   [96] Ibid.
[97] H. J. Cook, *Matters of Exchange: Commerce, Medicine and Science in the Dutch Golden Age* (New Haven: Yale University Press, 2007).

in nineteenth-century British India. Drugs that were preferred as reliable in the official files were often projected as exotic items. Such items were shown to bear strains of travel from distant places. Colonial officials often reported on 'local medicines' circulating in the interior bazaars of India. These reports claimed that because these drugs remained confined within the immediate locality, the charm associated with them was often depreciated by quotidian access. Easy rejections of these conveniently accessible drugs were based on the claim that their uselessness had been revealed or exposed.[98] In contrast, drugs that were advertised as exotic confidently carried with them the untested promise of offering more effective cure. One of the most common tropes in Bengali medical advertisements in the 1850s, for instance, involved stating the names of distant places from where certain drugs were imported. Such advertisements even mentioned the names of the ships and vessels that carried them into British Indian ports. The value of drugs was often asserted by hinting at the journeys they had undertaken.[99]

Similarly, the distant origins of cinchonas were recurrently reemphasised in course of the second half of the century. Increasing circulation across British Empire of sketches of the interiors of cinchona forests (see Figure 1.4) and maps of the extensive 'cinchona region' in South America converged with descriptions by geographers like Markham of various stages of the long, and often perilous journey which the plants underwent.[100]

...When the unprecedented length of the voyages and the numerous transshipments are taken into consideration, the wonder is that any of the plants should have been successfully conveyed from the slopes of the Andes in South America to the Ghats in Southern India, over thousands of miles, through every variety of climate, subject to the risk of crossing the isthmus of Panama, of changing steamers at the island of St Thomas, at Southampton, at Suez, and at Bombay, and of the journey through Egypt... The most important introduction of plants into India...[101]

[98] A. Smith, *Notes on the Principal Plants Employed in India, on Account of their Real or Supposed Febrifuge Virtues*, quoted in Markham, *Travels*, 546–565. See also J. Macpherson, *Quinine and Antiperiodics in Therapeutic Relations Including an Abstract of Briquet's Work on Cinchona and a Notice of Indian Febrifuges* (Calcutta: R. C. Lepage, 1856).
[99] For example see the following advertisements published in the Bengali newspaper *Sambad Purna Chandroday*. 'Messrs Nosky and Co Druggists', *Sambad Purna Chandroday*, (8 May 1850), 1 and 'D N Paul and Co', *Sambad Purna Chandroday* (25 December 1850), 1.
[100] 'Map showing Cinchona region of the Andes, South America' from C. R. Markham, *Peruvian Bark* (London: John Murray, 1880). Credit: Wellcome Library, London, L0025458.
[101] Markham, *Travels*, 324, 334–335.

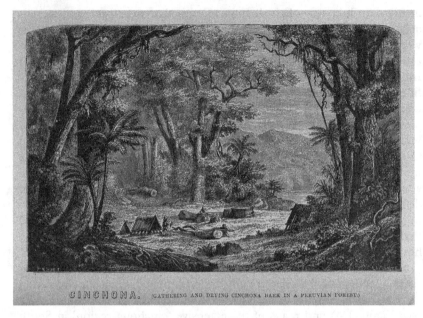

CINCHONA. [GATHERING AND DRYING CINCHONA BARK IN A PERUVIAN FOREST]

Figure 1.4 Wood-engraving by Charles Laplante, c. 1867. Credit: Wellcome Library, London.

Such narratives of global travel revealed the cinchonas as invaluable and mortal. The physical stresses suffered by these plants in circulation were elaborated rather than concealed. The transformation of these cinchonas' corporeal properties during transit upheld them as lively, responsive, sensitive organisms and not as eternally stable and vacuous objects. These travelling cinchonas were ascribed various anthropomorphic features in the official files: they often died, but when they didn't die, they lived; even if they barely survived, got injured, turned sickly and got their identities messed up.[102] At the same time, these hostilities encountered by the plants were indicative of the length of the difficult journey. For instance, Mr Pritchett, an agent engaged by Markham, had transmitted a 'valuable assortment of seeds', consisting of varieties denominated as cinchona *micrantha*, cinchona *nitida* and cinchona *peruviana* from Lima to Bombay. It was reported that the seeds had to wait at Lima for six weeks and at Bombay for another twenty-seven days, and in the process lost some of their vital properties. D. Macpherson, the Inspector

---

[102] Anderson to Grey. Home, Public, 22 February 1862, 54–58 A (NAI).

General of Hospitals, on special duty at Ootacamund found it difficult to distinguish between them.[103]

The reports conveyed a sense of precision involving the meagre numbers of plants that survived the journey. Such frequent reference to numbers reinforced the impression that cinchonas were not only therapeutically invaluable but also numerically rare and exotic items in British India. It was reported, for instance, that only 400 plants belonging to the *Cinchona Calisaya* species collected by Markham in South America made it to Ootacamund in South India. Even these died shortly thereafter. Amongst the first batch of plants and seeds shipped from South America by collectors Cross and Spruce only 463 of the *Succirubra* species and six belonging to the Calisaya species survived the journey and reached Ootacamund on 9 April 1861.[104] These indicated that plants which had shown extraordinary resilience to survive the vagaries of the journey were noteworthy, rare and valuable commodities, and commanded careful attention. Thus, the value of cinchonas seems to have been aggravated by awareness of the distance which they were made to traverse. The impression about the indispensability of the cinchonas in British India was produced and reconfirmed by the desperation of the government to access these plants despite such numerous difficulties.

Besides, the firmer recognition of cinchona in the official records as a valuable commodity was also closely linked to its feminisation. The ascription of feminine attributes to these plants was not restricted to William Dawson Hooker's description of the cinchonas as 'the fairest of Peruvian maids',[105] or to the designation of carefully showcased cinchona barks on display in London exhibitions as beautiful.[106] In bureaucratic correspondence they were often projected as delicate plants. This was the most recurrent trope to reinforce the femininity of the cinchonas. The value of cinchonas was reinforced by its representation as a delicate item. The word *delicate* could have multiple connotations: fragile and subtle; vulnerable and graceful. Thomas Anderson, the then Superintendent of the Botanic Gardens at Calcutta, for instance, seems to have had knowledge 'of the difficulties attending the transporting of so *delicate plants* by long sea voyages and especially of the trying journey in the Red Sea [emphasis mine]'.[107] However, the cinchonas could as

[103] D. Macpherson, to J. Boudillon, No. 7, 5 February 1861, Ootacamund. Home, Public, 25 April 1861, 34–35 A (NAI).

[104] Anderson to Grey. Home, Public, 22 February 1862, 54–58 A (NAI).

[105] Hooker, 'Title page', *Inaugural Dissertation*.

[106] Anonymous, 'The Cinchona Plant', *The Brisbane Courier* (Saturday, 8 February, 1868), 6 http://trove.nla.gov.au/ndp/del/article/1318474 [retrieved on 26 December 2012].

[107] Anderson to Grey. Home, Public, 22 February 1862, 54–58 A (NAI).

well display their delicate character whilst in transit through more tranquil waters. The image of cinchona as a delicate plant survived till the late 1860s. Captain W. J. Seaton, Conservator of forests, British Burma, informed: 'A fresh batch of plants was received from Ootacamund, and the glasses, in crossing, were again broken and the plants killed... finally 12 only reached Tounghoo alive, most of them having been killed by *over watering* on the way up the Sittang river... Eight were at last planted in Bogalay [emphasis mine]'.[108] In view of the 'delicate' nature of cinchona plants, Anderson had prescribed strict instructions for carrying them during inland transit. 'Each case requires *eight men*. It is of greatest importance that the plants should not be shaken in the transport, nor should be exposed to the sun [emphasis mine]'.[109] The delicate features of these plants were underscored by projecting them as 'sensible' to variations of temperature and altitude. 'They are extremely *sensible* to a greater or lesser degree of heat, humidity, shade etc so that the slightest departure from the mean of these influences (for example, a height more or less elevated by 500 feet) exercises a visible influence on the condition of trees, and this *sensibility* varies with each species of the Cinchona [emphasis mine]'.[110]

Cinchonas were designated as feminine plants, which required careful handling by imperial men almost at every step. The imperial gestures of possessing, rescuing, collecting, protecting, transporting and receiving cinchona plants, it was suggested, were chivalrous and masculine. The imperial projection of cinchonas as invaluable commodities was sustained and invigorated by the recurrent description of the physicality of these plants as distant, rare and delicate in myriad sources. The circulation of this 'Peruvian maid' to distant corners of the colonial world was advertised as an accomplishment more glorious than even the introduction of tea from China into India in 1849.

Geographies of Plantations: Anderson in Java

The imagining of cinchonas as rare and valuable was not restricted to narratives describing the journeys of these plants from South America to British India. Bags containing cinchona seeds and plants reached South India from different ports in Peru, Bolivia, Ecuador or New Grenada by

---

[108] W. J. Seaton to Secretary, Chief Commissioner, British Burmah, PWD. Home, Public, 4 July 1868, 57–63 A (NAI).

[109] T. Anderson to E. H. Lushington, 6 March 1862. Home, Public, 14 April 1862, 122–125 B (NAI).

[110] Dr Junghuhn to the Governor General of Netherlands India, 23 October 1861, Lembang. Home, Public, 16 December 1861, 26–30 A (NAI).

the early 1860s.The construing of the physicality of cinchonas as distant, sensitive and delicate persisted through the course of the 1860s. The enduring impression that these exotic mortals survived only in certain specific geographical situations meant that they could not be planted just anywhere in British India. The selection of suitable sites for the cinchona plantations was a long, complex and contested process. It preoccupied botanical debates, bureaucratic travels and plantation experiments over much of the decade. Such elaborate efforts to 'maintain'[111] cinchonas in British India conveyed the impression that these plants were not only fragile, but also invaluable.

The issue of where cinchona plantations could be established in British India became a contested topic. Thomas Anderson, the Superintendent of the Botanic Gardens in Calcutta, in an early official correspondence drafted in 1859, tended diligently to conform to the opinions of best known explorer-botanists in India who had visited the cinchona forests in South America.[112] This led to the search for localities in India that could be thought to resemble the landscapes and climates where cinchonas were 'indigenous'. This was preceded by two puzzling questions. The one asked what the climates prevalent in the natural cinchona forests were like, and the other, how could the landscape that was supposed to support such forests be accurately described.

The opinions of botanists, explorers and agents who had visited the natural cinchona forests in South America were solicited. The perceived delicate physicality of the cinchonas, in turn, conferred on Markham, Cross, Spruce, Pritchett unforeseen authority. Their roles did not end with despatching different varieties of cinchona plants and seeds to India. Instead, their status graduated from bearers of seeds and plants to custodians of knowledge about the cinchonas in British India. They were entrusted with locating sites in British India, which apparently resembled South American forests closest. In this process, Markham emerged as one of the most influential figures associated with cinchona planting endeavours in South India in the 1860s. Markham's travel accounts bore elaborate justifications for selecting certain locations in the Madras presidency as suitable for the survival of the cinchonas.

Meanwhile cinchonas continued to acquire newer sets of authorities. The expertise of explorers like Markham in the geographies of cinchonas was effectively contested since Thomas Anderson's return from his deputation to Java in February 1862. It began as a clash over authority

---

[111] Latour, 'Whose Cosmos'.
[112] T. Anderson to the Secretary, Government of Bengal, No. 193, 6 September 1859. Home, Public, 13 January, 1860, No. 18–27 A (NAI).

between explorers who had known the cinchonas in the 'natural forests' of South America and officials who were aware of the conditions in which artificial plantations in Dutch Java thrived. In 1862, Dutch Java was the only place in the world, other than South America, where cinchonas grew. Only in Dutch Java were cinchonas cultivated in plantations. In successive reports, Anderson revised his earlier opinions, emphasising the relevance of lessons acquired in the cinchona plantations in Java in deciding upon suitable sites in British India. Anderson was one of the very few British officials deputed to visit Java, and he underscored the relevance of this precious experience in determining the possible locations of plantations in British India.[113]

Anderson reported that as early as 1862 about 8000 plants of *Cinchona Calisaya* and more than half a million plants of the species *Cinchona Pahudiana* were already thriving in the Javanese plantations. He further noted that some of those, which had been planted five or six years earlier, had already grown up to acquire a height of about 25 or 30 feet. The successes witnessed in these plantations were explained in terms of the exceptional characteristics of Javanese landscape and climate. In his travel account, the cinchonas reappeared as a valuable breed of plants because the terrain that housed the plantations in Java was relatively rare. Anderson's journeys in search of the cinchona plantations in Java brought him to the foothills of volcanoes, and his narrative showed his experience of the interiors of Java as an engagement with an active landscape. While travelling between plantations he appeared to be moving from one volcanic site to another.[114]

The causes behind the proliferation of cinchona trees in Java, Anderson suggested, was inherent in the natural history of the region. The 'meteorology, botany and geology' of the Javanese mountains seems to have been characterised by strange blends. Such features appeared distant and different from Anderson's familiar world. These rare enmeshes, it was claimed, were typical of the regions where the cinchonas survived. The rarity of such regions in British India, it was suggested, made cinchonas a precious group of plants.

Anderson pointed out that the principal plantations were located on the Kendeng and Malabar range of mountains in the southern portion of the islands in the vicinities of the plateau of Bangdong. The altitude of such mountains varied from 2000 to 7000 feet above the sea.

---

[113] Anderson to Grey. Home, Public, 22 February 1862, 54–58 A (NAI).
[114] Ibid.; T. Anderson to W. Grey, No. 326, 4 December 1861. Home, Public, 16 December 1861, 26–30 A (NAI).

He found the landscape equally conducive for the sustenance of dense 'natural forests' and plantations. The 'natural' and the 'agricultural' conveniently merged to constitute the surrounding vegetations. Gigantic trees, typical of the Malayan archipelago, formed the bulk of the vegetations of these forests. Anderson thought that such trees were often 150 or 180 feet high. He found that 'beautiful and extensive coffee plantations' and craters of active volcanoes frequently broke continuities of these dense forests. Anderson noted that as he ascended along the plantations 'through the dripping forests', the eclectic features of the existing vegetations struck him. Tropical forms of trees appeared to intimately mingle with the temperate species like the rhododendrons. Trees ascribed to the American genus *Gaylussacia* and those apparently belonging to the Himalayan genus *Astilbe* appeared to closely coexist with 'gregarious volcanic plants'.

Anderson noted that such curious blends could also be witnessed in the weather prevalent usually in the cinchona plantations of Java. Anderson found them similar to what Karsten had written about the Andes or the way Mr Pritchett described the forests of Huanaco. 'At one moment, a raging tempest of rain and wind; at another, the calm, tranquil, laden atmosphere of chilling cloud and fog...' 'The misty regions of the Andes, where... constant rain is interrupted in the day by interchanging sun rays and fog clouds...'. It appears from Anderson's account that the weather prevalent in the Javanese plantations witnessed a constant interplay of light and shade: frequent rainfall, interrupted by dazzling beams of sunlight, followed once again by steady formations of gloomy clouds. The weather compatible with the sustenance of the cinchonas in the plantations, according to Anderson's engaging narrative, revealed such rigidly repetitive patterns.[115]

In the travel narratives of this British Superintendent of the Botanic Gardens in Calcutta, Javanese cinchona plantations thrived on a landscape which bore the scars of numerous volcanoes. It was represented as a rare region where apparently contradictory features in weather and vegetations could conveniently coexist. These features, he claimed, conformed to his readings of what botanists and explorers wrote about the 'natural cinchona forests' in South America. Anderson attributed the successes of the cinchona plantations in Java to these exceptional features in its landscape. Anderson's narrative suggested that the cinchonas were not merely a distant and delicate group of plants. The landscape, the weather and surrounding vegetation, which sustained their survival,

---

[115] Anderson to Grey. Home, Public, 22 February 1862, 54–58 A (NAI).

would be difficult to locate in British India. In the relative absence of such geographic characters, Anderson sounded uncertain about the prospect of cultivating cinchona in British India:

There can be no doubt that, on the whole, there will be greater difficulties to contend with introducing Cinchona into India than have been experienced by the Dutch in Java. Dense forests possessing a moist climate do not occur extensively in South India at elevations from 3000 to 6500 feet high, which may be taken roughly as the two extremes at which the cultivation of the species of Cinchona would be most successful.[116]

Tours of Ambition

Thus, on his return from Dutch Java, Anderson questioned the selection of Dodabetta and Neddivattum as sites for cultivating cinchonas in the Nilgiris in South India by Markham and his associates. Anderson argued that these selections followed neither the lessons learnt from the 'natural cinchona forests' in South America nor the plantations in Dutch Java. Opinions varied as to what were the ideal conditions for cinchonas to thrive. Anderson's understandings often clashed with those of Markham, Spruce or Cross, and he emphasised the relevance of the knowledge learnt from Java over the experiences of those others. Anderson considered, for instance, the practice initiated by Markham of planting the cinchonas in the open, without any form of shade to guard them from the scorching rays of the sun, unacceptable. He confirmed from the writings of travellers into South America like Weddell and Karsten as well as the experiences of the Dutch in Java that cinchona plants only survived when they were accommodated within an existing 'natural forest'. At Neddivattam, Markham had instructed the clearance of 50 acres of forest from trees to plant cinchonas without shade. Thus, Markham was about to deprive Neddivattam, feared Anderson, of one of the essential conditions for the survival of the cinchonas, that is, continuous luxuriant vegetation.[117]

Anderson argued that the selection of Dodabetta and Neddivattum as sites for plantations were based on 'a very erroneous idea of climate'. Unlike South American cinchona forests or the Javanese plantations, the vegetation in the Nilgiris, Anderson thought, suffered from long continued droughts. Here, Anderson missed the large luxuriant sections of *Dendrobium*, *Cymbidium* and *Vanda*, as well as the perennial terrestrial orchids of the moist Java forests. He found the climate in Dodabetta and

---

[116] Anderson to Grey. Home, Public, 16 December 1861, 26–30 A (NAI).
[117] Anderson to Grey. Home, Public, 22 February 1862, 54–58 A (NAI).

Nedivattam 'too dry' in comparison to the data furnished by Markham himself on the Caravayan forests in South America. The altitudes of the selected sites, noted Anderson, were much higher than what suited these plants. He alleged that the site selected for planting *Cinchona Calisaya* at Ootacammund by Markham was 1500 feet above the highest elevation at which that species survived in Bolivia, and 2000 feet above the highest limit at which it had been possible to cultivate it in Java.

Anderson's prediction about the fate of those plants was precise: 'The young plants will most certainly be lost'.[118] Similarly, he pointed out that plants belonging to the *Succirubra* species at the government garden at Ootacamund turned 'sickly'. Those were planted 'at least 2500 feet above their highest limit', he reasoned.[119] Anderson argued that exposure to adverse climatic conditions were reflected in the poor health of these plants. It was suggested that in comparison to the plants grown in Java, the South Indian cinchonas suffered from a lack of vitality. After having received a group of cinchona plants each from Java and Ootacamund in Calcutta in August 1862, Anderson wrote:

Out of fifty nine plants obtained from Java only one death occurred, while of the 170 plants from Ootacamund no less than thirty were completely lost. *This difference in the healthiness of the plants from the two places* becomes more striking when it is known that the plants from Java were brought by Coolies from the mountains in the interior of the Island to Batavia and thence by steamer to Calcutta; while those from Ootacamund were transported in twelve hours by Railway over most of the land journey, and the Sea voyage only lasted three days. The plants from Java were in addition exposed for two months longer than the others to the confinement of small pots and wardian cases as they arrived in Calcutta two months before them . . . [120]

Thus, Anderson's enchantment with cinchonas was, yet again, founded on the invocation of the delicate physicality of these plants. The puzzlement with locating suitable sites for rearing cinchonas in British India augmented them not only as an exclusive group of plants, but also as sensitive and living bodies which survived only in specific geographical conditions. The incorporation of the cinchonas within the colonial plantation economy, Anderson implied, was an intimately corporeal experience for these plants. As in the case of displaced indentured labourers, Indian soldiers in the British Indian army, or European colonisers, efforts to acclimatise cinchonas in an alien landscape was informed by

---

[118] Anderson to Grey. Home, Public, 16 December 1861, 26–30 A (NAI).
[119] Anderson to Grey. Home, Public, 22 February 1862, 54–58 A (NAI).
[120] T. Anderson, 'Report on the Cultivation of the Quineferous Cinchonae in British Sikkim from the 24 March to the 1 August 1862'. Home, Public, 13 September 1862, 30–31 A (NAI).

concerns of preventing deaths and sickness, and ensuring 'healthiness' and productivity. I will continue to explore in the following section how mystification of cinchonas persisted with attempts to assist these plants to survive in an unfamiliar landscape.

Anderson's scathing remarks regarding the efforts of Markham performed other functions. Such acts of contrasting the climates and landscapes of South India with Java and South America were not disinterested exercises in comparative geography or a selfless clash of botanical opinions. It also reflected a clash of ambitions in a struggle over whose expertise was best suited to the management of the cinchonas in British India.[121] Thus, cinchonas revealed tensions within the botanical establishment in British India.

Anderson's remarks were carefully framed towards contesting Markham's claims as the leading authority of knowledge about the cinchonas in British India. Dr Junghuhn was the Principal Inspector of the cinchona cultivation at Dutch Java. In view of the highly advertised successes in the Javanese plantations, he had begun to command enormous prestige in the world of knowledge about the cinchonas. He wrote the following letter in support of Anderson's abilities. Anderson attached excerpts from this letter ahead of the detailed account of his trip of Java.

... Dr Anderson, ... now understands the climate and the character of the forests in which the Cinchonas at Java grow in great fertility; ... is acquainted more than any other person in British India with all the peculiarities of our method of cultivating and transplanting the Quinine trees in the forests, and ... in consequence possesses all the necessary qualifications for the superintendence and general direction of the Quinine culture in British India.[122]

In response, Spruce, one of Markham's associates in South America wrote from Guayaquil in 1862 defending the latter. He implicitly alleged Anderson for his ignorance of the 'native conditions' that reared the cinchonas in South America.

... Mr Markham's notions on the cultivation of Cinchonae entirely coincide with my own ... If some empiric who has never seen the Cinchonae in their native country, has sufficient influence to inform the Indian government to attempt to cultivate Cinchona plants accordingly then let him be responsible for the result ...[123]

---

[121] Ibid.
[122] Junghuhn to Governor General of Netherlands India. Home, Public, 16 December 1861, 26–30 A (NAI).
[123] Mr Spruce, 'Note on the cultivation of Cinchonae', (Chandug near Guayaquil, June 1862). General, General. 14–16 A, September 1862 (WBSA).

Hetero-Genus: Cinchona 'Experiments' in British India

Published in the same year, Markham's *Travels in Peru and India* was much less polemical. He was more interested in the eclectic facets of the landscapes through which he travelled in and around the Nilgiris. Each new spot in the Nilgiris reminded him of different places he had encountered during his extensive travels as an explorer. As he travelled from the port at Calicut towards Ootacamund he felt that 'the whole scene bore a close resemblance to one of Sandwich or Society Islands'.[124] Further into the interior, rows of betel nut plants reminded Markham of palm trees on familiar settings in 'the South Sea Islands or the forests of South America'.[125] On reaching Dawson's hotel at Ootacamund he found it difficult to persuade himself that he was 'not again in England'. The hotel was located amidst gardens and plantations of Eucalyptus, with trees introduced from Australia around them.[126] However, such 'English associations' faded as he walked merely a few miles away from Ootacamund. Instead, 'there was much' that made him feel that he had returned amongst the Pajonales in the 'Chinchona region of Caravaya'.[127]

Bureaucratic exoticisation of cinchonas in British India converged with the realpolitik of plantations. In the process, the cultivation of cinchonas was projected as both difficult and yet plausible. Cinchona plants figured in the official files as both alien and yet increasingly adaptable in British Indian landscapes. Material properties of cinchonas as well as the textures of certain landscapes appeared suitably malleable.

In Markham's writings the Nilgiris figured as a landscape with myriad facets and possibilities, which the European investor could intervene and mould at his will. He mentioned that with the aid of 'an East Indian foreman and labourers from the Mysore plains', William G. McIvor, the Superintendent of the Botanic Gardens at Ootacammud, had converted 'the wild mountain sides into a beautiful public garden', consisting of English fruits, flowers, vegetables and grasses.[128] Similarly, Markham indicated how several extensive European estates of coffee had emerged near Coonoor. He therefore found no reason to doubt that the 'English capitalist would make large and rapid profits' by cultivating cinchonas in the Nilgiris.[129]

Such hope converged with attempts to characterise the cinchonas as a widely heterogeneous family of plants. It has already been shown how official narratives presented the cinchonas as delicate plants. They were shown to grow in climates that were relatively unfamiliar to British

---

[124] Markham, *Travels*, 341.   [125] Ibid., 349.   [126] Ibid., 356–357.   [127] Ibid.
[128] Ibid., 371.   [129] Ibid., 378.

officials in India. These plants appeared as rare and exotic in India. Such projections added to the aura associated with them. At the same time, officials continued to explore the possibility of cultivating cinchonas in British India. To that end, cinchonas figured as a botanical genus that comprised of different varieties of species, which survived in diverse conditions. Such understandings questioned the apparent rigidities within certain prevalent geographies of cinchona.

Official files mentioned at least twenty different varieties of cinchonas.[130] Basic physical attributes were supposed to vary extensively amongst the different species of cinchonas. Thomas Anderson was delighted to note the 'profusion of flowers' in certain varieties of cinchonas. He was, however, amazed by the absence of flowers in some others.[131] J. Broughton, the Government Quinologist at Ootacamund, pointed out a few years later that the vigour of growth, size of trees and content of quinine varied in the different varieties of cinchonas, adding that such qualities might manifest differently within the same species when exposed to different conditions.[132]

In official correspondence, such inherent diversities were frequently invoked. This enabled officials to assert that different varieties of these plants thrived in an extensive range of climatic conditions.[133] There could hardly, then, be any specific locality in British India that could rear every variety of cinchonas within the shared space of a single plantation. However, different localities in British India, it was hoped, might prove suitable for the survival of different species of cinchona. The difficult task confronting the officials was to suggest comfortable localities for every species considered rich in quinine.

A report was solicited in September 1859 from W. Jameson, the Superintendent of the Botanic Gardens, North Western Provinces, on the 'best localities for cultivating cinchonas in North Western Provinces'. He recommended a range of different sites suitable for each variety of cinchona.[134] Anderson was also drawn into these discussions and speculated on possible sites for different varieties:

There is an abundance of localities obtainable in the Neilgherries for the cultivation of the less temperate species of Cinchona, such as *C Succirubra*,

[130] W. Jameson to F. B. Outram, No. 439, 11 September 1859. Home, Public, 13 January 1860, 18–27 A (NAI).

[131] T. Anderson to Secretary, Government of Bengal, 30 June 1868, Home, Public, 29 August 1868. 34–35 A (NAI).

[132] J. Broughton to Government Fort St George, Revenue department, 31 August 1870, Ootacamund. Home, Public, 13 May 1871, 99–100 A (NAI).

[133] Jameson to Outram. Home, Public, 13 January 1860, 18–27 A (NAI).

[134] Ibid.; Anderson to Grey. Home, Public, 22 February 1862, 54–58 A (NAI).

C Calisaya, and probably *C Nidita* and *Peruviana,* as well as *C Pahudiana.* For the temperate species of which we now possess *C Micrantha* and *C Lancifolia,* . . . *C Peruviana* . . . that will almost withstand a slight fall of snow, we must look for a proper home in the moist region of Darjeeling and the damp deep inner valleys of Eastern Kumaon.[135]

Such confident and precise recommendations were often followed by cautious caveats. Once again, various 'idiosyncrasies'[136] of the material life of these plants were elaborated to suggest how the sustenance of cinchona plants in British India continued to be both plausible and difficult. Various reasons were extended to explain why the identification of suitable sites for cultivating different species of cinchonas in British India remained arduous. First, knowledge about the physical characteristics of different varieties of cinchonas was shown as far from clear. It made the search for suitable localities appear as difficult. For example, D. Macpherson, the Inspector General of Hospitals, Madras Presidency, was amazed by the striking differences amongst 'authorities' and 'best informed writers' regarding the altitude where the species *Josephiana* thrived.[137] The cinchona trees were described as extremely sensitive to changes in altitude. An error of 500 feet could have had an adverse impact on the health of the trees.[138] Such varied understandings of the altitude conducive to the survival of these plants, Macpherson predicted, would make the search for suitable sites in India prolonged and difficult. Secondly, these converged with considerable confusions involving the precise identities of the seeds and plants that were transmitted to British India. Such confusions were manifested in official accounts in different ways. Superintendents of different botanical gardens in India or Ceylon tended to doubt the projected identities of certain varieties of cinchonas they received. It appears from the official correspondence that different species of cinchonas were not always absolutely rigid, inflexible categories. Instead, these appeared more as subjective labels. The identities of different varieties of cinchonas could often be a subject of debate amongst contending officials.[139] Thirdly, it was suggested that the

---

[135] Anderson to Grey. Ibid. (NAI).

[136] G. E. Shaw, *Quinine Manufacture in India* (London: Institute of Chemistry of Great Britain and Ireland, 1935), 3.

[137] Anderson to Grey. Home, Public, 22 February 1862, 54–58 A (NAI); Anderson to Grey. Home, Public, 16 December 1861, 26–30 A (NAI); D. Macpherson to J. Boudillon, No. 7, Fort St George Ootacamund, 5 February 1861. Home, Public, 25 April 1861, 34–35 A (NAI).

[138] Junghuhn to Governor General of Netherlands India. Home, Public, 16 December 1861, 26–30 A (NAI).

[139] T. Anderson, 'First Annual Report on the Experimental Cultivation of the Quiniferous Cinchona in British Sikkim from 1 April 1862 to 30 April 1863', 'Appendix'. Home Public, 19 August 1863, 85–87 A (NAI).

'vital properties' of seeds and plants were often lost in transit. This was mainly caused by unexpected delays during the long journey from South America. As principal distinguishing features became obscured by these changes, the identities of different groups of seeds in bags or Wardian cases often blurred.[140] Finally, careless receiving officers in the Calcutta or Bombay ports were often warned against ignoring labels and mixing up different species of cinchonas together. These made the selection of suitable sites difficult as 'the locality that suits one species may be quite unfitted for another'.[141]

Government files therefore predicted inevitable delays in the selection of suitable sites for cinchona plantations. It was proposed that the planting of every variety would be tried in different locations.[142] Sites, which were found unsuitable for most species would be discarded, and the trials would shift to another location. These trials would be pursued until the most suitable sites for the different species of cinchonas were identified. These efforts to locate 'suitable spots' for cultivating different varieties of cinchonas in the 1860s were shown to constitute a series of 'experiments'. As part of these experiments (see Figure 1.5), Anderson suggested the 'immediate establishment of nurseries on all the mountain ranges...where large tracts of forests are available, such as the Khasia hills, Eastern Himalayas, the mountains extending from Chittagong down to the Malayan peninsula'.[143] He got sheds erected at three different altitudes in Darjeeling.

Sheds have been erected at the plantation at three different heights, at 3743, 2500 and 1760 feet above the sea. In these I have placed a considerable number of all species i.e. *Succirubra* 100, *Officinalis* 100, *Micrantha* 50, *Calisaya* 2, *Pahudiana* 21; a total of 273 plants...They will afford at the same time some data concerning the comparative rate of growth of the species at different altitudes.[144]

In British Sikkim as well as the Nilgiris several sites were chosen and then discarded in the early 1860s. In search of compatible altitude, temperature, humidity, shade and vegetation, the 'experiment' travelled from Sinchan in British Sikkim to neighbouring Sinchal. 'Cold of the

---

[140] Macpherson to Boudillon. Home, Public, 25 April 1861, 34–35 A (NAI).

[141] Anderson to the Secretary, Government of Bengal. Home, Public, 13 January, 1860, 18–27 A (NAI).

[142] Anderson to Grey. Home, Public, 16 December 1861, 26–30 A (NAI); T. Anderson, 'Report on the Cultivation of the Quineferous Cinchona at Darjeeling from the 1 April 1863 to 15 July 1864.' Home, Public, 31 January 1865, 94–98 A (NAI).

[143] Anderson to Grey. Home, Public, 16 December 1861, 26–30 A (NAI).

[144] Anderson, 'Report on the Cultivation.' Home, Public, 31 January 1865, 94–98 A (NAI).

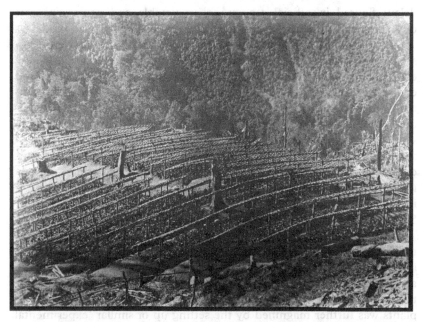

Figure 1.5 Photograph of a cinchona nursery at Munsong in British Sikkim set up a few decades later. Credit: Wellcome Library, London.

winter' enforced a shift from Sinchal to Lebong.[145] The plantations further moved to a more 'suitable spot' on the 'south eastern slopes of a long spur from Sinchal' in June 1864. It was called Rungbee.[146] Anderson and his colleagues kept exploring newer locations for the experiment in eastern and northeastern British India. Similar experiments were organised in the Nilgiris. The search for suitable sites began almost simultaneously in Dodabetta, Neddivattam, Avalanche, Mercara, Annamalai and Coorg forests.[147] Markham proposed similar 'trials and experimental cultivation' of cinchonas in Mahabaleshwar, the 'high hills east of Goa', Wynaad, the Shervaroys and 'mountains between Tinnevelly and Travancore'.[148]

Officials cautioned that such elaborate and widespread trials might involve a considerable length of time. Possible setbacks or definite

---

[145] Anderson, 'First Annual Report.' Home, Public, 19 August 1863, 85–87A (NAI).
[146] Anderson, 'Report on the Cultivation.' Home, Public, 31 January 1865, 94–98 A (NAI).
[147] Macpherson to Boudillon, No. 7, Fort St George Ootacamund, 5 February 1861. Home, Public, 25 April 1861, 34–35 A (NAI).
[148] Markham, *Travels*, 509–520.

delays figured in official reports as predictable and necessary costs of a long and difficult experiment. Thus, possible setbacks or delays could now appear as imminent and even necessary. These were foreseen as useful revelations in a long-standing scientific trial. These experiments, it was hoped, would be followed by more sustained and confident investments in the plantation of cinchonas; culminating eventually in the establishment of factories for the manufacture of quinine. Macpherson predicted that the project would require seven more years before it began to yield 'remunerative returns'.[149] In 1862, Anderson referred to his conversations with the Dutch managers of the cinchona plantations in Java. They were not expecting 'to obtain quinine in its full proportion until trees have acquired their full development in thickness as well as stature. That will not be attained under 40 or 50 years...'.[150]

Thus, profitable re-colonisation of cinchonas in British India, not unlike the journey of these plants from South America, was foretold as a very long and tedious process. Such elaborate arrangements to govern and make sense of the cinchonas seem to have reconfirmed them as distant, delicate and difficult plants. The enigma about these recalcitrant plants was further magnified by the setting up of similar 'experimental trials and cultivation' not only in the Nilgiris, but also in various sites across the British Empire including Peradenia and Nuwera Ellia in Ceylon, Sikkim, Bhutan and Khasia Hills in the Eastern Himalayas, Yoonzaleen Hills in British Pegu and various spots in Trinidad and Jamaica.[151]

'Indian Plantations'

Experimental plantations also emerged as sites for the relative profanation of cinchonas. Here, through the everyday acts of handling, trenching, planting, carrying, shedding, enclosing, discarding and replacing them, the cinchonas gradually became more mundane in the mid-1860s.[152] Private investments in cinchona experiments began in 1862

---

[149] Macpherson to Boudillon, No. 7, 5 February 1861. Home, Public, 25 April 1861, 34–35 A (NAI).

[150] Anderson to Grey. Home, Public, 22 February 1862, 54–58 A (NAI).

[151] Markham, *Travels*, 509–520.

[152] Government of Madras to Secretary of State for India, No. 57, 24 August 1869, Madras in Anonymous (ed), *East India, Chinchona Cultivation (Copy of All Correspondence Between the Secretary of State for India and the Governor General, and the Governors of Madras and Bombay, Relating to the Cultivation of Chinchona Plants from April 1866 to April 1870)* (London: House of Commons, 1870), 218 http://books.google.co.uk/books?id=bfxKAAAAYAAJ&printsec=frontcover#v=onepage&q&f=false (retrieved on 1 May 2013).

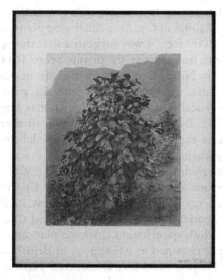

Figure 1.6 Photograph of a cinchona tree in British Ceylon, 1882. Reproduced by kind permission of the Syndics of Cambridge University Library, Shelfmark: Ms. ADD. 7957_6_55. F.H.H. Guillemard Photographs.

in Ceylon[153] and extended subsequently to Kangra valley, Assam,[154] Darjeeling[155] and Malabar.[156] The supposedly exclusive status of cinchonas was compromised when in the private estates these thrived in the intimate company of tea, teak and coffee plants.[157]

Besides, expediencies of private planters revised the geographies of certain species of cinchonas. These plants (see Figure 1.6), it was now argued, could survive in more eclectic geographical conditions than it was previously assumed. Private experiments examined, for example, whether cinchonas could be accommodated within previously acquired tea estates. In such cases geographies of cinchonas began to follow the set

---

[153] Markham, *Travels*, 511.

[154] 'Appointment of a Committee for Conducting Experiments with the Alkaloids, besides Quinine, which the Cinchona contains', Home, Public, 26 February 1866, 58 A (NAI).

[155] T. Anderson, 'Report on the Cultivation of Cinchona at Darjeeling from 1 April 1865 to 31 March 1866', Home, Public, October 1866, 21–22 (NAI).

[156] A. Fraser to the Secretary, Government of India, P.W.D, No. 139–7 F, 6 May 1868. Home, Public, 4 July 1868, 57–63 A (NAI).

[157] T. Anderson to the Secretary, Government of Bengal, 30 June 1868, Botanical Gardens Calcutta. Home, Public, 29 August 1868, 34–35 A (NAI).

trajectories of existing tea plantations. In contrast with conventional wisdom, which had set the ideal habitat of *Cinchona Succirubra* plants at altitudes varying from 2000 to 3000 feet, it was suggested that this species could thrive, as well, along with tea plants on the private Selim Tea Estate at the foot of the Terai hills in North Bengal at an altitude of 350 feet above the level of sea.[158] Thus, when confronted with the realpolitik of private plantations the physical attributes of the cinchonas began to surface as much more flexible. By managing to survive in diverse geographical terrains these plants exposed themselves as less delicate and more robust than previously imagined.

At the same time, greater numbers of colonial officials were asserting themselves as spokespersons and experts of cinchonas. By the early 1870s, it was acknowledged on behalf of the government in British India that the phase of 'fair, patient, attentive and prolonged trials' was over.[159] Already in the mid-1860s government cinchona plantations had been set up at Rungbee (later renamed as Mungpoo) in British Sikkim and at various sites in the Nilgiris including Dodabetta, Neddivattam and Malkoondah. C. B. Clarke, who succeeded Anderson as the Superintendent of the Botanic Gardens in Calcutta and In-Charge of the Cinchona Cultivation in Bengal as well as his counterpart in Ootacamund, W. G. McIvor, asserted that these emerging 'Indian plantations'[160] were sites where newer knowledge about the cinchonas was being produced. The establishment of cinchona plantations in globally dispersed sites across various European colonies had diversified the prevalent geographies of these plants. These officials rejected the tendency to describe cinchonas in general or universal terms. Instead, they insisted that knowledge about cinchonas should incorporate the specific experiences of the managers of these colonial plantations.

Whether debating the appropriate techniques or suitable altitudes for planting cinchonas, Clarke or McIvor claimed to correct or add nuance to the existing insights of established botanists like Howard, Hooker or Junghuhn.[161] Clarke and McIvor alleged that these existing authorities from their distant locations in London, The Hague or Dutch Java

---

[158] Anderson, 'Report on the Cultivation', Home, Public, October 1866, 21–22 (NAI).

[159] W. Jameson to C. A. Elliott, Secretary to Government, North Western Provinces, No. 90, 10 May 1873, Saharanpur. IOR/V/23/131 No. 6 Art 30 (BL).

[160] C. B. Clarke to Secretary, Government of Bengal, No. 202, 1 July 1870, Rungbee. Home, Public, 17 December 1870, 123–125 A (NAI).

[161] Anderson, 'First Annual Report.' Home, Public, 19 August 1863, 85–87 A; Clarke to the Secretary, Government of Bengal. Home, Public, 17 December 1870, 123–125 A (NAI).

could not have immediate exposure to the specific vagaries experienced in the 'Indian plantations'. These managers of the emerging plantations in British India contested some of their generalisations about cinchonas. For instance, Clarke wrote an engaging review of Howard's second major book about the cinchonas, *The Quinology of East Indian Plantations* in 1870. Clarke criticised Howard's ignorance of the conditions in which cinchonas thrived in Bengal, while questioning his speculations about the most suitable altitudes in which these plants could survive.

The conclusions, though stated as general do not in many important points hold as good as regards the Bengal plantations... Howard opens the discussion of the proper elevation at which to grow Cinchonas in India in these words: 'Recent observations on this point may save the apparently useless attempt to cultivate these plants at a level below 4000 feet above the ocean', Upon this I remark that the whole of the 1,000,000 plants of *C Succirubra* at Rungbee are below that level. The species appears to thrive best at about 2000 feet elevation, and grows very well down to the river at 800 feet elevation.[162]

Thus, Indian plantations did not witness the straightforward application of instructions conveyed from the distant 'centres of calculation' in Europe or Dutch Java. Instead, these were emerging as sites where conventional wisdom about cinchonas could be reexamined, and where newer claims to knowledge about cinchonas could be asserted. Unsurprisingly, experiences derived by managers in these colonial plantations soon formed the basis of a series of books on the art of cultivating cinchonas.[163]

By the late 1860s, 'Indian plantations' began to feature as new destinations for training future managers of neighbouring plantations. When cinchona experiments were about to be initiated in British Burma in 1868, officials who required training like the Conservator of Forests in Burma, Captain W. J. Seaton, were not made to travel to distant 'natural' cinchona forests in South America or the plantations in Dutch Java. Instead, Seaton was deputed to the South Indian plantations in Ootacamund and the Nellumboor Teak plantations in Malabar

---

[162] C. B. Clarke to the Secretary, Government of Bengal, No. 165, 10 February 1870, Botanic Gardens Calcutta. Home, Public, 12 March 1870, 157 A (NAI).

[163] W. G. McIvor, *Notes on the Propagation and Cultivation of the Medicinal Cinchonas, or Peruvian bark Trees* (Madras: Graves, Coodson, 1863); G. King, *A Manual of Cinchona Plantation in India* (Calcutta: Office of the Superintendent of Government Print, 1880).

for receiving training and acquiring knowledge in the art of managing cinchonas.[164]

'A Botanical Curiosity'

Thus various cultures of plantations from the mid-1860s hinted at the gradual transformation of cinchonas into more tameable, accessible and everyday objects in British India. Still, the predominant image of the plants as invaluable rarities persisted. Cinchonas were constructed not only as objects of botanical knowledge and plantation capital, but also as materials which could arouse and sustain curiosities across an expansive imperial world. In course of the decade and beyond, these plants found themselves empowered to reinforce various imperial protocols, processes, desires and hierarchies.

Cinchonas were amongst the few objects which bound up the distant corners of the British Empire into a globally interconnected political entity. Cinchonas brought officials in British India into immediate contact with counterparts in other parts of the Empire. As we will see, the journeys of British officials posted in Burma like Captain Seaton were not exceptional events. Cinchonas necessitated correspondence between Anderson, the Superintendent of Botanic Gardens in Calcutta, McIvor, the Superintendent of the Botanic Gardens in Ootacamund in the Nilgiri hills, Mr Thwaites, the Director of the Royal Botanic Gardens of Peradenia, Dr Brandis, the Conservator of Forests in Pegu, and Mr N. Wilson, the Superintendent of the Botanic Gardens in Jamaica. Discussions concerning techniques of managing cinchonas were often followed by exchanges of plants as well as officials located at different sites.[165] In a letter Anderson thanked the Director of the Royal Botanical Gardens at Kew, William Hooker, for nominating Gustav Mann as the head gardener in charge of the cinchona experiments in Darjeeling. 'Mann had just returned from the West Coast of Africa, where he had greatly distinguished himself in the capacity of Government Botanist...'.[166] These routine interactions between personnel inhabiting dispersed locations and disparate contexts were amongst the many ways the British Empire was crystallised not only as an ideological configuration, but also as an extensive machinery of governmental enactments.

---

[164] Fraser, to Secretary, Government of India, Public Works Department. Home, Public, 4 July 1868, 57–63 A (NAI).

[165] Markham, *Travels*, 511, 518.

[166] Anderson, 'Report on the Cultivation.' Home, Public, 31 January 1865, 94–98 A (NAI).

At the same time, these exchanges were not confined within the British Empire. Figure 1.7 and Figure 1.8 indicate that cinchonas also figured as objects of exchange between empires. Such exchanges could take either the form of gifts or collaborations. In the early 1860s, different colonial governments exchanged cinchona seeds and plants as gifts. Cinchonas began to feature as valuable plants that symbolised good will. In the early 1860s, the English government reportedly placed up to 800 plants at the disposal of the French Governor General in Algeria.[167] Again in June 1866, a consignment of many thousands of cinchona seeds was despatched by the Madras Government to be sown in Mexico.[168] Similarly, the Dutch Government in Java presented cinchona seeds and plants to British India in different moments in the 1860s.[169] The Governor General of Dutch Java, for instance, wrote to the Governor General of British India from Buitenzorg in June 1861: '...The successful issue of the cultivation of the Peruvian bark in the Island of Java enables me to place at the disposal of the British Government 500,000 seeds, about 100 or 200 seedlings of the Chinchona *Encumaefolia*, and from 50 to 100 plants of the Chinchona *Calisaya*...'.[170] In April 1865, the Botanical Gardens in Calcutta was reported to have received an assortment of 200 seeds belonging to the *Cinchona Calisaya* variety from Dr Junghuhn, the Principal Inspector of the cinchona cultivation at Dutch Java. Anderson revealed a brief history of those seeds; the seeds were produced in Java in one of the cinchona trees Junghuhn had brought from the Botanic Gardens in Leiden. Those trees, it was claimed, had been raised from seeds presented to the Dutch Government in the early 1850s from Bolivia by Weddell, the French botanist.[171] Such gift giving was often reciprocated by the British Indian officials.[172]

Cinchonas enabled collaborations between competing empires. From the early 1860s senior officials from British India travelled into Dutch Java to study proliferating cinchona plantations. Most significant amongst them were Thomas Anderson, the Superintendent of the Botanical Gardens in Calcutta and D. Macpherson, the Inspector Generals of Hospitals, Madras Presidency. In his account of his trip to Java,

---

[167] Planchon, *Peruvian*, 46.

[168] Government of Madras to Secretary of State for India, No. 7, 26 June 1866, in Anonymous (ed), *East India, Chinchona Cultivation*, 15.

[169] Junghuhn to Governor General of Netherlands India, Home, Public, 16 December 1861, 26–30 A (NAI).

[170] Ibid.

[171] Anderson, 'Report on the cultivation'. Home, Public, 31 January 1865, 94–98 A (NAI).

[172] Anderson to Grey. Home, Public, 22 February 1862, 54–58 A (NAI).

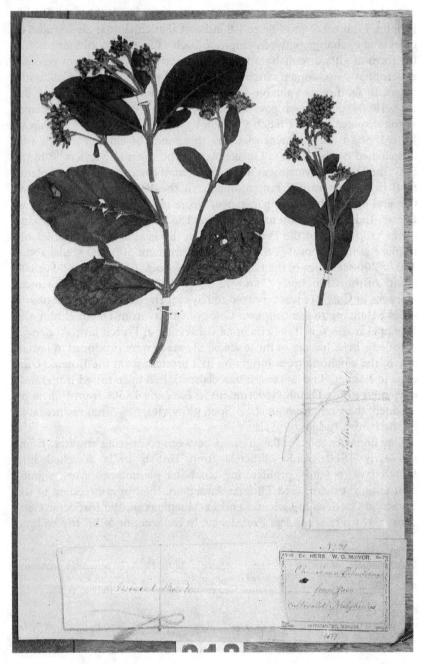

Figure 1.7 A sample of *Cinchona Pahudiana* from Java cultivated in Nilgiris, 1877. Credit: Wellcome Library, London.

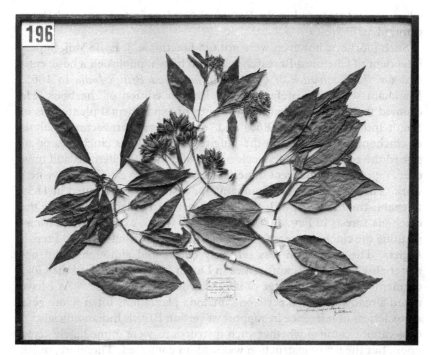

Figure 1.8 A sample of *Cinchona Officinalis* from Madras cultivated in Java. Credit: Wellcome Library, London.

Anderson devoted an entire section towards acknowledging the support he received from the Dutch government in Java. He claimed to have received assistance 'at every step': These included arrangement of rest-houses in the interiors, supply of 'ample relay of coolies', 'trained plant collectors', 'servants', horses and wardian cases. He recounted how he received generous logistical support from the Acting Governor General of Netherlands India, The Resident of the Preanger Regencies and the Regent of Bandong. In his journeys into the interiors of Dutch Java, Anderson was joined by the Geologist to the Prussian embassy in Java, Baron Von Richthofen, as well as leading Dutch experts of the Javanese plantations, de Vrij and Junghuhn. These Prussian and Dutch officials accompanied Anderson almost 'on all occasions satisfying' his 'curiosity on every point'. Anderson claimed to benefit from the inputs he received about the possible geographies of cinchona plantations from these officials. On his return in February 1862, he reported to have brought 40000 seeds and 412 plants belonging to the *Cinchona Calisaya*, *Cinchona Pahudiana* and *Cinchona Lancifolia* species from Dutch Java which were distributed in the Botanical Gardens in Calcutta and Oota-camund.[173]

Such journeys, however, were not unidirectional. J. E. de Vrij, Super-intendent of Chemical Researches in Dutch Java, published a book enti-tled *On the Cultivation of Quinine in Java and British India* in 1865. Markham wrote the preface to the English edition of the book. He claimed that de Vrij had visited the sites of experimental plantations in South India in the early 1860s and 'made a very satisfactory analysis of cinchona bark grown on the Nilgiri hills'.[174] Thus cinchonas occa-sioned the convergence of an eclectic set of botanists, chemists and trav-ellers representing different imperial formations into a collaborative net-work. The Ecuador Land Company, for instance, was formed in 1859 to enable the French and British governments to collectively explore the cinchona forests in Ecuador. The company was to extend help in trans-planting the cinchona trees from Ecuador to the British India and French Algiers. The suggestion was seriously considered although it did not materialise.[175] Besides, authorities in Dutch Java often advised the Gov-ernment of India on a range of issues involving cinchonas.[176] As I have noted already, Dutch experts on cinchona plantations often wrote gen-erous letters of reference in support of certain British Indian officials.[177] One cannot confirm whether such instructions were immediately acted upon, but the act of instruction was seldom contested. Therefore, much like cinchona plants and seeds, botanical officials, administrative instruc-tions, and proposals for collaborations travelled beyond particular impe-rial boundaries. Planting cinchonas in the colonies seem to have been a shared project where the delineating protocols of imperial formations went blur. At the same time, however, such cultures of exchanging gifts and efforts of collaboration between designated imperial officials rein-forced the French, Dutch and British Empires as distinctively tangible entities. These recurrent rituals of trans-imperial exchanges and collab-orations, in turn, contributed in sustaining the image of cinchonas as invaluable plants.

Within British India, enthusiasm about cinchonas was not confined to the botanical establishments and the planters' communities within

---

[173] Ibid.

[174] J. E. de Vrij, 'Notice,' *On the Cultivation of Quinine in Java and British India* (London: G. E. Eyre & W. Spottiswoode, 1865).

[175] D. Williams, 'Clements Roberts Markham', 433.

[176] The Governor General of Netherlands India to the Viceroy and Governor General of British India, No. 185 A, 13 June, 1861, Buitenzorg. Home Public, 19 July 1861, 8–10 A (NAI).

[177] Dr Junghuhn to the Governor General of Netherlands India, 23 October 1861, Lembang. Home, Public, 16 December 1861, 26–30 A (NAI).

Madras and Bengal presidencies. By 1862 different provincial governments within British India had begun to consider organising cinchona
experiments a matter of dignity. They often hankered for their share of
cinchona seeds and plants even when supplies were not forthcoming.
For instance, W. Jameson, the Superintendent of the Botanical Gardens
in North Western Provinces, wrote to his counterpart in Calcutta, Dr
Thomas Anderson, soliciting some cinchona plants in a ward's case.
He received no reply. Jameson wrote again, this time to Mr A. Grote,
a member of the Sudder Board of Revenue in Calcutta. Grote turned
his request down. Thereafter, Jameson made similar requests to the
Madras government. Jameson claimed that he had located suitable sites
for experimental cultivation in the province, long before any seeds were
promised to him.[178] In these letters, Jameson mentioned that two sites
selected for the experiment in the province belonged to the territory of
one Tiree Raja. Apparently, the Raja had agreed to 'make land available'
for experiments. One cannot be sure from Jameson's letters whether the
Raja willingly volunteered to be part of the project.

However, cinchona plants and seeds had emerged widely amongst
local Rajas of the native states as objects of collections in the 1860s. The
Madras government in June 1866 published a long list of individuals and
agencies who on request, were distributed samples of cinchona plants
growing in the Nilgiris.[179] The list, amongst other suggestive information, reveals that the Rajas of Travancore and Poonganoor had requested
and were then supplied with cinchona plants from the emerging plantations in the Nilgiris. A closer study of the list suggests that cinchonas
had by the mid-1860s aroused the curiosities and commercial ambitions of a range of individuals and institutions located in distant sites.
Requests for cinchonas were received not only from different stations
within British India particularly South India, Central Provinces, Punjab, Cachar and Assam, but also from places situated as far as Rangoon,
Java, Melbourne, Wellington, Mauritius, Reunion, Algiers and Jamaica.
Amongst the applicants were those we have already encountered in this
chapter: noted botanists Dr Thomas Anderson, Superintendent of the
Botanical Gardens in Calcutta, Dr W. Jameson, the Superintendent of
the Botanic Gardens in North Western Provinces, and Dr Junghuhn, the
Principal Inspector of cinchona cultivations at Java. Requests appeared
to have been made on behalf of institutions of state as well as private business groups, for example, Royal Gardens at Mauritius, French

---

[178] W. Jameson to G. Couper, No. 524, 20 September 1862, Kumaon. Home, Public, 15
October 1862, 14–16 A (NAI).
[179] Home Public, July 1866, 129 B (NAI).

government at Algiers, Messrs Thompson Shaw and Company amongst others. Similar applications were also received from the Governor Generals of Java and Goa, Governors of Vizagapatanam, Bombay and Madras, Chief Commissioner of Nagpore, Collectors of Belgaun and Honore. The list bore names of hundreds of other individuals. Those names were preceded by a wide range of titles: Mr, Professor, Dr, Reverend, Colonel, Captain, Major, General and so on. These suggest that individuals interested in acquiring cinchonas could be private individuals or personnel employed in different positions in the colonial military establishments or civil administrations. They could be academics, physicians or missionaries.[180] It appears that collecting cinchonas had emerged as an obsession across the colonial world. Possessing cinchonas figured not only as a symbol of significant status and prestige, but also as an expression of many attributes of Victorian respectability ranging from commercial enterprise and scientific inquisitiveness to benevolence.

Unsurprisingly therefore British Indian cinchonas attracted the attention of antiquarians, artists and keepers of imperial museums. Since very early in the 1870s different varieties of cinchonas growing in India appeared to make their ways as 'botanical curiosities'[181] to museums and exhibitions in Europe and the United States.[182] Cinchonas also began to circulate as objects of contemporary global news. Apart from recurrently finding expression in the sketches by Anglo-Indian artists (see Figure 1.9 and Figure 1.10), the progress of 'Indian plantations' was commented on in newspapers published from places as distant as Singapore, Brisbane and Wellington in the 1870s.[183] In vernacular medical marketplaces across British India, for example in Bengal, the arrival of cinchonas witnessed many publications in its praise as well as a series of advertisements about indigenous substitutes for quinine.[184]

---

[180] Ibid.

[181] Home, Medical, May 1886, 37–38 A (NAI); Anderson to Grey. Home, Public, 22 February 1862, 54–58 A (NAI).

[182] Home, Public, 11 March 1871, 36–37 A; Home, Medical, April 1882, 20–22 A (NAI).

[183] Anonymous, 'The Cinchona Plant', The Brisbane Courier (Saturday, 8 February 1868), 6 http://trove.nla.gov.au/ndp/del/article/1318474 [retrieved on 26 December 2012]; Anonymous, 'The Cultivation of the Cinchona Plant', Wellington Independent, 22, 2667 (14 April 1868), 5. http://paperspast.natlib.govt.nz/cgi-bin/paperspast?a=d&d=WI18680414.2.25&e=----10-1--0WILLIAM+EDWARD+KNOWLES-all [retrieved on 18 March 2013]; Anonymous, 'Cinchona Culture', The Straits Times (4 June 1870), 1, http://newspapers.nl.sg/Digitised/Article/straitstimes18700604.2.7.aspx [retrieved on 18 March 2013].

[184] See for instance, Anonymous, 'Cinchona', Swasthya, 3, 5 (1899), 145–148; Anonymous, 'Sarvajvarankusha,' Education Gazette and Saptahik Vartabaha (9 March 1888), 733; G. Nandi, 'Malaria Jvarey Dasyadi Pachan.' Chikitsak 1, 1 (1889), 70–72.

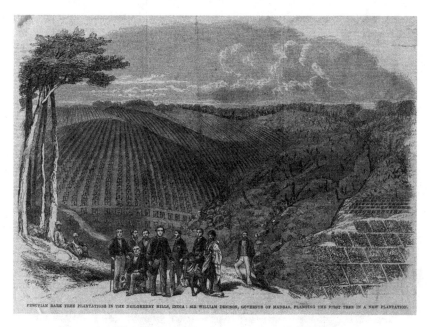

PERUVIAN BARK TREE PLANTATIONS IN THE NEILGHERRY HILLS, INDIA : SIR WILLIAM DENISON, GOVERNOR OF MADRAS, PLANTING THE FIRST TREE IN A NEW PLANTATION.

Figure 1.9 Wood-engraving of the planting of the first cinchona tree in
a new plantation in the Nilgiris. Credit: Wellcome Libary, London.

The establishment of cinchona plantations in the eastern Himalayas provided one of many occasions in which the Bengali *bhadraloks* came in immediate contact with the interiors of British Sikkim. Over time, destinations like Mungpoo became conceivable as locations for *bhadralok* livelihood, memoirs and nostalgia.[185]

Earliest photographic images (see Figure 1.11 and Figure 1.12) of cinchona plantations show keen local inhabitants engaged in voluntary labour in the misty landscapes of British Sikkim or Peradeniya in Ceylon. However, these photographic projections about eager labourers framed by the colonial state need to be read with caution. It is possible to argue that these photographs captured individuals who were often described in the published official correspondences as members of dispossessed 'hill tribes', discredited 'jhoom cultivators', 'Nepalese coolies', 'Lepchas' and convict labourers.[186] Introduced in South Asia in the immediate

[185] M. Devi, *Mungpoote Rabindranath (Rabindranath in Mungpoo)* (Calcutta: Prima Publications, 1943).

[186] T. Anderson to Secretary, Government of Bengal, 30 June 1868, Botanical Gardens Calcutta. Home, Public, 29 August 1868, 34–35 A (NAI); Veale, *A Historical Geography of the Nilgiri Cinchona Plantations*, 252, 261–275.

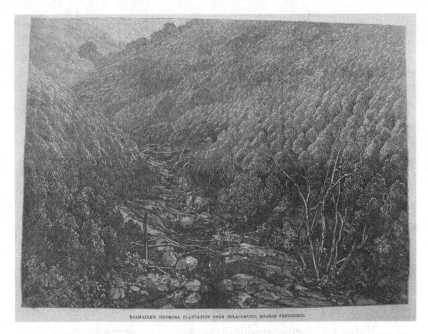

BALMADIE'S CINCHONA PLANTATION NEAR DOLACAMUND, MADRAS PRESIDENCY.

Figure 1.10 Wood-engraving showing 'Balmadie's Cinchona Plantation Near Dolcamund, Madras Presidency' from the *Illustrated London News*, (10 February 1872), 132. Credit: Author's Copy.

aftermath of the munity of 1857 as a hallmark of humanitarianism, these plants quite soon found themselves implicated within broader histories of dispossession and incarceration.

Conclusion

The history of circulating and planting cinchonas in British India in the initial decades of 1850s and 1860s reveals the imbrications of imperial governance, botanical knowledge, materiality of plants and processes of commodification. Collapsing the distinction between biographical objects and public commodities proposed by Janet Hoskins, I have argued that the bureaucratic construction of cinchonas as a commodity was founded on assertions about their intense physicality.[187] This could take two apparently contradictory forms. At one level, cinchonas figured

[187] J. Hoskins, *Biographical Objects: How Things Tell the Stories of People's Lives* (New York and London: Routledge, 1998), 7–9.

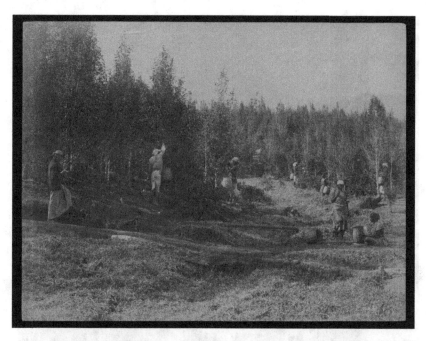

Figure 1.11 Reproduced by kind permission of the Syndics of Cambridge University Library. Royal Commonwealth Society Library, Photograph collection of John Abercromby Alexander. (No infringement of copyright intended.) Shelfmark: RCS/Y303E_46. Circa 1880–1896. Photograph of local inhabitants engaged in cinchona plantations in Ceylon.

as lively objects which were sensible, delicate and feminine. Because they were projected as exotic and fragile beings, it was predicted that it would be difficult for them to be transported to and to thrive in British India. At the same time, the exigencies of economic botany shaped the projection of cinchonas as plausible objects of plantation, which could survive, grow and proliferate in British India. The physical properties of cinchonas were upheld as suitably malleable. Cinchonas appeared adaptable to the textures of landscapes, and the emerging expertise of planters, botanists, labourers and bureaucrats in British India.

The history of cinchonas in British India unfolded in the wider context of extensive engagement of British imperial actors with a range of plants. These engagements were often structured by the interactions between metropolitan institutions like the Royal Botanic Gardens at Kew, on the one hand, with emerging plantations and botanical gardens

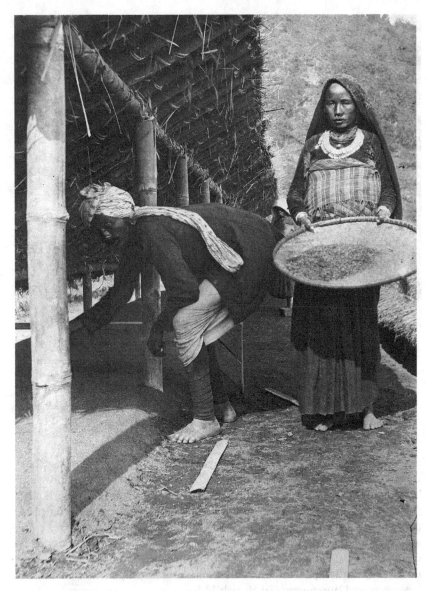

Figure 1.12 Photograph of local inhabitants labouring at Munsong cinchona plantations in British Sikkim, India. Credit: Wellcome Library.

in distant corners of the colonial world, on the other.[188] The entanglement of imperial power, botanical knowledge and plantation economy, as explored in this chapter, bears resonance with what existing histories have indicated in relation to other botanical commodities including indigo, cotton and rubber in South Asia and beyond.[189]

While imperial rule predominantly occasioned and mediated the sustenance of the commodity status of cinchona in British India in these decades, Empire itself, following an expression of Donna Haraway, was 'becoming with' cinchonas.[190] It is possible to suggest that various organisms, materials and institutions which shaped the history of cinchonas in the late 1850s and 1860s (for example, plants, barks, trees, bottles, photographs, sketches, bureaucratic correspondence, travel narratives, wardian cases, steamers, herbariums, nurseries or plantations) were as much tools of a preordained Empire as they were ingredients of an imperial apparatus in the making.

While being shaped as objects of governance and knowledge, as commodities and as materials, cinchonas, as I have noted, held together an extensive imperial network of bureaucrats, botanists, explorers, private planters, local Rajas, distant newspaper reporters, contending vernacular advertisements, photographers and illustrators amongst others. In the process, cinchonas consolidated as well as revealed fissures within what Richard Drayton calls an 'improving plantocracy'.[191] Apart from figuring as subjects of routine bureaucratic correspondence, cinchonas also engendered more spectacular circulation of personnel, gifts and ideas within and between the British, Dutch and French Empires. These plants emerged as one of the various objects which crystallised the British Empire as a globally dispersed and yet interconnected machinery of administrative predicaments and enactments.[192]

---

[188] Drayton, *Nature's Government*; Brockway, *Science and Colonial Expansion*.

[189] A. Ramesh, 'Scientific Commodities, Imperial Dreams', *Studies in the History and Philosophy of Biological and Biomedical Sciences* (2016), http://dx.doi.org/10.1016/j.shpsc.2016.04.006 [retrieved on 10 July 2016]; P. Kumar, *Indigo Plantations and Science in Colonial India* (New York and Cambridge: Cambridge University Press, 2013); S. Hazareesingh, 'Cotton, Climate and Colonialism in Dharwar, Western India, 1840–1880', *Journal of Historical Geography*, 38, 1 (2012), 1–17; B. Kar, 'Historia Elastica: A Note on the Rubber Hunt in the North-Eastern Frontier of British India', *Indian Historical Review*, 36, 1 (2009), 131–150.

[190] D. Haraway, *When Species Meet* (London: University of Minnesota Press, 2008), 2, 23–27.

[191] Drayton, *Nature's Government*, 115.

[192] For a recent work which comments on the makings of the British Empire through everyday practices of governance, see J. Wilson, *The Domination of Strangers: Modern Governance in Eastern India, 1780–1835* (Basingstoke: Palgrave Macmillan, 2008), 4, 9–18, 183–185.

Cinchonas exposed not only some of the commercial temptations of British Empire, but also featured as amongst Empire's many ideological justifications. Particularly, in the immediate aftermath of the Sepoy mutiny of 1857, cinchonas were upheld as emblematic of benevolent Victorian governance. The arrival of cinchonas in British India was presented as ushering in 'the pleasantest episode of British rule' which would be characterised by the charitable dispensation of medical relief to the colonial poor.

Such ideological talk about colonial munificence, however, was linked intimately with the reinforcement of a series of imperial prejudices and violence. The early efforts of planting cinchonas in British India reveal how in imperial history processes of anthropomorphism and dehumanisation happened hand in hand. Cinchonas were ascribed with lively as well as human-like attributes of being sensible,[193] delicate,[194] feminine[195] and idiosyncratic.[196] Resonating with the wider literature about indentured labourers, colonising administrators and soldiers, it was feared that these plants turned 'sickly' while undergoing acclimatisation in an alien climate.[197] At the same time, the beginning of cinchona experiments provided an excuse to label the Peruvian Indians of South America, or 'hill tribes' in British India or colonial 'primitives' more generally as lesser humans. Apart from being accused of 'barbarous meddling',[198] they were often denounced variously as people associated with 'rude cultivation',[199] or as inhabitants of the 'state of nature',[200] who deserved colonial tutelage because of their 'reckless short-sightedness.'[201] The planting of cinchonas in British India, it was hoped, would sustain the transformation of 'wild mountain sides into beautiful public garden(s)'.[202] Underscoring the deeper commercial and symbolic relevance of these plants, such aesthetic appeal appeared to justify the enforced employment in the emerging Nilgiri plantations of

---

[193] Junghuhn to the Governor General of Netherlands India. Home, Public, 16 December 1861, 26–30 A (NAI).
[194] Anderson to Grey. Home, Public, 22 February 1862, 54 to 58 A (NAI).
[195] Hooker, *Inaugural Dissertation*, 'Title Page'.
[196] Shaw, *Quinine Manufacture in India*, 3.
[197] Anderson to Grey. Home, Public, 22 February 1862, 54–58 A; Anderson, 'Report on the Cultivation'. Home, Public, 13 September 1862, 30–31 A (NAI).
[198] Philip, *Civilising Natures*, 260.
[199] Anderson to Secretary, Government of Bengal. Home, Public, 29 August 1868, 34–35 A (NAI).
[200] T. Wilson, *An Enquiry Into the Origin and Intimate Nature of Malaria* (London: Henry Renshaw, 1858), 14, 106, 107.
[201] Markham, *Travels*, 338.   [202] Ibid., 371.

Chinese convict labour from the Straits Settlements,[203] and the displacement of Nepalese coolies and Lepchas from forest lands and traditional livelihoods to make room for the plantations in British Sikkim.[204] Thus, like most other objects of plantations the cinchonas were entangled within broader regimes of marginalisation. The augmentation of these plants to the status of lively valuable beings was founded upon the persistence of dehumanising colonial prejudices reflected in expressions such as primitives, wild, hill tribes and barbarous.[205]

A new geography of cinchonas emerged by the 1860s. Between the late seventeenth and early nineteenth centuries, the history of cinchonas was shaped, to a considerable extent, by explorers, traders, apothecaries, alkaloid chemists and pharmacologists across the Atlantic.[206] As objects of knowledge and commerce, the cinchonas were confined predominantly (if not exclusively) to the networks of circulation between 'natural forests' in Spanish America and sites within Europe and North America. With the integration of the cinchonas into the emerging global plantation economy in the mid-nineteenth century, comparable to the case of rubber transplantation, these plants began to circulate more widely than ever before.[207] Their circulation now extended to the distant corners of the colonial world engendered by British, French and Dutch Empires. Colonial plantations in Java, Ceylon, Jamaica, St Helena, Chiffa in Algeria,[208] Bhutan and Khasia Hills in the Eastern Himalayas; Yoonzaleen Hills in British Pegu[209] emerged as new homes of cinchona plants. Those associated with planting cinchonas in Bengal and Madras presidencies in British India were locked increasingly in correspondence with institutions and individuals located across the Indian Ocean world and beyond in Jamaica, Java, Wellington, Mauritius, Algiers, Ceylon, Reunion and

[203] Veale, *A Historical Geography*, 261–275.
[204] Anderson to Secretary, Government of Bengal. Home, Public, 29 August 1868, 34–35 A (NAI).
[205] For colonial constructions of the 'wild', see K. Sivaramakrishnan, *Modern Forests: Statemaking and Environmental Change in Colonial Eastern India* (Stanford: Stanford University Press, 1999), 49, 83; A. Skaria, *Hybrid Histories: Forests, Frontiers and Wildness in Western India* (New Delhi: Oxford University Press, 1999), 39–41. For the significance of the 'primitive' in modern imperial history see for instance, J. Fabian, *Time and the Other: How Anthropology Makes its Object* (New York: Columbia University Press, 2002); P. Banerjee, *Politics of Time: 'Primitives' and History-Writing in a Colonial Society* (New Delhi: Oxford University Press, 2006).
[206] Bleichmar, 'Atlantic Competitions', 242–244.
[207] W. Dean, *Brazil and the Struggle for Rubber: A Study in Environmental History* (Cambridge: Cambridge University Press, 1987), 4.
[208] J. Broughton, to Acting Secretary, Government Fort St George, Revenue Department, 31 August 1870, Ootacamund. Home, Public, May 13 1871, 99–100 A (NAI).
[209] Markham, *Travels*, 509–520.

Rangoon.[210] In the next chapter, I will explore corresponding shifts in the geographies of the disease, which the cinchonas were most consistently attributed to heal. Projected shifts in the geographies of malaria appeared to coincide with relocations within geographies of the cinchonas.

[210] Home Public, July 1866, 129 B (NAI).

2   'An Imponderable Poison'
Shifting Geographies of a Diagnostic Category

> Malaria can be found everywhere and should be found nowhere. Malaria is entirely and completely under human control. Give me the healthiest locality in the world, and I will develop there malaria in twenty-four hours. Give me the most malarious district of the globe, and in time I will remove from it every trace of malaria.[1]

By the second quarter of the nineteenth century, as I have suggested, quinine began to signify the collective curative properties attributed to cinchona barks. In different moments in the century, across dispersed locations, quinine was recognised as the cure of a variety of maladies including fevers, dysentery, sore throat, headache, toothache and impotence.[2] Mostly such debilities were projected as results, preconditions or expressions of exposure to malaria. It has been shown in existing histories that malaria remained an ambiguous diagnostic category through most of the century. The word malaria could mean a fever-disease as well as a cause behind many diseases.[3] It surfaced as a commodious label, and was variously flexed and eclectically invoked.[4] Quinine was cited as the most consistent and effective remedy of maladies associated with malaria. Quinine and malarial diseases were often projected as invariably connected. Quinine was employed as a pharmacological agent in quick-fix diagnostic tests. Whether a malady was malarial could be determined, it appears, from how the suffering body responded to quinine.[5]

---

[1] J. F. Edwards, *Malaria: What it Means and How Avoided* (Philadelphia: P. Blakiston, 1881), 28.

[2] See Chapter 1.

[3] M. Harrison, '"Hot Beds of Disease": Malaria and Civilization in Nineteenth-Century British India', *Parassitologia*, 40 (1998), 11–18.

[4] For a detailed discussion on the range of maladies attributed to malaria in the nineteenth century and the various contradictory meanings associated with it see, R. Deb Roy, 'Mal-areas of Health: Dispersed Histories of a Diagnostic Category', *Economic and Political Weekly*, 42, 2 (January 2007), 13–19; also M. Worboys, 'From Miasmas to Germs: Malaria 1850–1879', *Parassitologia*, 36 (1994), 61–68.

[5] A. Christie, 'On Latent Malarial Disease', *Medical Times and Gazette London*, 1 (May 11, 1872), 550; G. De Pascale, 'Curious Effects of Malaria on the Body', *BMJ*, 1, 58 (February 8, 1862), 141–142.

Writings about malaria in the nineteenth century were certainly not confined to the English language, but the bulk of it emerged from English-speaking parts of the world, particularly North America, Great Britain and its colonies. One of the recurrent themes in most of these writings was to describe malaria as an insensible, imperceptible, invisible, imponderable 'mystery'.[6] Any form of physical unease witnessed almost anywhere could be potentially attributed to malaria. Such projections, however, coexisted with attempts to delimit malaria as tangible and perceptible.

Many existing histories either extend twentieth-century (or even more recent) medical understandings about malaria by analysing the political and economic causes behind historical outbreaks, or draw on these recent medical insights about malaria to retrospectively chart out the patterns of mortalities and events in earlier centuries.[7] This chapter focuses on the nineteenth century to trace the ways in which malaria itself was reconsolidated as a widely accepted diagnostic category across the imperial world. An analysis of English medical journals, government correspondence, physicians' memoirs, treatises and books reveals the cultural and political history of how during this period malaria was reinforced as an object of knowledge and governance. Malaria was re-inscribed and sustained in the course of the century through, what Gregg Mitman calls an 'ecology of knowledge,'[8] which was occasioned considerably by burgeoning imperial formations. Malaria was not only shaped by, but also, in turn, held together an extensive imperial network. The recurrent nodes which constituted this network included: *places* dispersed across the distant corners of the colonial world; *objects* ranging from decaying plants to sun-baked rocks; *careers* of geologists, meteorologists, chemists, economic-botanists, colonial administrators amongst others; and *processes* including the production of races[9] and regions,

---

[6] Quoted in M. Worboys, 'Germs, Malaria and the Invention of Mansonian Tropical Medicine', in D. Arnold (ed.), *Warm Climates and Western Medicine: The Emergence of Tropical Medicine, 1500–1900* (Amsterdam-Atlanta: Rodopi, 1996), 187; J. MacCulloch, *Malaria: An Essay on the Production and Propagation of this Poison; and On the Nature and Localities of the Places by Which it is Produced, with an Enumeration of the Diseases Caused by It and the Means of Preventing or Diminishing Them, Both at Home and in the Naval and Military Service* (London: Longman, Rees, Orme, Brown, Green, 1827), 53–55; R. La Roche, *Pneumonia: Its Supposed Connection, Pathological and Etiological, with Autumnal Fevers; Including an Inquiry into the Existence and Morbid Agency of Malaria* (Philadelphia: Blanchard and Lee, 1854). 118.

[7] These significant trends in the historiography of malaria have been discussed in the introduction.

[8] G. Mitman, 'In Search of Health: Landscape and Disease in American Environmental History', *Environmental History*, 10, 2 (April 2005), 202.

[9] D. Arnold, '"An Ancient Race Outworn': Malaria and Race in Colonial India, 1860–1930", in Waltraud Ernst and Bernard Harris (eds.), *Race, Science, Medicine, 1700–1960*

circulation of labour, intervention of the state, and the governance of compensation, architecture, pedagogy and revenue. In disparate ways, therefore, Empire and malaria were both co-consolidated by an assemblage of interconnected places, processes, objects and careers. As in the case of cinchona plants I would note here that imperial networks were hardly preordained and inflexible, but were instead 'becoming with' the categories they were themselves putting together.

Particularly significant are the various perceived material configurations of malaria. Malaria was often described as invisible and imponderable. At the same time, a range of entities and organisms such as decaying vegetation, friable granite rocks, water casks, mouldy bed sheets, stale mushrooms, dusty old books, refuse of indigo factories and groups of humans described pejoratively as tribes, aborigines, negroes and primitives were shown to personify malaria in contemporary texts. Although themselves immune, they were believed to affect their immediate vicinities with malaria. The material and physical configurations of malaria thus transgressed human–nonhuman binaries.

A history of malaria enables an engagement with continuing scholarly efforts to narrate the relevance of materials and objects in imperial history while retaining a critique of the ways in which scientific knowledge was put together.[10] Nineteenth-century malaria alerts us to the need for bringing histories of ideas and histories of material inscriptions into a sustained dialogue. While resisting the temptations of biological determinism and denying any possibility for accessing straightforward materiality of objects, historians need to examine the obsessive invocations of materials and objects in contemporary published discourse about malaria.

Such an approach also builds on considerably the literature about spatial history more generally and the production of colonial disease ecologies in particular.[11] Indeed, malaria reveals the ways in which the various constituents of the nineteenth-century colonial world were conceived as parts of a wider geographical, ecological, medical and environmental

(London and New York: Routledge, 1999), 122–143; W. Anderson, *Colonial Pathologies: American Tropical Medicine, Race and Hygiene in the Philippines* (Durham: Duke University Press 2006), 207–225.

[10] For example Mitman, 'In Search of Health', 184–210.

[11] See for example A. Bewell, *Romanticism and Colonial Disease* (Baltimore: Johns Hopkins University Press, 1999); W. Anderson, 'Geography, Race and the Nation: Remapping "Tropical" Australia, 1890–1930', in N. A. Rupke (ed.), *Medical Geography in Historical Perspective, Medical History, Supplement No. 20* (London: Wellcome Trust Centre for the History of Medicine at UCL, 2000), 146–159; D. N. Livingstone, 'Tropical Climate and Moral Hygiene: The Anatomy of a Victorian Debate', *The British Journal for the History of Science*, 32, 1 (March 1999), 93–110.

paradigm. Distant and diverse locations in Australia, Batavia, Ceylon, India, Sierra Leone or the West Indies were shown to share characteristics peculiar to colonial landscapes. The 'imaginative geographies'[12] of colonial landscapes drew upon the extant nineteenth-century stereotypes ascribed to the tropics, the East, hot climates, Torrid Zone, Indian Ocean region and so forth. Yet the recurrent invocation of materials such as rocks, casks, decaying leaves and the politics of race, regions, class or governance in contemporary literature about malaria suggests that the colonial landscapes, as Alan Bewell alerts us, 'were not simply the product of the ethnocentric inscription of pathologies onto blank spaces'.[13] Colonial landscapes figured not only as imagined recalcitrant spaces, but also as lived places which various subjects and objects of Empire inhabited and negotiated.[14]

This is certainly not to reduce all histories of malaria to episodes within colonialism. Rather this chapter explores the historical specificities in which malaria acquired exceptional currency in nineteenth-century public cultures within imperial Britain and in the wider colonial world. In so doing, it interrogates the conventional chronologies of scientific knowledge production by revealing the ways in which cures like cinchona plants and the drug quinine did precede and shape understandings about the diagnostic category, malaria. First, the discovery of quinine in the 1820s was followed by the beginnings of unprecedented circulation of the category malaria in English language sources. Secondly, with the establishment of cinchona plantations in European colonies in the mid-nineteenth century, malaria shifted from being considered a predominantly European preoccupation to an almost exclusively colonial concern.

'Insensible and Imponderable Poison'[15]

By the late 1820s, quinine manufactured commercially in Europe began reaching colonial outposts in India. A letter written by James Low from Calcutta in June 1828 to his brother Alexander Low in Jersey confirms this.[16] The letter suggests that Alexander Low had followed Pelletier and

---

[12] E. W. Said, 'Invention, Memory, and Place', *Critical Inquiry*, 26, 2 (Winter, 2000), 181.

[13] Bewell, 29.

[14] For the relationships between space and place, see S. Ramaswamy, 'Catastrophic Cartographies: Mapping the Lost Continent of Lemuria', *Representations*, 67 (Summer, 1999), 95; T. Unwin, 'A Waste of Space? Towards a Critique of the Social Production of Space', *Transactions of the Institute of British Geographers*, New Series, 25, 1 (2000), 25–26.

[15] MacCulloch, *Malaria*, 53.

[16] James Low in Calcutta to Alexander Low in Jersey, dated 2 June 1828. ACC-1037/853/2D. Howard Private Papers [LMA].

Caventou's footsteps in extracting quinine from cinchona barks. Quinine manufactured by Alexander Low in Jersey was shipped to Calcutta, where his brother received it. James Low, who otherwise worked for a bank, invested considerable energy in distributing quinine in Calcutta on behalf of European manufacturers. The letter also indicates that James Low acted as a local agent in Calcutta representing a European quinine dealer named Pelletier. It is not entirely unlikely that James Low's employer was the same Frenchman who co-discovered quinine in 1820, and who by the late 1820s was running a business venture known as the Pelletier pharmacy, and had undertaken commercial manufacture of quinine.[17]

James Low noted that the simultaneous arrival of various vessels carrying quinine into Calcutta had led to a 'glut of that article', which threatened to bring down the selling price of quinine from Rs. 25 per ounce to Rs. 4 per ounce. Under such circumstances, James Low found it difficult to profitably sell all the quinine he had received from various sources. Thus the commercial interests of Pelletier clashed with those of British manufacturers of quinine like Alexander Low. James Low mentioned that he was caught between his commitments to his brother and obligations towards his employers. The letter also indicates how the East India Company's government in British India had, by then, emerged as a convenient site for disposing of excess quinine. It hints at strategic alliances between higher officials in the colonial government, distributors of quinine in Calcutta, commercial manufactures of quinine in Europe and possibly phytochemists.

A single letter perhaps provides inadequate archival foundation for reconstructing the complex history of trade in quinine in the late 1820s, but it does offer certain revealing suggestions. Within eight years of its discovery, apart from being considered as an alkaloid confined to European phytochemical laboratories, quinine acquired the status of a lucrative item in distant colonial markets. An extensive network of European manufacturers, shipping corporations, colonial distributors and administrators had begun investing in quinine. This converged with a plethora of publications about malaria from within Britain and its colonies. The geologist John MacCulloch's 500-page book was one of the most detailed works on malaria to be published in the wake of the recognition of quinine as a lucrative commercial item. This book was published by Longman, Rees, Orme, Brown and Green in London a year before James Low's letter was written.

[17] G. E. Trease, 'Pierre-Joseph Pelletier (1788–1842): The Discoverer of Quinine', *British Journal of Pharmaceutical Practice*, 2, 7 (1980), 32–33.

Here malaria figures variously as the cause behind myriad expressions of physical unease.[18] At the same time, MacCulloch defined malaria as an 'invisible',[19] 'insensible and imponderable poison...'[20] '...which has hitherto eluded all chemical investigation'.[21] MacCulloch identified malaria along with odour and contagion as the three mysteries that confronted contemporary chemistry,[22] and lamented the inability of chemical tests to detect its presence as 'easily as oxygen or carbonic acid'.[23] The existence of malaria could be gauged retrospectively from its perceived effects on the human body.[24] Once a particular 'situation' was framed as malarial, every form of physical unease witnessed there, MacCulloch argued, could be confidently attributed to malaria.[25]

Malaria, MacCulloch suggested, could remain latent within a body, and manifest itself several years or decades after the body had imbibed it or been exposed to it.[26] Even when one travelled away from 'malarial situations', the body once exposed to malaria, could retain and manifest it.[27] In MacCulloch's narratives, malaria figured as both invisible and mobile or portable. Malaria could durably attach itself to tangible materials and be transported to distant places along with them.[28] By referring to theories of motions and currents, and meteorological observations, MacCulloch suggested that "migration or dispersion" of malaria did not necessarily follow horizontal routes.[29] Like currents, malaria could descend or move vertically upwards.[30] It rarely moved in a straight line and often adopted capricious and curvilinear paths.[31] Depending upon the various degrees in strength and direction of winds, MacCulloch argued, malaria could travel varying distances. If malaria did manage to cling on to winds that were rapid, singularly steady, linear and horizontal, MacCulloch argued, it could cover a distance far greater than that between Holland and England.[32]

Malaria was thus perceived as a highly malleable, commodious and fluid category. Diverse varieties of maladies witnessed in eclectically dispersed locations could be conveniently attributed to malaria. MacCulloch thus suggested that malarial diseases could appear anywhere. However, he tried to identify certain 'situations' as more malarial than others. Although malaria could travel and cause ill health anywhere, it was generated in specific locations which he termed as most notoriously 'malarious'. 'Accurate and minute knowledge of the exact spot and of every

---

[18] MacCulloch, *Malaria*, 2–4, 11–13, 22–25, 49–50. See also the last chapter 'On General Effects of Malaria'.
[19] Ibid., 14.   [20] Ibid. 53.   [21] Ibid. 14.   [22] Ibid. 421.   [23] Ibid. 26.
[24] Ibid. 14.   [25] Ibid. 24.   [26] Ibid. 27–29.   [27] Ibid. 32–33.
[28] Ibid., 217, 234.   [29] Ibid., 213, 309, 310, 239–240.   [30] Ibid., 240.   [31] Ibid.
[32] Ibid., 325–326.

spot, productive of malaria', MacCulloch thought, was the first necessary step towards ensuring protection from malarial diseases.[33]

'Wetness' emerged as a constant feature, which in MacCulloch's narrative defined malarial spots. Landscapes bearing tangible traces of
water were almost obsessively labelled as malarial; to the extent that
a contemporary reviewer suggested that the author might be suffering from 'professional hydrophobia'.[34] MacCulloch began by identifying marshlands – whether saline or stagnant – as potential sources of
malaria.[35] He was meticulous in his description of 'malarial marshlands'.
Such marshes, MacCulloch suggested, were characterised by the co-
existence of water and living vegetation. Malaria emerged when living
vegetation went through the process of decay. He defined 'decay' as an
intermediate stage 'between life and absolute decomposition'.[36] Mac-
Culloch argued that different plants as well as different parts of the
same plant were more prone than others were towards decomposition
or putrefaction. In the process, these generated poisonous exhalations
with varying degrees of impact. By claiming to track the chemical action
of decaying vegetations over moist soil, he appeared simultaneously to
engage with different disciplines – geology, chemistry and botany.[37]

Malaria, MacCulloch claimed, could also be witnessed in many situations which were not, 'in a usual lax sense', defined as a 'marsh'.[38] The
generation of malaria did not require extensive space,[39] but could happen in 'smallest fragments of wet lands',[40] in a 'thousand, unsus-
pected places...'[41] '...obscure as well as innumerable'.[42] Thus, various 'undrained spots', 'wet woods', 'moist meadows',[43] 'rushy pools',
'petty swamps',[44] 'peaty bogs',[45] vicinities of mobile water bodies
such as mountainous rivers, tide rivers, mangrove rivers,[46] 'smallest
streams',[47] urban drains,[48] ditches[49] and canals[50] were labelled as potential non-marshy sources of malaria.

Examples of 'malarial situations' were extended to include locations
which were devoid of any form of vegetation. Malaria provided Mac-
Culloch an opportunity to also pathologise a range of quotidian and
negligible sites, spaces and objects such as vicinities of ponds in gravel
pits,[51] milldams,[52] water casks,[53] the refuse of indigo factories,[54] garden dunghills,[55] flax and hemp in the stage of soaking,[56] bilge water

[33] Ibid., 12.
[34] C. Caldwell, 'Appendix', *Essays on Malaria and Temperament*, (Lexington, Ky.: N. L.
Finnel and J. F. Herndon, 1831), 162–164.
[35] MacCulloch, *Malaria*, 35–38.   [36] Ibid., 61–62.   [37] Ibid., 57, 58, 59.
[38] Ibid., 63, 69.   [39] Ibid., 63.   [40] Ibid., 67.   [41] Ibid., 63.   [42] Ibid., 68.
[43] Ibid., 20–21.   [44] Ibid., 67.   [45] Ibid., 65–66.   [46] Ibid., 77–79.
[47] Ibid., 80.   [48] Ibid., 86–87.   [49] Ibid., 84.   [50] Ibid., 83.   [51] Ibid., 108–109.
[52] Ibid., 103–105.   [53] Ibid., 143.   [54] Ibid., 142.   [55] Ibid.   [56] Ibid., 140.

produced from the leakage of sugar in the voyaging ships at the sea[57] and mud laid bare by the summer heat.[58] One commentator subsequently hinted that in malaria MacCulloch found a euphemism for 'fenny or marshy' counties as well as urban conditions such as 'neglected drains, ill-conditioned sewers, imperfectly trapped cesspools and overflowing dead wells'.[59]

MacCulloch invoked not only the sciences of chemistry, geology, meteorology, natural history and botany, but also the 'practical wisdom' of doctors and farmers.[60] This meshed with his claim of having access to narratives involving distant places. MacCulloch distinguished himself from 'domestic and untravelled' writers.[61] He frequently cited travelling authors like Francis Buchanan Hamilton,[62] Volney[63] or Captain Smyth.[64] His narrative thus could engage, for instance, anecdotes involving malaria in Lombardy with those relating to Bengal,[65] China,[66] the West Indies[67] or North America.[68]

Whence else should fevers come? Do they not thus come in Italy and in Africa? Have they other causes in Rome or Mantua than here? The Thames indeed is not the Congo, nor can we parallel Ostia or Terracina; the fevers do not slay in three days; but the disease is the same, the poison the same, and the same is the cause.[69]

MacCulloch began one of his eleven chapters by advocating: 'To detail the geography of malaria for the whole world, would be little else than to write a general grammar of geography'.[70] He intended to construct a 'map of malaria of the world'[71] to contribute to the processes of 'war, colonisation and commerce', and to the disciplines of political economy and statistics. Despite these grand programmatic statements, his detailed engagement with 'malarial situations' drew upon examples predominantly from England and different parts of continental Europe. This is certainly not to overlook his numerous invocations of malarial locations beyond Europe. Such citations, however, were stray and sporadic. Europe appears to have been the focus of his work. He elaborately projected familiar features within British or continental landscapes as potentially malarial. 'I must almost limit myself to Europe ... by such a detail, I may perhaps at length convince our incredulous countrymen that there is such a thing as Malaria under blue skies and amid the perfume of orange flowers'.[72]

---

[57] Ibid., 145.   [58] Ibid., 151.
[59] T. Wilson, *An Enquiry into the Origin and Intimate Nature of Malaria* (London: Renshaw, 1858), 4.
[60] MacCulloch, *Malaria*, 64.   [61] Ibid., 17.   [62] Ibid., 40.   [63] Ibid., 71.
[64] Ibid., 373.   [65] Ibid., 25, 26, 40.   [66] Ibid., 48.   [67] Ibid., 97.   [68] Ibid., 71.
[69] Ibid., 280.   [70] Ibid., 366.   [71] Ibid., 372.   [72] Ibid., 368.

Much of his chapter on the geography of malaria was based on one Captain Smyth's accounts of towns located on the shores of the Mediterranean. This geography revealed a long 'statistical catalogue of towns'[73] located in France, Sardinia, Sicily, Portugal, Italy, Greece and Spain.[74] Macculloch located 'malarial spots' even in certain parts of Switzerland,[75] Denmark, Poland, Russia,[76] Moldavia, Wallachia and Hungary.[77] Commenting on the prevalence of 'malarial situations' in the interiors of France, MacCulloch wrote, 'so numerous are the tracts and spots of this nature ... that an entire catalogue would form almost a geographical grammar of the country.'[78] The Mediterranean shore of France figured in MacCulloch's narrative as 'one entire range of malaria from the Pyrenees to the Alps.'[79] He attributed low life expectancy rates in contemporary Europe (that is, twenty-five in Holland, fifty in England, and twenty-two in certain districts in France) to malaria.

He argued that England continued to remain under the sway of malaria. England's malarial past, he suggested, was enshrined in the statistical and medical history of the two preceding centuries. Malaria was a 'scourge' for London as it was for the rest of the country. Oliver Cromwell apparently died of malaria.[80] In relation to England, MacCulloch described malaria as a 'Destroying Angel'.[81] England was 'comparatively freed from malaria, by industry and attention. However, it was not yet exempt'.[82] His narrative on the geography of malaria bore extensive references to English parishes, 'unwholesome districts',[83] and 'fenny peaty counties'.[84] MacCulloch identified various sites on the borders of the Thames,[85] river banks about Reculver, on Heron Bay,[86] Kent in the Isle of Thanet,[87] Epping Forest in Essex,[88] and Sussex, Kent, Hampshire,[89] Cambridgeshire, Somersetshire, Lancashire and Huntingdonshire[90] more generally as malarial.

He associated malaria with some of the most beautiful European landscapes, and his descriptions reveal considerable poetic moments in the narrative. These scenic landscapes could be deceptive, MacCulloch suggested. Malaria, he thought, could easily mingle with European prosperity, beauty and grandeur. Thus, for example,

...Amidst the splendor and fragrance of the walnut, the olive, the vine, the fig, and the almond, intermixed with jessamines, aloes, roses, myrtles, oleanders, and a thousand aromatic shrubs, in the very bosom of beauty and luxuriance, amid the delights of a spot which poetry would lose itself in celebrating, the miserable and cadaverous natives drag out a wretched existence; dying rather than living

[73] Ibid., 381. [74] Ibid., 373–411. [75] Ibid., 412. [76] Ibid., 413.
[77] Ibid., 414. [78] Ibid., 411. [79] Ibid., 406. [80] Ibid., 4. [81] Ibid., 8–9.
[82] Ibid., 5. [83] Ibid., 3, 5. [84] Ibid., 66. [85] Ibid., 74, 309. [86] Ibid., 39.
[87] Ibid., 74. [88] Ibid., 42. [89] Ibid. [90] Ibid., 74.

where the vegetable world spreads all its colours and odors to summer airs and bright skies.[91]

Italy, the fairest portions of this fair land is a prey to this invisible enemy, its fragrant breezes are poison, the dews of its summer evenings are death. The banks of its refreshing streams, its rich and flowery meadows, the borders of its glassy lakes, the luxuriant plains of its overflowing agriculture, the valley where its aromatic shrubs regale the eye and perfume the air, these are the chosen seats of this plague, the throne of Malaria.[92]

Commenting on the insalubrities associated with the 'most romantic lakes' of Switzerland, MacCulloch remarked:

The general purity of the waters of a lake, added to its brilliancy, often to its romantic or picturesque character, and not a little aided by poetical feelings or metaphysical prejudices, commonly remove all suspicion ... the physician ... the painter or the geologist will discover or even see, along the shores of such a piece of water, the particular ground which is a cause of suspicion or a source of disease ... he will see reasons of suspicion, even in the most romantic lakes of an alpine region ...[93]

MacCulloch linked malaria to European aesthetics, opulence and splendour, apart from landscapes and demographics. Small wonder then the capitals of various aggrandising European empires in different centuries figured as seats of malaria. MacCulloch projected 'Imperial Rome' – the 'eternal city',[94] Athens – 'the Wapping of Greece,'[95] Babylon,[96] Paris,[97] and London – 'our own capital'[98] as victims of malaria. He did not invariably associate malaria with poverty. On the contrary, he understood malaria as 'death knocking at the door of the opulent to spare the mean'.[99] Overcrowded situations, streets or habitations, MacCulloch showed, were capable of neutralising the effects of malaria.[100]

He pointed out that residence across successive generations in European 'malarial districts' in France and Italy could produce a 'degeneracy of the races'. The inhabitants of such districts often appeared to suffer from rickets and deformities.[101] The colour of their skin mostly turned sallow or yellow, or appeared stained with different hues and livid.[102] 'Personal beauty' in women, MacCulloch thought, dwindled prematurely. They appeared unhappy, stupid, apathetic, melancholic and insensible.[103] These adversely affected the 'moral conditions' of the people, and the 'moral life' of the inhabitants of such districts, MacCulloch argued, was 'frightful'. Infanticides, abortion, drunkenness, want of

---

[91] Ibid., 383.   [92] Ibid., 6.   [93] Ibid., 94–95.   [94] Ibid., 7.   [95] Ibid., 294.
[96] Ibid., 255.   [97] Ibid., 294.   [98] Ibid.   [99] Ibid., 293.
[100] Ibid., 292–294.   [101] Ibid., 430.   [102] Ibid.   [103] Ibid., 432.

religion, gross superstitions and assassinations were frequently encountered in these European 'malarial districts' as a result of enduring exposure to malaria.[104]

Malaria thus featured in this 1827 book as an elusive and invisible diagnostic category which could be deployed to ascribe medical connotations to a diverse range of predominantly European sites and situations including stagnant marshes, industrial wastes or spectacular Swiss lakes. Malaria could be invoked to explain not only a variety of debilities like fevers, impotency or idiocy, but also moral and racial degenerations, ugliness and the general absence of public order.

The 'First Book' and Its Author

MacCulloch's book was published at a time when the invocation of malaria as a diagnostic category in the English language was acquiring unprecedented recurrence. A foray into the overlapping worlds of bureaucratic correspondence, journal articles, reports on the health of the army, medical manuals, treatises and monographs uncover such trends. It is possible to locate stray references to the expression malaria in medical literature written in the English language before the nineteenth century. However, most medical historians who have written on malaria in early-modern England and North America continue to engage in conscious acts of retrospective diagnosis. These works have tended to ascribe malaria with connotations, which the category acquired in the late nineteenth and early twentieth centuries, and were hardly known or in use earlier.[105] Such histories suggest that 'chills and fever', 'fever and ague', 'estivo-autumnal fever', 'marsh fever' and 'jungle fever' were different ways to describe the same disease.[106] Thomas Sydenham, Robert Talbor, James Lind, John MacCulloch and experts on the germ theory figure in these works as characters, who in different centuries contributed collectively towards knowledge of a continuous and unchanging disease.[107] These works have been authored by various scholars ranging from social historians of demography like Mary Dobson[108] to a group of archaeologists, who by conducting DNA tests, claim to have excavated traces of plasmodium falciparum and malaria in a Roman villa in

---

[104] Ibid., 437.
[105] Dobson, 'Marsh fever'; A. Murray Fallis, 'Malaria in the Eighteenth and Nineteenth Centuries in Ontario', *Bulletin of the Canadian History of Medicine*, 1, 2 (1984), 25–38; J. R. Palmero and A. R. Vega, 'Spanish Agriculture and Malaria in the Eighteenth Century', *History and Philosophy of Life Science*, 10 (1998), 343–362.
[106] E. Ackerknecht, 'The Development of our Knowledge of Malaria', *Ciba Symposia*, 7, 3/4 (1945–46), 38.
[107] Dobson, 'Marsh fever'.   [108] Ibid.

the mid-fifth century AD.[109] It might be misleading anachronistically to situate commentators invoking various categories in different contexts as part of the same teleological narrative on malaria. Failing to appreciate the changing meanings ascribed to a category in specific historical periods is equally problematic. This chapter recognises malaria as a commodious category of knowledge, a flexible diagnostic label and a significant ordering principle. Unprecedented textualisation, circulation and firmer entrenchment of the word malaria in English language sources beginning in the late 1820s should have a history of its own. The publication of John MacCulloch's *Malaria* in 1827, seven years after the discovery of quinine, constitutes a crucial moment in that history. In the next year MacCulloch published another book on the same subject.[110]

Malaria, which surfaced in English texts from the 1820s onwards, inherited the older meanings associated with the Greek word miasma and Italian word mal'aria in vogue in the earlier centuries.[111] This was enabled in a decade marked variously by a 'revival of interest in Hellenistic culture'[112] in Britain, 'a revival of classical humoral aetiological theory'[113] and a 'renewed Hippocratism,'[114] and an appreciation for its foundational tenets of 'Airs, Waters and Places'. At the same time, the increasing relevance of malaria as a credible category in the following decades was further enabled not only by the global proliferation of print markets, but also by concerns about agricultural improvement, labour circulation, colonial governance and stagnation in industrial Britain. The

---

[109] D. Soren, 'Can Archaeologists Excavate Evidence of Malaria?', *World Archaeology*, 35, 2 (October 2003), 193–209; see also, Sallares, *Malaria and Rome*.

[110] MacCulloch, *Malaria*; J. MacCulloch, *An Essay on the Remittent and Intermittent Diseases, including Generically Marsh Fever and Neuralgia*, London: Longman, Rees, Orme, Brown, and Green, 1828.

[111] R. Wrigley, 'Pathological Topographies and Cultural Itineraries: Mapping Mal'aria in Eighteenth- and Nineteenth-Century Rome', in R. Wrigley and G. Revill (eds.), *Pathologies of Travel*, (Amsterdam and Atlanta: Rodipi, 2000), 207–228; C. M. Cipolla, *Miasma and Disease: Public Health and the Environment in the Pre-Industrial Age* (New Haven: Yale University Press, 1992); M. Harrison, *Medicine in an Age of Commerce and Empire: Britain and its Tropical Colonies, 1660–1830* (Oxford: Oxford University Press, 2010), 47–88; Bewell, *Romanticism*, 31, 37–39; P. B. Mukharji, 'The "Cholera Cloud" in the Nineteenth-Century "British World": History of an Object-without-an-essence', *Bulletin of the History of Medicine*, 86 (Fall, 2012), 311–313.

[112] M. Harrison, 'Differences of Degree: Representations of India in British Medical Topography, 1820–c. 1870', in Rupke (ed.), *Medical Geography in Historical Perspective, Medical History, Supplement No. 20* (London: Wellcome Trust Centre for the History of Medicine at UCL, 2000), 55.

[113] H. Deacon, 'The Politics of Medical Topography: Seeking Healthiness at the Cape during the Nineteenth Century', in Wrigley and Revill (eds.), *Pathologies of Travel*, 280.

[114] C. B. Valencius, 'Histories of Medical Geography', in Rupke (ed.), *Medical Geography in Historical Perspective*, 10.

emerging disciplines of economic botany, geology, chemistry, meteorology and medical topography found in malaria a problem worth exploring.

A reflection of this wider interest was the claim both in contemporary history and in historiography about malaria being a relatively new category in the early nineteenth century. Historians who have written on malaria in early modern England, Spain or North America have themselves acknowledged the rarity of the 'term malaria' in contemporary medical literature. Juan Riera Palmero and Anastasio Rojo Vega have suggested that the 'term malaria was totally unknown in eighteenth-century Spain'.[115] Erwin H. Ackerknecht has pointed out that the 'Italian word malaria was not introduced into English medical literature until the first half of the nineteenth century'.[116] Mary Dobson and Richard Wrigley have in their own works suggested that 'the word achieved popular usage in the English language'[117] after the publication of MacCulloch's work on malaria. One of MacCulloch's biographers has called him 'the precursor of the discipline of Malariology', and credited him with 'the introduction of the word malaria' into English scientific writing.[118]

Quite curiously, MacCulloch projected himself as the pioneer of English writings about malaria. According to him, 'the truest account of the nature of malaria would be an acknowledgment of utter ignorance'.[119] He suggested that malaria could have been sporadically invoked in the past. However, it remained an 'unseen and unknown' category.[120] He claimed to be the author of the first full book-length study of malaria in English.[121] Malaria constituted a 'subject', he argued, that had 'never before been submitted before an English public'.[122]

Soon after publication, MacCulloch's work was widely reviewed and cited in essays written or published from distant locations. One Dr Hardy published an article titled 'On the Malaria and the Medical Topography of Oudypoor' (in British India) in the *Transactions of the Medical and Physical Society of Calcutta* in 1831.[123] In the same year Transylvania-based physician Charles Caldwell's *Essays on Malaria and Temperament* was published from Kentucky in the United States.[124] Otherwise considerably critical of MacCulloch's work, these authors reconfirmed his

[115] Palmero and Vega, 'Spanish Agriculture and Malaria', 343.
[116] Ackerknecht, 'The Development of Our Knowledge of Malaria', 38.
[117] Dobson, 'Marsh Fever', 371; Wrigley, 'Pathological Topographies', 207.
[118] L. J. Bruce-Chwatt, 'John Macculloch (1773–1835): The Precursor of the Discipline of Malariology', *Medical History*, 21 (1977), 164–165.
[119] MacCulloch, *Malaria*, 419.   [120] Ibid., 2.   [121] Ibid., 11.   [122] Ibid., 14.
[123] Dr Hardy, 'On the Malaria, and the Medical Topography of Oudypoor', *Transactions of the Medical and Physical Society of Calcutta*, 5 (1831), 1–37.
[124] Caldwell, 'Appendix', 157–160.

claim to being one of the earliest to write on malaria in English. Much later in the century, Thomas Wilson, an official working for the Dutch government, authored a treatise called *An Enquiry into the Origin and Intimate Nature of Malaria*. Describing MacCulloch as the proponent of 'the theory of universal malaria'[125], Wilson showed how 'prior to the appearance of MacCulloch, no one had given to the theory of malaria any definite form'.[126] 'It can scarcely be said that any author prior to MacCulloch ever considered this matter from a philosophical or physiological point of view...'.[127] In the 1880s and even later, journals published in Bengali from distant Calcutta continued to recognise MacCulloch as the first English author about malaria.[128]

Engendered by contemporary commercial, political and institutional cultures, the nineteenth century thus witnessed not only a new energy of writing and publishing about malaria, but also the need to discover a first original author. Emphasising the originality of the 'first' author, citing him as an inheritor of received knowledge, revealing him as respectable, and constantly referring back to him; all these taken together underscored the credibility and significance of MacCulloch, of the subsequent authors and of the category malaria itself.

Biographical entries on MacCulloch published in the nineteenth century and later projected him as a man of many facets. Perhaps it was helped by the fact that he had established himself as a prolific author much before his works on malaria were published. It is possible to suggest that his enduring credibility as an author provided the category malaria renewed currency in nineteenth-century Britain and beyond. The work on malaria was published eight years before his death, and was one of his last works.

Writing on malaria was one amongst his several other significant identities. One of his biographers has pointed out how he was eclectically trained in different disciplines.[129] Although he studied medicine at Edinburgh University in the 1790s, he developed considerable interest in chemistry, natural history, geology, botany, mineralogy, mathematics and zoology. Despite his formal training as a doctor, he was for much of his professional career a geologist, at a time when geology was being institutionalised in industrial Britain with the participation of mining interests, land surveyors, canal builders, coal prospectors, drainage experts, mineral assayers, quarrymen and civil engineers. MacCulloch joined the Geological Society of London in 1808. In 1811

---

[125] Wilson, *An Enquiry*, 7.   [126] Ibid., 124.   [127] Ibid., 11.

[128] R. Mitra, 'Malaria', *Chikitsa Sammilani*, 2 (1885–1886), 311; N. Majumdar, 'Malaria Rahasya' ('The Malaria Mystery'), *Hahnemann*, 9, 11 (c. 1910), 576 and 583.

[129] Bruce-Chwatt, 'John Macculloch', 158.

he was commissioned by the Board of Ordinance to locate alternate sources of limestone for use in British gunpowder mills to those in Belgium. He returned to Scotland to determine the most appropriate types of rocks, searching for silica-free limestone for millwheels. In 1814, he was appointed geologist to the Trigonometrical Survey, which was then engaged in preparing a one-inch topographical map of Scotland. Between 1814 and 1821, he was engaged in examining the geology of about hundred Scottish peaks and compiling a geological map of West Scotland. He narrated his activities and revelations as a geologist in a series of publications. Much before the publication of his first work on malaria in 1827, he had already published most of his seminal works on geology. These included *A Description of the Western Isles of Scotland, including the Isle of Man* (1819), *A Geological Classification of Rocks* (1821) and *The Highlands and Western Isles of Scotland* (1824). The second book acted as a textbook of geology in the East India College for ten years.[130] A 4-mile-to-an-inch geological map of Scotland prepared by MacCulloch appeared posthumously in 1836. It is considered to be the first official geological survey of any country in the world.[131] Although intensely criticised for considerable topographical and geological inaccuracies, it was not superseded for many years.[132] Two years after his death while on honeymoon to Cornwall in 1835, his *Proofs and Illustrations of the Attributes of God* was published, which revealingly argued that geological evidence revealed the work of God in creation.[133] This image of the pioneer English writer about malaria as a God-fearing man of science is comparable to the devout Christian beliefs of John Eliot Howard, the most widely celebrated Victorian authority on quinine.

MacCulloch's career bore revealing overlaps with contemporary colonial projects. He was an industrial geologist employed by the British government to work in Scotland. He suggested in *The Highlands and Western Isles of Scotland* (1824) that the Highlanders were 'indolent and lazy', lacked 'military propensities' and should be cleared from the land.[134] This met with vigorous criticism. He taught chemistry and geology to the cadets of the East India Company at the East India College at Addiscombe from 1814 until his death in 1835, and received financial support from the East India Company towards publishing his books, including *A Geological Classification of Rocks* (1821) and *A System of Geology* (1831). These were intended as practical reference works for engineering field

[130] D. A. Cumming, 'MacCulloch, John (1773–1835)', *Oxford Dictionary of National Biography*, Oxford University Press, 2004 [www.oxforddnb.com/view/article/17412, retrieved on 25 August 2013].
[131] Bruce-Chwatt, 'John Macculloch', 160.   [132] Cumming, 'MacCulloch, John'.
[133] Ibid.   [134] Ibid; Bruce-Chwatt, 'John Macculloch', 158–159.

officers in India, and acted as textbooks for the courses he offered at Addiscombe.[135]

Writing about Macculloch in the late 1850s, Thomas Wilson recalled that he 'moved in the best circles'.[136] As early as 1801, he was elected fellow of the Linnean Society.[137] He served as the president of the Geological Society of London between 1816 and 1818, and was elected Fellow of the Royal Society in 1820.[138] Well before the publication of his work on malaria, he had thus established himself as a versatile and prolific writer. In addition to his nine major books, he had written about seventy-nine scientific papers. These addressed topics as diverse as geology, the art of making wine, marine fishes and crabs, Greek fire and indelible ink.[139]

His reputation lent significant currency to the category malaria in the English language. This shows why his work on malaria was reviewed in locations as distant as Kentucky in the United States and Rajputana in British India within two years of its publication. The significance ascribed to men like MacCulloch in contemporary British culture is explained by the curious ways in which these careers linked apparently disparate worlds of natural history, geology, medicine, Industrial Revolution, romanticism and colonialism.[140] Perhaps this is why within thirty years of its publication, as the Dutch official Thomas Wilson suggested, MacCulloch's book had found many sympathisers in different departments of the English government including the sanitary board.[141] MacCulloch's views on malaria found acceptance amongst a network of diverse interests represented by the government, medical faculty and sewer makers.[142] 'Supporting and maintaining the theories of MacCulloch', Wilson suggested, emerged as one of the viable ways of ensuring 'lucrative official appointments'.[143] Inspired by MacCulloch's analysis of malaria, the government had launched extensive schemes in the late 1850s towards 'improving' the drainage of the city of London.[144] MacCulloch's theory of malaria, Wilson observed, had received

---

[135] D. A. Cumming, 'John Macculloch at Addiscombe: The Lectureships on Chemistry and Geology', Notes and Records of the Royal Society of London, 34, 2 (February 1980), 178.

[136] Wilson, An Enquiry, 7.   [137] Bruce-Chwatt, 'John Macculloch', 157.

[138] Cumming, 'MacCulloch, John'.   [139] Bruce-Chwatt, 'John Macculloch', 158.

[140] For the links between colonialism, science, medicine and romanticism, see J. A. Secord, 'John MacCulloch: Geology and the Appreciation of Landscape' [Unpublished manuscript], 2–18; Bewell, Romanticism, 14; Arnold, Tropics and the Travelling Gaze. For the links between the emerging discipline of geology and the British Empire, see J. A. Secord, 'King of Siluria: Roderick Murchison and the Imperial Theme in Nineteenth-Century British Geology', Victorian Studies, 25, 4 (Summer 1982), 413–442.

[141] Wilson, An Enquiry, 5.   [142] Ibid., 7, 11.   [143] Ibid., 8.   [144] Ibid., 8–11.

significant government appreciation since his death in 1835. MacCulloch was very uncertain about the effectiveness of his denunciation of open sewers, undrained streets, untrapped cesspools and overflowing dead-wells. Execution of such projects entailed damage to the proprietors of London residences. MacCulloch had even solicited counsel from a 'distinguished barrister' apprehending legal retaliation from propertied interests in London.[145] Contrary to his apprehensions, Wilson showed, MacCulloch's book on malaria had begun enjoying patronage from the political establishment in London by the 1850s.

Thus, both MacCulloch and his book resonated in a range of publications about malaria in the decades that followed. Even when reviewed, contested and ridiculed, MacCulloch's work featured as a point of reference for the next half-century.[146] Many of the impressions conveyed in the book were modified over the course of the century, but the category malaria was retained as a credible way of defining land, landscape and people in distant locations. The use of the expression malarial in the English language proliferated. This converged with the crystallisation of the image of MacCulloch as the author who published the first full-length book on malaria. The book was followed by publications from a dispersed network of authors on the subject. These authors hailed from diverse contexts and pursued different sets of interests. They included medical professors based in Kentucky,[147] British Indian bureaucrats from Rajputana,[148] officials working for the Dutch government,[149] physicians working for the US army,[150] and editors of medical journals in the vernacular.[151] Such authors published in scientific journals,[152] bureaucratic correspondences,[153] book-length treatises,[154] medical reports of national armies,[155] and Bengali journals.[156] Most of these authors were engaged in reciprocal acts of quoting and citing from one another's works, and in the process they appeared to endorse each other's credibility as authors on malaria. These in turn vindicated the proliferation of malaria as a medical term. Recurrent projections of MacCulloch as the first English author on malaria were related to such efforts of deriving legitimacy.

At last one man, a shrewd, intelligent and influential observer, a man of genius, gave to the whole question a new phasis. Since his day his hypothesis has

---

[145] Ibid., 7.   [146] Caldwell, 'Appendix', 187–189.   [147] Ibid.
[148] Hardy, 'On the Malaria'.   [149] Wilson, An Enquiry.
[150] G. M. Sternberg, Malaria and Malarial Diseases (New York: Wood, 1884).
[151] Mitra, 'Malaria', 311.   [152] 'Malarial Fever', IMG, 8 (August 1, 1873), 215.
[153] Home, Public, 12 March 1870, 167–170 A (NAI).   [154] Wilson, An Enquiry.
[155] Sternberg, Malaria and Malarial Diseases.   [156] Mitra, 'Malaria', 311.

undergone a variety of modifications, as was to be expected, in no way, however, affecting the practical deductions originally drawn from it by its author.[157]

Retention of the category malaria by subsequent authors, by itself, was related to such efforts to establish legitimacy. These authors appeared to cling on to a word associated with an established figure. MacCulloch himself, however, began both his books on the subject by referring to two closely related terms, that is, malaria and miasma. According to MacCulloch, his consistent use of the Italian word, malaria, instead of the 'Greek expression miasma' was one of 'preference'.[158] However, he did not provide justifications behind such preference. Nor did he elaborate on any technical distinction between these two terms. He appeared uncertain and was silent about the distinctions between them. From the 1830s onwards he was recognised as an authority on malaria and not miasma. Similarly, authors in English who claimed to follow MacCulloch's pioneering lead projected themselves as experts on malaria and not miasma. Later in the century, some of these authors tried to distinguish between these two categories. They tried to justify the recurrent usage of one term over the other. Malaria according to these authors conveyed certain connotations which could not be subsumed within the expression 'miasma'. Most of these efforts were witnessed from the 1850s.[159] As late as 1881, Joseph Edwards, a physician based in Philadelphia, wrote:

The word *malaria* has been derived from the two words *mal aria* i.e. bad air ... the word miasm has a different origin, being derived from the Greek ... a *stain, I contaminate* ... although Dunglinson in his medical dictionary refers the definition of the word malaria to *miasm or miasma* and so confound the two ... they are distinct ... while malaria ... is a comprehensive term for atmospheric impurities of various kinds; miasma conveys the idea of an effect and not a cause, it is a stain, a contamination of some portion of the human body ... the only relation that they can possibly hold together is that of cause and effect, malaria or bad air being the cause and miasma or contamination being the effect of this cause ...[160]

MacCulloch remained an archetypal writer on malaria in English for much of the nineteenth century in other ways. His claims to being the first author on malaria in English ironically converged with his attempts to project it as an established explanatory category in Europe.[161] 'Hundreds of writers' including 'Lancisi, Sennert, Orlandi, Platner,

---

[157] Wilson, *An Enquiry*, 6.

[158] J. MacCulloch, *An Essay on the Remittent and Intermittent Diseases*, xviii.

[159] Wilson, *An Enquiry*, 89–98; T. H. Barker, *On Malaria and Miasmata* (London: John W. Davies, 1859), 1–3.

[160] Edwards, *Malaria*, 13–14.   [161] MacCulloch, *Malaria*, 224–231.

De Baumes, Zimmerman, Pringle, Lind, Blane, Jackson', he argued, 'explained this subject...sufficiently'.[162] He associated malaria with certain significant events in European military history.[163] Malaria figured not only as a cause of disease, but also as a factor which determined the fates of decisive battles and expeditions. Discussions about malaria, Macculloch pointed out, were not confined to the savants in Europe, but had occurred across classes and beyond Europe. 'Through out the world it is a fact known to the vulgar, and even to less enlightened nations; familiar to the Negroes of Africa, familiar to the lower orders of France, Italy, Holland and not less known to at least our own rural population'.[164]

Similarly, subsequent writers followed MacCulloch to project malaria as a credible diagnostic category which had endured several centuries. Narrating long histories of malaria seems to have been one recurrent way of achieving this. These writers appeared able to trace the category in the writings of legendary medical writers and literary figures of previous centuries. For example, a Philadelphia-based physician R. La Roche described malaria as a 'long admitted efficient agent' and devoted a chapter towards locating the 'antiquity of this opinion'.[165] Medical writers from Hippocrates and the Galenics,[166] down to Ramazzini and Lancisi[167] in the seventeenth century, argued La Roche, had commented on the same disease-causing entity, which in the nineteenth century was known as malaria. Thus, while MacCulloch's narrative on the 'antiquity' of thinking about malaria began with Lancisi, La Roche's ended with him.

Like MacCulloch himself, many subsequent writers who published in the first half of the century, appeared simultaneously invested in many disciplines.[168] Knowledge about malaria was thus accessed, framed and articulated in the language of different disciplines. Thomas Herbert Barker, a British physician based in Bedford, won the Fothergillian Prize Essay for 1859 from the Medical Society of London for *On Malaria and Miasmata*.[169] It summarised the different ways in which geologists, meteorologists and the organic and inorganic chemists were engaged in addressing the 'profound mystery' called malaria. This explains how different definitions of malaria could co-circulate around the nineteenth

---

[162] Ibid., 225.   [163] Ibid., 224–231.   [164] Ibid., 1.
[165] Roche, *Pneumonia*, 101.   [166] Ibid., 101–107.   [167] Ibid., 107–109.
[168] D. Drake, *A Systematic Treatise, Historical, Etiological and Practical, On the Principal Diseases of the Interior of North America As They Appear in the Caucasian, African, Indian and Esquimax Varieties of Its Population* (Cincinnati: Winthrop B. Smith & Co., 1850), ix–xiv, 719–723.
[169] Barker, *On Malaria*.

century. Barker pointed out, for instance, that chemists like Samuel Metcalfe defined malaria as inorganic poisons, which resulted from the decomposition of organic matters.[170] Metcalfe appeared to add that malaria constituted organic matter in the gaseous state, in the forms of carbonic acid, carburetted hydrogen, phosphuretted hydrogen and ammonia. Malaria then, according to these chemists, could reveal itself to chemical analyses.[171] Barker's book suggested how the 1850s witnessed beginnings of the cell origin or germ theories of malaria. He referred to Pettenkofer and Grainger, who explained malaria in terms of animal effluvium. 'Effluvium consists of organic matter, a protein compound in a most minutely divided form and therefore adapted, in a special manner to enter the blood, to diffuse itself rapidly and extensively'.[172] Amongst the geologists, Barker referred to Sir Ranald Martin, who projected high temperature in a ferruginous soil as favouring the generation of malaria.[173] Martin also appeared to explain malarial situations in terms of the electrical conditions of the atmosphere.[174] Such coupling of meteorological observations with geological references was, according to Barker, reflected in other writings as well.[175] Most meteorologists appeared to explain malaria in terms of season, climate, barometrical pressure, hygrometrical state, temperature and elasticity.[176] MacCulloch, as I have already noted, claimed to derive insights from chemistry, botany, geology, meteorology and geography. Following him, subsequent writers on the subject pursued the definition of malaria through different disciplines and arrived at diverse answers.

Colonising Malaria, Malarial Colonies

To understand malaria, MacCulloch suggested, one needed to explore its possible geographies. In his narrative, he frequently cited anecdotes about malaria relating to various places. Some of these locations and landscapes kept recurring in MacCulloch's account as particularly malarial. Throughout his book he projected continental Europe and England as the heartland of malaria, although sporadically and rarely he referred to Africa, West Indies, and certain sites in India, North America and even China.

Many later nineteenth-century authors adopted his anecdotal style of writing about various places, peoples and objects. That the geographies of malaria were undergoing significant mutations, however, had become evident by the 1850s. Published geographies of malaria began gradually

[170] Ibid., 10.   [171] Ibid., 13–15, 20.   [172] Ibid., 42.   [173] Ibid., 51.
[174] Ibid.   [175] Ibid., 52.   [176] Ibid., 9.

to shift away from Europe and to bear uncanny overlaps with the emerging geographies of colonial cinchona plantations. The global geographies of European empires, cinchonas and malaria seem to have overlapped to a considerable extent and in significant ways by the third quarter of the nineteenth century. Until the1840s, as I have suggested, cinchonas were predominantly confined to the networks of circulation between 'natural forests' in South America and sites within Europe and North America. Surviving images and relics associated with cinchonas and malaria from the first half of the nineteenth century or even earlier invoke objects, landscapes and people related almost exclusively to Europe.

The jar (see Figure 2.1) is amongst a collection of containers of cinchona barks that have survived from the eighteenth and early nineteenth centuries, and which were in use in different parts of Europe.[177] Similarly, the sketch (see Figure 2.2) published in the *Penny Magazine* and the lithograph (see Figure 2.3) drawn by Français in the first half of the nineteenth century refer to European landscapes, figures and attires while describing malaria. By the time Maurice Sand (1823–1889) painted his allegorical work 'The ghost of the swamp' (Figure 2.4), explicit references to European people and landscapes had begun to fade at least in certain sectors of visual culture, even as the iconography of malaria continued being dominated by European artists.

The 1840s witnessed the beginnings of most sustained proposals for the establishment of cinchona plantations in the Dutch, French and British colonies.[178] In the 1850s, cinchona seeds and plants from the 'natural' cinchona forests in South America had been transported to many of these colonies. By the 1860s, experimental plantations had been set up in Dutch Java, French Algeria and British India, Jamaica and Ceylon (see Figure 2.5). These enabled unprecedented circulation of the cinchonas between different parts of the colonial world.[179] Such locations included Algiers, Burma, Ceylon, India, Java, Jamaica, Mauritius and Wellington. These newer destinations of cinchonas and quinine were described as places precisely in need of such commodities. In the emerging medical geographies, these locations appeared to abound in particularly malarial situations. The official files which documented the transfer of cinchona plants and seeds were one of the earliest and most consistent

---

[177] See for example photographs of 'Clear glass shop round for Quinine, England, 1801–1850' and 'Drug jar for cinchona bark, Italy, 1701–1730'. Credit: Wellcome Library, London.

[178] D. Williams, 'Clements Roberts Markham and the Introduction of the Cinchona Trees into British India, 1861,' *The Geographical Journal*, 128, 4 (December 1962), 432; C. R. Markham, *Travels in Peru and India* (London: John Murray, 1862), 46–47.

[179] See Chapter 1.

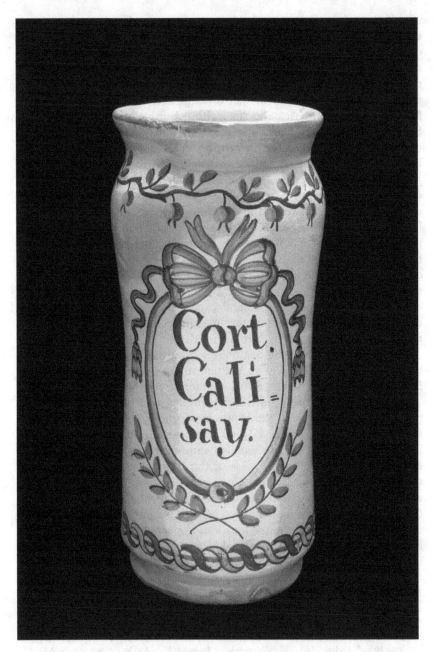

Figure 2.1 Image of 'Albarello drug jar used for cinchona bark, Spain, 1731–1770'. Credit: Wellcome Library, London.

ARRIVAL OF REAPERS IN THE PONTINE MARSHES

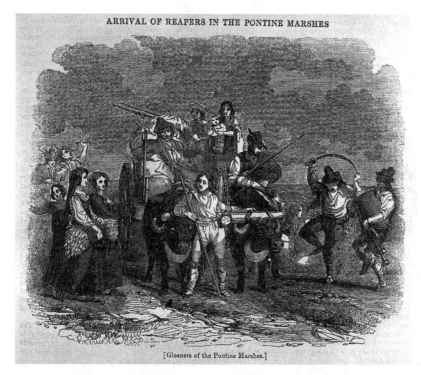

[Gleaners of the Pontine Marshes.]

Figure 2.2 Sketch with the note 'Gleaners of the Pontine Marshes. These people suffered from malaria when working on the Marshes', *Penny Magazine*, 1837, vol. 6, 337. Credit: Wellcome Library, London.

sites projecting, for instance British India, as a predominantly 'malarial' landscape – a land of death, fever and disease.[180]

This is however not to suggest that the mid-nineteenth century indicated an absolute shift in the perceived geography of malaria. References to sites within Europe did not disappear altogether.[181] Nor was every colonised location described as absolutely exempt from the effects of malaria before the colonial transfer of cinchona seeds and plants.[182]

---

[180] Home Department, Medical Board, 21 October 1858, 14A; Home Department, Medical Board, 28 October 1858, 52A; Home Department, Medical Board, 2 December 1858, 58A, (NAI); Home, Medical, January 1884, 9–11 A (NAI).

[181] See for example, F. M. Snowden, *The Conquest of Malaria: Italy, 1900–1962* (New Haven and London: Yale University Press, 2006), 7–52.

[182] Hardy, 'On the Malaria'; Harrison, *Medicine in An Age of Commerce*, 47–88. See also, J. Lind, *An Essay on Diseases Incidental to Europeans in Hot Climates with the Method of Preventing their Fatal Consequences* (London: T. Beckett and A. De Hondt, 1768); J. Bontius, *An Account of the Diseases, Natural History, and Medicines of the East Indies*,

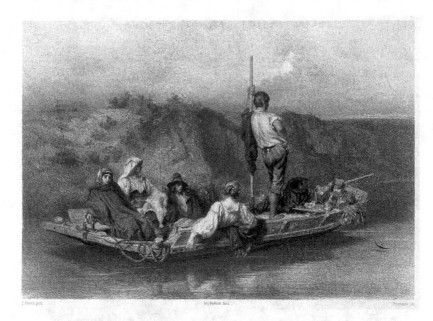

Figure 2.3 Lithograph of 'A group of people adrift in a boat, perhaps suffering from malaria'. Lithograph by Français after A. E. Hébert, 1850. Credit: Wellcome Library, London.

MacCulloch himself made tangential references to non-European sites. It has been already suggested how MacCulloch's career as a writer, geologist and lecturer were intimately tied to the East India Company. Such associations could not have left his world view unaffected. Many of his books were published with support from the East India Company. In the nineteenth century, then, writing about malaria in English was never completely dissociated from colonial concerns.

However, mid-century onwards malaria found itself unprecedentedly entangled with colonial lands, landscapes and people. In contemporary texts which commented on malaria, references to the 'mountainous jungles of India', 'impenetrable mangrove forests' in the West Indies, alluvial plains in Algiers,[183] 'natural prairies of French Guiana', 'arid deserts of Peru and Spanish Guiana', Antigua, Barbados, Dominica, Bahamas, Tobago, the Pigeon Islands, Senegal, the coasts of Coromondal,

---

Translated from the Latin of James Bontius, Physician to the Dutch Settlement at Batavia (London: T. Noteman, 1769); J. Johnson, *The Influence of Tropical Climates on European Constitutions* (London: Thomas and George Underwood, 1827).

[183] Roche, *Pneumonia*, 129.

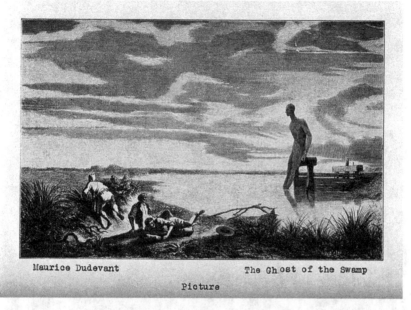

Maurice Dudevant   The Ghost of the Swamp

Picture

Figure 2.4 'An allegory of malaria'. Reproduction of an engraving after M. Sand (1823–1889) c. 1850s. Credit: Wellcome Library, London.

Malabar, the deserts of Arabia,[184] the coasts of Africa,[185] 'vessels engaged in the West Indian, South American or African trades',[186] winds blowing along the coasts of Ceylon or Sierra Leone or Batavia[187] featured more regularly than ever before.

Even while promising to comment on malaria in Europe, most texts in the 1850s lost focus and ended up devoting substantial parts towards describing colonised situations. Thomas Wilson, for instance, began by promising to write about malaria which he had observed in Belgium and Holland. However, he devoted significant parts of the book to describing the Ionian Islands, the Ireland Islands in the Bermudas, and lakes and the margins of streams in Upper Canada and the West Coast of Africa.[188]

As in the case of cinchona plants, malaria began to acquire a wider variety of colonial authorities from the 1860s. The decade witnessed the resurgence of a gush of publications about malaria from colonies such as British India. At the same time, the projection of most colonised locations as malarial landscapes acquired overwhelming consistency. Most of

---

[184] Ibid., 135.   [185] Ibid., 143–145.   [186] Ibid., 204.   [187] Ibid., 216–217.
[188] Wilson, *An Enquiry*, 34–36.

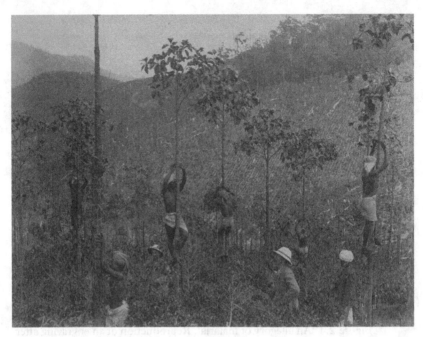

Figure 2.5 Reproduced by the kind permission of the Syndics of the Cambridge University Library. Royal Commonwealth Society Library, Photograph collection of John Abercromby Alexander, Shelfmark: RCS/Y303E_47. (No infringement of copyright intended.) This photo describes local inhabitants engaged in the cinchona plantations in Ceylon (most probably in Peradeniya), circa 1880–1890.

these texts were written in the colonial world, and their authors claimed recurrently to have known malaria in its 'hotbeds'. The germ theories of malaria, for instance, were established by officials working for colonial governments in Formosa, Amoy, parts of Algeria and India in the 1870s. C. F. Oldham's *What is Malaria? And Why Is It Most Intense in Hot Climates?*,[189] William Moore's 'Malaria vs. More Recognisable Causes'[190] and Joseph Fayrer's 'Malaria'[191] were amongst the most significant contributions on malaria in the 1870s and 1880s. It is perhaps

---

[189] C. F. Oldham, *What is Malaria? And Why Is It Most Intense In Hot Climates?* (London: H K Lewis, 1871).

[190] W. Moore, 'Malaria versus More Recognisable Causes of Disease', *Transactions of the Epidemiological Society of London*, New Series 9 (1889–90), 23–46.

[191] J. Fayrer, 'Malaria', Text of the paper read before the Epidemiological Society of London on 1 February 1882 (WL).

not entirely accidental that all these authors had been highly placed colonial officials, serving the British government in India. Revealingly, Oldham's book was dedicated to the then Secretary of State for India, the Duke of Argyll.

From the early 1870s, malaria attracted the attention of medical journals published from British India, such as the *Indian Medical Gazette*, with remarkable regularity. Distant corners of the British Empire and beyond – Queensland, Northern Australia, Virginia, Bengal,[192] Massachusetts, Natal,[193] French Algeria,[194] Assam, British Guiana[195] – figured in these articles, as significant spots in an eclectically dispersed and yet intimately connected world of malaria. These articles configured, compared and publicised such locations as abound in malarial situations, which could be rescued precisely through regimes of improvement and circulation of quinine.[196]

These simultaneous invocations of distant place-names, it may be argued, were enabled by intricate overseas colonial, commercial and military networks, which reinforced a spectacular circulation of personnel and texts in the second half of the nineteenth century. Dispersed geographies of malaria resulted from journalistic reports, scholarly articles and memoirs written by diverse groups of mobile men: physicians in charge of ships carrying immigrant labourers from Calcutta to Port Natal;[197] transferable officials like John Meredith and G. Dodds, who held assignments in places ranging from British Guiana to Assam, from Borneo to Hong Kong;[198] physicians and soldiers travelling with the British army, who were engaged in British America, the Mediterranean, Ceylon, Australasian colonies, China, Japan, India, West Indies, Western Africa, St Helena, Cape of Good Hope and Mauritius.[199] These reports were eventually published in widely circulating and extensively cited journals, Annual Medical Reports of the British Army and bureaucratic correspondence. A report, an article or a memoir concerning dispersed

---

[192] Anonymous, 'Malaria', *IMG*, 8 (September 1, 1873), 241.

[193] Anonymous, 'Marsh Fever Produced by Obstruction of the Outlets of Subsoil Water', *IMG*, 8 (October 1, 1873), 279–280.

[194] Anonymous, 'Selections: Report on the Causes of Reduced Mortality in the French Army Serving in Algeria', *IMG*, 8 (May 1, 1873), 139–140.

[195] J. Meredith, 'On Malarial Sites and Fevers, Relating Chiefly to Assam,' *IMG*, 6 (1 September 1871), 175–177.

[196] Bewell, *Romanticism*, 34.

[197] J. Para, 'Cases of Fever Treated Successfully by Hypodermic Injection of Bromide of Quinine', *IMG*, 17, (1 February 1882), 45–46.

[198] Meredith, 'On Malarial Sites'; note 182; G. Dodds, 'Malaria', *IMG*, 17 (April 1, 1882), 111.

[199] *Army Medical Department Report for 1866*, Volume viii (London: Harrison and Sons, 1868).

colonial frontiers could be read and invoked in distant locations. Thus, by the 1870s malaria aroused the curiosities of an ever-growing variety of publishers, authors and readership spread across the colonial world. There malaria was alleged to acquire forms, extents, ferocities and resilience unthinkable elsewhere.

The persisting imagination of malaria as a flexible diagnostic category was reinforced and extended further in scholarly treatises, books, journal articles, journalistic accounts, bureaucratic reports which were produced in the colonies from the 1870s onwards. In his book on malaria published in 1871, C. F. Oldham, who had been an Assistant Surgeon to Her Majesty's Indian Forces and Surgeon In-charge of the Dalhousie Sanatorium, proposed a distinction between the prevalence of malaria in hot and cold climates.[200] In cold climates, Oldham suggested, malaria was prevalent in 'certain situations, specific localities and particular seasons';[201] mostly in autumn[202] and in 'low and swampy' areas.[203] In hot climates, Oldham suggested, malaria knew no bounds, and could reveal itself in diverse landscapes in every part of the 'habitable globe' and beyond.[204]

Malaria is found in the swamp and in the sandy desert; in the dense forest and the cultivated plain; on the lofty mountain and in the alluvial delta, scarcely raised above the level of the sea; in the fertile valley and amongst bare, sun-baked, rocks; in an atmosphere saturated with moisture and where the air is so hot and dry that no dew is formed, all vegetation are burnt up.[205]

Most of Oldham's examples of 'hot climatic conditions' were derived from colonised or previously colonised locations. Referring to a range of travel writings, Oldham suggested that in Ceylon, Java, the Malayan Archipelago, New Guinea, Gilolo, Orinoco[206] and at an altitude of 4000 feet and upwards in the Himalayas,[207] malaria could be most prevalent in the rainy season. In contrast, he showed that in the lower ranges of the Himalayas, the hill ranges or table lands of Southern India or in the 'oases of the Sahara, as in Algiers' the effects of malaria were most intense in the 'hottest and driest seasons'.[208] Quoting David Livingstone's account on the 'elevated regions of Central Africa', Oldham pointed out how malarial fever was found to be prevalent amongst the 'negroes' in the 'middle of winter'.[209] Unlike MacCulloch, Oldham labelled 'dry' locations devoid of any vegetation as potentially malarial situations. He believed that malaria could 'coexist with barrenness and intense drought'. Oldham thus extended the geography of malaria to

---

[200] Oldham, *What is Malaria?*, 13.   [201] Ibid., 13–14.   [202] Ibid., 14.
[203] Ibid., 20.   [204] Ibid., 19.   [205] Ibid., 14.   [206] Ibid., 18.   [207] Ibid., 17.
[208] Ibid., 17–18.   [209] Ibid., 19.

include 'hot and arid' regions of Venezuela,[210] desert tracts of Western Rajputana including Marwar, Jaisalmir, Bickaneer,[211] the flat, dry and sandy military stations at Jacobabad and Mean Meer,[212] and the sun-baked rocks of Aden,[213] Gibraltar and the Ionian Islands.[214] Malaria in the hot colonial climates, according to Oldham, revealed itself indiscriminately across an eclectic variety of seasons, weather, landscapes, altitudes and soil textures.

Malaria, it was argued, could thrive extensively in the colonies independent of vegetation and conditions of wetness. Malaria began being associated with a myriad range of colonial objects. Oldham described friable granite rocks encountered in Hong Kong and Amoy, magnesium limestone in Sindh and ferruginous rocks in Southern India as particularly generative of malaria.[215] Such suggestions were elaborated further in successive articles published in the *Indian Medical Gazette*. An anonymous reviewer of Oldham's work acknowledged the prevalence of not one but several malarial poisons: marsh poisons, granite poison, sandstone poison, limestone poison, clay poison and black soil poison.[216] In July 1874, C. A. Gordon, a Deputy Surgeon General working for the British Indian Government, published an article titled, 'The Hygiene of Malaria' in the same journal. He mentioned how malarial fevers could be contracted from inspecting musty hay or consulting old books.[217] Similarly, James Henry Salisbury associated 'malarial germs' with damp and mouldy bed sheets, bedding and clothes tightly packed in trunks, dust that adhered to old books and edible objects like mushrooms.[218] Malaria was construed as an enigmatic and usually invisible diagnostic category, which could nonetheless be embodied in a variety of forms and objects in the colonies. Malaria not only occupied place-names inscribed on the surface of medical texts, but also allegedly inhabited the depths of colonial landscapes, permeating the spectacular worlds of minerals, rocks, forests, deserts, coasts, winds, vessels, as well as everyday objects.

Salisbury's Macnaughton Prize-winning book, *Malaria*, was published in 1885 in New York, where he was a practicing physician. It laid the foundation of what was eventually known as 'the Cryptogrammic origin of malarial fevers'. A reading of his book suggests that writing about malaria in the colonies did not necessarily entail residence in such locations. Nor were such writers always officials in the colonial bureaucracy.

---

[210] Ibid., 43.   [211] Ibid., 44.   [212] Ibid., 43–45.   [213] Ibid., 46.
[214] Ibid., 45.   [215] Ibid., 47.
[216] Anonymous, 'Review of C. F. Oldham's 'What is Malaria? And Why is It Most Intense In Hot Climates?' *IMG*, 6 (1 May 1871), 101.
[217] C. A. Gordon, 'The Hygiene of Malaria', *IMG*, 9 (1 July 1874), 192.
[218] J. H. Salisbury, *Malaria* (New York: W. A. Kellogg, 1885), 17, 21, 22.

Even figures like Salisbury who worked in Cleveland and New York seems to have had access to stories narrated by travelling physicians and officials spread across the colonial world. His book drew upon narratives about Kingston in the West Indies, Nepal, Malwa, Peru, Brabant, New South Wales, the Southern Ocean, Tongataboo, Ovalau, the island of Soloo in the West coast of Africa, lower Egypt, Singapore, Sierra Leone, Batavia and Malacca, Zanzibar, St Lucia, Ceylon, Barbados and Mauritius.[219]

Publishing about malaria in the colonies and in Europe did not necessarily constitute mutually exclusive worlds. The same authors often wrote in journals published in Europe as well as in its colonies. European journals like *Edinburgh Medical Journal*,[220] the *British Medical Journal*[221] and the *Lancet*[222] frequently published articles about colonial malaria, as much as journals published from within the colonies. British officials serving the Empire in India often published medical memoirs from London-based firms. A. T. Macgowan, a physician with the British army, for instance, wrote about malaria in Kanpur during the Sepoy Mutiny in 1857. It was published and distributed by the same firm in London.[223] In 1880, E. G. Russell published an extensive treatise on malaria encountered while on duty in Assam. This book was eventually distributed from London, Madras, Bombay and Calcutta.[224] It is clear that publishers based in London were committed to circulating narratives about malaria involving different corners of the Empire. Similarly, authors based in the colonies appeared keen to share their insights with an informed home audience. Thus Joseph Fayrer, J. W. Moore and George Dodds, all colonial officials, often read out essays on colonial malaria to the Epidemiological Society of London or the Medico-Chirurgical Society of Edinburgh.[225]

By the 1870s, malaria was projected as an exclusively colonial concern. This converged with attempts to describe locations within Europe

---

[219] Ibid., 3–12.
[220] J. Bettington, 'On Decaying Vegetable Matter in Wells and Nullahs as Productive of Disease', *Edinburgh Medical Journal*, II (1856–1857), 556–559.
[221] Pascale, 'Curious Effects of Malaria'.
[222] J. Fayrer, 'Troonian Lectures on the Climate and Fevers of India', *Lancet*, 119, 3055 (18 March 1882), 423–426.
[223] A. T. Macgowan, *Malaria, the Common Cause of Cholera, Intermittent Fever and its Allies* (London: John Churchill and Sons, 1866).
[224] E. G. Russell, *Malaria: Cause and Effects, Malaria and the Spleen: An Analysis of Thirty-Nine Cases* (Calcutta: Thacker, Spink, 1880).
[225] Fayrer, 'Malaria'; Moore, 'Malaria vs More Recognisable Causes of Disease'; G. Dodds, 'Tropical Malaria and its Sequels', *Edinburgh Medical Journal*, 33 (1887–1888), 1090–1097.

as almost free from malaria. Malaria was shown as a contemporary reality for much of the colonial world in the 1870s. In contrast, malaria figured as an attribute of an embarrassing past, which England had left behind. To get rid of malaria, it was suggested, the colonies had to experience a similar set of historical processes. These included regimes of improvement and the circulation of different varieties of cinchonas. Articles published in the English journals from British India tended to associate malaria with known figures and periods in British history. An editorial published in the *Indian Medical Gazette* in October 1873 claimed that malarial fevers 'raged like a plague' during the sixteenth century reformation and during Thomas Sydenham's lifetime, a century later.[226] In 1876, T. E. Brown, the Principal of the Medical School in Lahore, published an article titled, 'On the References to Intermittent Fever in Shakespeare'. He noted frequent allusions to the diseases attributed to malaria and expressions like 'marsh-air on a dewy night' or 'bogs and fens' in the writings of Shakespeare. This he contrasted with the relative absence of such references in contemporary English literature.[227] He attributed such change to the 'improvements' of the drainage network initiated in Elizabethan England.[228] Such impressions were also conveyed in articles published in England. In 1885, *The Medical Times and Gazette of London* published an anonymous article titled, 'The Improvement of Malarious Countries'. It suggested in detail how measures of 'improvement' had substantially diminished the effects attributed to malaria all over Italy.

It is noteworthy in connection with the malaria in Rome that only one case of actual perniciosa was admitted into the Santa Spirito hospital during the year 1884; only two during 1883, and that only one case of malarious melanaemia has been available for research there during the past winter showing very clearly the improvement of late years in regard to malaria.[229]

However, the most detailed and overt statement came from Joseph Fayrer in a paper read out to the Epidemiological Society of London. Malaria, he observed:

In the tropics as they are now...have been in Europe in past times. Read Pringle's valuable work, Lind, Ferguson, Macculloch, and others of that time and at a subsequent date; or go back further, and read Lancisi and Sydenham,

---

226 Anonymous, 'Malaria', *IMG*, 8 (1 October 1873), 266.
227 T. E. Brown, 'On the References to Intermittent Fever in Shakespeare's Works', *Indian Annals of Medical Science*, 19 (1877) 217–226.
228 Ibid., 221.
229 Anonymous, 'Special Correspondence: The Improvement of Malarious Countries', *The Medical Times and Gazette*, 1 (1885), 626.

and you will see that not the coast of Guinea or the Nepal Terai can give you anything much worse than Europe did in those times . . . [230]

Fayrer added:

Once we were a very suffering people, and lost two kings, a queen, a cardinal, a lord Protector, and many other great people, from a disease that is now almost unknown, . . . Why this change? It comes of better drainage, better houses, better food, better personal and general hygiene, and therefore it is full of encouragement for other countries; and are we not now profiting by this experience, and gradually diminishing disease everywhere?[231]

Thus malaria figured as one of the cultural tropes which emboldened imperial discourse to argue that the colonies were characterised by a temporal lag. Imperial literature about malaria tended to reconfirm the notion that contemporary British India was a reenactment of historical predicaments which Europe had already encountered and resolved in the past. To that extent, the spectre of malaria empowered imperial ideologies to condemn the colonies to what Dipesh Chakrabarty calls 'the waiting room of history'.[232]

Such impressions were not always confined to texts written by British authors located in India or elsewhere. English articles written by Bengalis employed in the colonial government's medical service shared similar insights.[233] Similar claims were also put forward in certain books and journals published in the vernacular. For example in the late nineteenth century, Bengali medical journals like *Swasthya* and *Chikitsa Sammilani* began projecting contemporary England as completely free of malaria, while admitting its intense malarial past.[234]

In contrast, in successive editorials the *Swasthya* described malaria as a relatively recent feature in the history of Bengal, unknown 'thirty to thirty five years earlier.'[235] Suburban locations like Burdwan, Katwa or Kalna, which until recently were considered healthy places had over time, they argued, emerged as malarial localities.[236] Such articles tended to situate malaria within the emerging historical geographies of Bengal. One such article published in *Chikitsa Sammilani* described the recent

---

[230] Fayrer, 'Malaria', 17.   [231] Ibid., 16.

[232] D. Chakrabarty, *Provincializing Europe: Postcolonial Thought and Historical Difference*, (New Jersey: Princeton University Press, 2000), 8–10. See also, P. Banerjee, *Politics of Time: 'Primitives' and History-Writing in a Colonial Society* (Delhi: Oxford University Press, 2006), 1–39.

[233] K. D. Ghose, 'A Plea for Malaria', *IMG* 17 (1 June 1882), 150–154.

[234] P. C. Sanyal, 'Health in Bengal', *Chikitsa Sammilani* 8, 1(1891–1892), 9; R. Mitra, 'Malaria', *Chikitsa Sammilani*, 2 (1885–1886), 287–288.

[235] Anonymous, 'The Preponderance of Malaria', *Swasthya*, 3, 1 (1897), 5–6.

[236] Anonymous, 'Miscellaneous', *Swasthya*, 2, 7 (1896), 164.

decline of urban centres at Gaud, Lakshanabati, Subarnagram, Jessore and Birbhum, and ascribed it to malaria.[237]

Such overlapping conceptions about the shifting geographies of malaria in accounts written in different languages might appear startling.[238] However, writings in Bengali did not necessarily indicate a radical act of dissent. Nor did they inevitably constitute a counter-discourse to official correspondence. Writing about malaria in Bengali, as I will explore in the epilogue, addressed a different set of audiences and cultural assumptions; pursued dissimilar political purposes, and, adopted a unique set of stylistic approaches and linguistic strategies. Nonetheless, most of these nineteenth-century Bengali authors were part of the colonial bureaucratic and pedagogical network. The editor of the journal *Swasthya*, Durgadas Ghosh, for instance, had been a colonial Civil Surgeon based in Cooch Behar. Many of the contributors to these journals held medical degrees from the Medical College of Calcutta.[239] Doyal Krishen Ghosh who was an Assistant Surgeon in Hooghly published one of the very few Bengali books on malaria in the late nineteenth century.[240]

In the same year, 1878, Amritalal Bhattacharya's *Jvar Chikitsa (The Treatment of Fevers)* was published. It was written as a textbook for Bengali medical students at the Campbell Medical College, one of the very few medical schools set up in nineteenth-century Calcutta, which taught aspiring doctors in the Bengali language. Bhattacharya had been trained at the Medical College in Calcutta. He acknowledged in his preface that his comments on malaria were entirely based on class lectures delivered by one of his professors at the Calcutta Medical College, Dr Smith.[241] Unsurprisingly then Bengali authors acknowledged MacCulloch as the first author on malaria in English.[242] Most nineteenth-century Bengali authors about malaria were drawn from amongst those who had been co-opted within the entrenched networks of British colonial bureaucracy. As local custodians of knowledge about malaria, they asserted themselves as 'medical authorities' in relation to their intended vernacular audiences. Their limited polemics with European authors were overshadowed by the rather consistently pedagogical stance they adopted towards their potential readers in Bengali.

---

[237] Mitra, 'Malaria', 286.
[238] See for instance P. B. Mukharji, *Nationalizing the Body: The Medical Market, Print and Daktari Medicine* (New York and London: Anthem Press, 2009).
[239] Sanyal, 'Health in Bengal', 9–11; Mitra, 'Malaria', 284–292.
[240] D. K. Ghosh, *Malaria* (Sultangachi, Hooghly: Doyal Krishen Ghosh, 1878).
[241] A. Bhattacharya, *Jvar Chikitsa* (Calcutta: Valmiki Press, 1878).
[242] Mitra, 'Malaria', 311; Majumdar, 'Malaria Rahasya'.

Malarial Governance: Intervention, Compensation, Circulation

By the mid-nineteenth century, malaria was increasingly embroiled not only with colonial places – landscapes, objects, climates – but also implicated within networks of governance and the global circulation of labour. Malaria, on various occasions, enabled the deeper penetration of the colonial state into the interiors of British India to appear legitimate. In 1856–1857, for instance, the *Edinburgh Medical Journal* published an article by one J. Bettington, who was engaged in the task of drafting revenue reports in Western India. Bettington recommended certain measures of 'improvement' in resisting the effects of malaria in the jungle talooks of the southern Mahratta country. These included the construction of wells in the jungle districts of Dharwar, Belgaum, Kolapoor, Sattara, Puna, Nagur and Candeish and bringing these areas under cultivation.[243] This, he predicted, would result in a 'great improvement of the revenue'.[244] However, he observed that the wells required regular cleaning to remain free from the accumulation of noxious plants, refuse and mud. Effective cleaning, he argued, would necessitate European supervision: 'Experience proves that neither the people, nor the heads of villages, nor the heads of districts, will trouble themselves about such matters, unless compelled by standing-orders, rigidly enforced under the personal supervision of *European officers* in their tours through the country'.[245]

Further, the need to identify severely malarial localities provoked state-initiated efforts to measure the size of organs internal to the human body.[246] The Indian government published a report titled 'Prevalence of organic disease of the spleen as a test for detecting malarious localities on hot climates' in 1868, written by T. E. Dempster, a Surgeon of the 1st Brigade Horse Artillery. The object of inquiry was whether irrigation canals in northern India left their immediate vicinities 'malarious', by comparing the 'irrigated' and 'unirrigated' districts on both banks of the river Jumna, from Hardwar to Meerut.[247] The difficulties of this investigation, Dempster thought, 'were insurmountable'.[248] He found the 'native's account' of the healthiness of his own town or village, even

---

[243] Bettington, 'On Decaying Vegetable Matter', 558.
[244] Ibid., 557.   [245] Ibid., 559.
[246] J. Bailkin, 'The Boot and the Spleen: When Was Murder Possible in British India?' *Comparative Studies in Society and History*, 48, 2 (April, 2006), 462–493.
[247] T. E. Dempster, *The Prevalence of the Organic Disease of the Spleen as a Test for Detecting Malarious Localities in Hot Climates* (Calcutta: Office of the Superintendent of Government Printing, 1868), 7.
[248] Ibid., 19.

for a season, 'the loosest and most vague.' Nor could he access 'the medical statistics of several localities under examination'. He lamented the absence of any record of diseases, deaths, births and population to which he could refer. However, he claimed that he compensated for such difficulties by 'touching the body'[249] of the inhabitants in the relevant localities. He observed, 'The native inhabitants of unhealthy districts in India, often carry in their own persons a record of past suffering, which can at all times be easily read, and which no one can falsify or suppress. This is the enlargement of the spleen . . . '.[250] The connection between malarial diseases and the size of the spleen, Dempster believed, was close to mathematical precision. About his revelations during the examinations he wrote:

Although the intimate connection between malarious fevers and organic disease of the spleen is established beyond doubt, it never was supposed that these diseases bear an exact proportion to each other, or that the number of enlarged spleens in any particular situation should correspond precisely with the number of attacks of fever suffered by its inhabitants.[251]

At each place, Dempster and his colleagues selected 20 children and 20 adult males. These included members of 'all castes' and a group of agricultural labourers.[252] They classified five different degrees of size of spleen in every locality. Based on such classifications they identified some localities as more malarial than others.[253] Dempster mentioned that enlargement of the spleen seldom carried any form of visible external manifestation. He described enlargement of the spleen as the 'least formidable of all organic diseases of the viscera . . . it may consist with every outward appearance of health and vigour . . . strikingly healthy looking men and children were found with decided enlargement of the spleen'.[254] The subjects were selected, Demspter wrote, not from amongst the sick, but the 'going about population of the town or village under inspection.' In the absence of any external manifestations, the detection of an enlarged spleen or the identification of a malarial locality became almost entirely the examining physician's prerogative. 'No case was ever registered as "spleen", unless I had so *distinctly felt* the enlarged organ . . . '.[255] The suspicion of malaria thus empowered the administrative apparatus of the state to intervene into the depths of colonised bodies.

---

[249] D. Arnold, 'Touching the Body: Perspectives on the Indian Plague' in R. Guha and G. Spivak (eds.), *Selected Subaltern Studies* (New York: Oxford University Press, 1988), 391–426.
[250] Dempster, *The Prevalence of Organic Disease*, 19.   [251] Ibid.,20.
[252] Ibid., 23.   [253] Ibid., 24.   [254] Ibid., 21.   [255] Ibid., 23.

The identification of interior localities within British India as malarial brought its obvious benefits for the colonial state: Malaria legitimised various degrees of government intervention, reinforced the relevance of myriad projects of agricultural improvement, enabling in turn the unhindered functioning of the revenue machinery. At the same time, protecting the 'native subjects' as well as officials from malaria in such localities began to be considered as amongst the responsibilities of the colonial governments. By the 1870s, officials posted in 'isolated stations in malarious districts' began to demand diverse forms of monetary compensation from the government.[256] The fear that the effects of malaria were most harmful close to the soil inspired particular forms of architecture in the colonial frontiers by the 1860s.[257] In the 1940s, the living quarters of managers of tea plantations in Assam, for example, continued to be raised substantially above the ground to provide security to the vulnerable residents from the collective threats of wild animals and malaria.[258] These were presumably inspired by existing practices in other parts of the world where tabernacles were raised for the shared purpose 'to avoid malaria and for watching against robbers who rob the crops'.[259]

Malaria featured in narratives of circulation of migrant labour from one British colony to another. This is revealed in the various ways in which the Mauritius fever – an epidemic attributed predominantly to malaria in that colony in late 1860s – was reported. In a mammoth report drafted for the Sanitary Commission of Mauritius, Charles Meldrum explained Mauritius fever in terms of the excessive immigration of 'coolies' from India. Immigrants from British India were considered crucial to the economy of Mauritius. They were employed as cheap labourers in the sugar estates, as domestic servants, gardeners, hawkers, carriers and grazers.[260] Meldrum claimed that from 1834 to 1865, the population of Indian immigrants had increased from 84 to 245700.

---

[256] Home, Public, 10 September 1870, 33–35 A (NAI).

[257] J. Sutherland, to H. M. Macpherson, No. 51, Fort William, 13 April 1868. Municipal, Sanitation, Prog 14–15, June 1868 (WBSA).

[258] See the photograph entitled, 'The Manager's bungalow, Panitola Tea Estate [Upper Assam]' taken by photographer P. Bose in c. 1950. Shelfmark: Photo 451/1(4) [India Office Select Materials, BL]. The photograph carries the following note: 'An Assam bungalow of the old style. The roof is thatched for coolness and the living quarters are raised on stilts, originally with the idea of escaping malarial miasma and the attentions of wild animals'.

[259] For instance see the photographs entitled 'Tabernacles Raised to Avoid the Malaria, Paestum, or for Watching Against Robbers who Rob the Crops', Samuel Butler Collection, IX/Albums/5/40/1–2, St John's College, Cambridge.

[260] C. Meldrum, *Weather, Health and Forests: A Report on the Inequalities of the Mortality from Malarial Fever and Other Diseases in Mauritius* (Port Louis: Mercantile Record Co. Printing Establishment, 1881), 97.

This increase, he pointed out, corresponded with the greater prevalence of malarial fever in the island. Fifty-six vessels had carried 20283
Indian coolies into Mauritius from Calcutta, Madras and Bombay in
1865 alone.[261] Meldrum quoted one Dr Reid, who claimed to observe
the 'notorious proclivity of the Indian race to febrile disease, and the
special tendency brought from their own land of many of them to malarious fever'.[262] Earlier reports written by government officials in Mauritius also cited immigration of labourers from British India as a cause
of Mauritius fever. Health officers based in Port Louis frequently suggested that the 'coolies' brought their propensity towards malaria from
home. Such propensities were nurtured and further intensified in the
'dangerously overcrowded depots' in the ports at Bombay, Madras and
Calcutta.[263] The 'coolies' were each allowed a space of 24 superficial
feet in the depots. It resulted in overcrowded conditions in the depots.
These conditions, it was suggested, continued during the voyage. Thus,
malarial fever was carried into the island along with the immigration
of labourers from India. Such impressions were even shared by higher
officials representing the British Indian government. In 1864, for example, Dr Leith, the Secretary to the Government of India wrote to the
Secretary of State recommending the extension of the minimum space
allocated for each labourer in the depots from 24 to 54 superficial
feet.[264]

Such recommendations met with stiff resistance from the Colonial
Office, the Emigration Board and the War Office Sanitary Commission.
Officials representing the Emigration Board did not consider the recom-
mendation economically viable.

I feel bound, in the interest of the West Indian Colonies and Mauritius, to submit
that no sufficient grounds have been shown for requiring them to provide depot
accommodation to an extent that would necessarily add largely to the cost of
emigration, and might eventually make it too expensive to be continued.[265]

Officials within the Emigration Board tried to argue that the allocated
space for emigrant labourers was sufficient. Prisoners in British India
were each allocated a space of 36 superficial feet, while the 'native servants in military cantonments' were offered a minimum space of 50 feet.
The emigrant 'coolies' were thus allowed a space, which was much more

---

[261] Ibid., 104.   [262] Ibid., 91.
[263] E. C. Bayley, to The Colonial Secretary, Government of Madras, 16 July 1869, Simla.
Home, Public, 17 July 1869, 109–112 A (NAI).
[264] S. Walcott to T. Eliot, 17 October 1868, Emigration board. Ibid.
[265] Ibid.

constricted in comparison to 'servants and prisoners' in India. However, such discrepancy was defended on behalf of the Emigration board.

> In one case... occupation is more or less permanent, and in the other it lasts only a few days... when a migration depot is not full the people have the advantage of the unoccupied space. They are unrestricted in their movements during the day and night... An Indian prisoner, on the other hand, although he may have 36 superficial feet of superficial space, yet from necessary condition of security is less favourably placed.[266]

Officials in the Emigration board suggested that the minimum superficial spaces allocated for the emigrant Indian labourers in the depots in Bombay, Calcutta or Madras were in parity with related provisions in other contexts. For instance, the London common lodging houses apparently allowed a minimum space of 33 superficial feet by 6.5 feet in height, or 115.5 cubic feet. The Imperial Passenger's Act required on board-ship allowance of 15 superficial feet by 6 in height or 90 cubic feet per adult. British depots in Plymouth and Birkenhead allowed about 222 cubic feet per adult. The Indian Emigration Act of 1864 made provisions on board-ship of only 10 superficial feet by 5.5 feet in height, or 55 cubic feet per adult, while West Indian Emigration made 12 superficial feet mandatory. These figures were elaborately quoted in correspondence between different members of the Emigration board. Emigrant coolies leaving Indian ports for Mauritius were allocated a minimum space of 24 feet by 12 in height or 288 cubic feet. Officials representing the Emigration board argued that it was not only sufficient, but also 'more than five times the minimum cubic allowance on board-ship'. Such allocations of space for Indian coolies bound for Mauritius was not only projected as sufficient, but also desirable. Writing to a colleague in the Emigration board, S. Walcott referred to one Dr Pearse. He described Pearse as one of the 'most experienced and able medical officers', a veteran of twelve voyages to Australia in medical charge of emigrants, and six voyages with upwards of 2570 'coolies' from India to the West Indies. In a letter written to Walcott, Pearse argued that 'the warmer and closer (within reason) the coolies lie at night the better for them'.[267]

Officials representing the War Office Sanitary Commission and the Emigration Board differed from the health officers at Port Louis and certain senior bureaucrats serving the government of India. They suggested that Mauritius fever and conditions of accommodation for the labourers

[266] Ibid.   [267] Ibid.

in the depots were unrelated. Instead, they argued that the fever could be attributed to local malarial situations within Mauritius itself.[268]

Correspondence about Mauritius fever reveals how a malarial event could be explained in terms of both local circumstances as well as mobile and portable agents. A particular event associated with malaria could be analysed differently by diverse sets of officials. Thus the aetiology of a malarial epidemic both sustained and was produced by questions of race, class and labour, and the exigencies of colonial economy. The epidemic further occasioned fault-lines and tensions between different colonial governments within the British Empire to be exposed, when Mauritian and Indian bureaucrats blamed one another for the event.

Regions and Races

Malaria was not just ascribed to local circumstances or circulating labourers. Widely dispersed locations across the extensive colonial world were believed to share myriad malarial situations. In contemporary bureaucratic correspondence or scientific writings, such locations converged to constitute overlapping geographical 'regions'. These regions stood for both geopolitical zones and disease ecologies. Distant constituents within such regions, it was claimed, shared propensities towards similar diseases. Thomas Barker in 1859 described how 'regions of disease corresponded with seasons and zones of climate'. He divided 'the surface of the globe' into three 'belts or zones'. Malarial diseases appeared most intense and concentrated in what he called 'the torrid zone or belt'.[269] Within the 'torrid zone', Barker identified the Gulf of Mexico, the West India islands, the northern portion of South America, India, Borneo, Ceylon, the Gulf of Guinea, Madagascar and Mozambique as 'the principal centres' of such diseases.[270] Barker appeared less certain about the 'perpendicular distribution' of malarial diseases. However, he observed that in Mexico they were prevalent at an elevation of 7000 or 8000 feet; and in South Eastern Asia they ceased at an elevation of 6000 or 7000 feet above the sea level. Barker proposed a connected and shared natural history of diseases which recurred across the torrid zone when he argued that the manifestation of malarial diseases at one location could indicate the beginnings of similar outbreaks in distant locations.

---

[268] G. B. Malleson to J. Geoghegan, No. 141, 5 March 1869. Home, Public, 17 July 1869, 109–112 A (NAI).
[269] Barker, *On Malaria*, 62.   [270] Ibid., 59–63.

The same morbid appearances are reproduced with the utmost constancy and regularity in a thousand places at once, wherever the same causes of insalubrities are met with, only they are more intense, continuous and prolonged in some places than in others... Similarity of geological formation indicates a similarity in the diseases of a country, as seen in the localities visited by malarial fevers.[271]

Such insights found reflection in Meldrum's collection of reports describing the causes of the Mauritius fever. The malarial epidemic was attributed to meteorological conditions, which were not peculiar to the island, including absence of floods, prevalence of intense periods of drought and fluctuations in rainfall. The period from 1864–1868, it was reported, was characterised by a 'remarkable absence of hurricanes' all over the Indian Ocean region. Meteorological conditions witnessed in Mauritius were also prevalent 'in other places bordering on the Indian Ocean'. Potentially malarial situations, it was suggested, could be almost simultaneously witnessed in places as far as Mauritius, Rodrigues, India, South Africa and the Australian colonies.[272] Such regions did not only share with Mauritius the 'abnormal weather' supposedly prevalent in the island between 1864 and 1868, but also experienced like Mauritius remarkable death rates.[273] These reports suggested that during this period conditions of ill health were not confined to islands bordering on the Indian Ocean region, but extended to 'considerable portions of the globe' including Malta, Gibraltar, the West Indies and certain parts of Southern Europe.[274] Such extensive manifestation of malarial diseases, it was conjectured, could be attributed to periodic mutations on the solar surface, which simultaneously affected meteorological and demographic conditions in different parts of the world.[275] Mauritius fever, it was suggested, could hardly then be described as a 'local' event.

By the mid-nineteenth century, composite geographical categories designated collectively as regions were thus constituted of distant and diverse forms of landscapes. The literature about malaria drew upon and consolidated contemporary regional formations. Malaria was consistently associated with some amongst these overlapping regional categories, including, as I have noted, 'torrid zones', 'hot climates' and 'Indian Ocean region'. The tropics constituted another such category.[276] George Dodds, a British doctor who held various official assignments in Asia, read out a paper entitled, 'Tropical Malaria and its Sequels' to the Medico-Chirurgical Society of Edinburgh on 4 April 1888.[277] Dodds' description of tropical malaria echoed Oldham's comments

---

[271] Ibid., 59. [272] Meldrum, *Weather, Health and Forests*, 105–111.
[273] Ibid., 152. [274] Ibid., 109. [275] Ibid., 152–157.
[276] See Arnold, *Tropics and Travelling Gaze*.
[277] Dodds, 'Tropical Malaria', 1090–1097.

about malaria in hot climates. In the tropics, Dodds argued, malaria was most intense and omnipresent, and could acquire vigorous and various forms.

It has the power of drifting along from its source for a considerable distance, and to be able to roll up the sides of mountains and along ravines, and yet can be stopped by a high hedge, a grove of trees or even by a mosquito curtain. It prefers low levels and yet can be found also on the tops of mountains. It coexists with vegetation, and is found in arid wastes, utterly devoid of any vegetable growth.[278]

Malaria was tied intimately to notions of race as much as conceptions of region. Malaria sustained the perceived correlations between composite geographical categories and racialised collectives of humans. Writers on malaria such as Dodds began by commenting on the vulnerability of Europeans in the tropics. He described malaria as more or less confined to the tropics, and in so doing proposed a radical shift from the geography of malaria conceived by MacCulloch half a century earlier. He considered Europe as almost free from malaria. Most malarial patients in Europe, Dodds thought, were those who had returned from Europe's various 'tropical and subtropical possessions'. Most of them appeared to carry 'malarial taints' in their bodies. Thus, malaria in Europe, Dodds argued, was a predominantly 'Anglo-Indian' disease.

As long as the European lives within the tropics... that asthenic condition inevitably overtakes every European or at least every Anglo Saxon... He never gets acclimatized, and is as liable to sunstroke after a residence of a dozen years as he was during the first week of arrival. Almost everyone who has resided in the East has imbibed the malarial poison...[279]

Colonialism necessitated, it was argued, the uncontrolled exposure of Europeans to myriad malarial situations in the tropics. The vulnerability of Europeans to malaria, according to authors like Thomas Wilson, was an effect of Europe's many imperial ventures in the nineteenth century. Wilson compared nineteenth-century European empires with ancient Rome, which had also ruled over 'many nations and races'. However, 'they met with no race with whom the Romans could not freely amalgamate'.[280] Malaria, argued Wilson, was thus unknown in ancient Rome. Unlike the ancient Roman Empire, nineteenth-century European colonialism involved 'the attempt to occupy by a white race a tropical country, and a land inhabited by coloured men'.

The problems presented by the modern history of a European race attempting to hold India by the sword, to colonise the American world from the Polar sea

[278] Ibid., 1091.   [279] Ibid., 1090.   [280] Wilson, *An Enquiry*, 106.

to the Land of Fire, to inhabit if not to cultivate, the insalubrious Antilles, the banks of the Orinoco, or of the still more dreadful Senegal, Gambia and Niger, nowhere occur in Roman or Grecian history... [281]

... However distant these lands lie, their malarious condition has an influence over the European family of nations, an influence... though originating in the obscure and unknown East, has shown itself at times at Rome and Moscow, London and Paris... [282]

Such exposure to the landscape, climate and people in tropical India, Africa and America, Wilson feared, would eventually result in the extinction of the European race. Behind this fear lay an implicit emphasis on the superiority of the 'European race'. European bodies were projected as sophisticated, tender and delicate. In hostile and rough tropical situations, the exalted forms of European life, it was apprehended, could undergo decay and degeneration. 'Extinction seems the sure result of all their efforts, whether they unite with the native races or not. If they unite, their purer blood soon disappears in the stream of a darker population; if they spurn the union... malaria speedily exterminates their race and name'.[283]

Nineteenth-century English scientific literature rarely referred to the colour of malaria, but stray references indicate how malaria was associated with different colours in the course of the century. MacCulloch did not refer to the colour of malaria. He however suggested that malarial patients in Europe turned flabby and acquired yellow stains on the body.[284] From the mid-nineteenth century, malaria was increasingly projected as brown or black in various sources. For instance, Justin von Liebig described water-bearing taints of malarial putrefaction as brown.[285] An anonymous editorial published in the *Indian Medical Gazette* in 1873 referred to marshy water in the vicinities of Melbourne as 'brown as brandy'.[286] In the late 1880s, Dodds claimed that Europeans, who lived long in 'malarious districts' acquired 'anaemia with brownish tint of skin'.[287] E. A. Parkes, Professor of Hygiene in the Army Medical School at Netley, published an article in the Annual Report of the Medical Department of the British Army in 1868. He referred to one Dr Massey, who was employed by the Army Medical Department in Jaffna, and claimed to have tracked the colours of 'particles of malaria'. 'Massey observed... the well known power trees exert in stopping the transit of malarial particles. He found the leaves of these trees greatly

---

[281] Ibid., 105.   [282] Ibid., 109.   [283] Ibid., 106.
[284] MacCulloch, *Malaria*, 429–430.   [285] Barker, *On Malaria*, 20.
[286] Anonymous, 'Malaria', *IMG*, 8 (1 September 1873), 241.
[287] Dodds, 'Tropical Malaria', 1094; See also W. D. Foster, *A History of Parasitology* (Edinburgh and London: E&S Livingstone Ltd, 1965), 159.

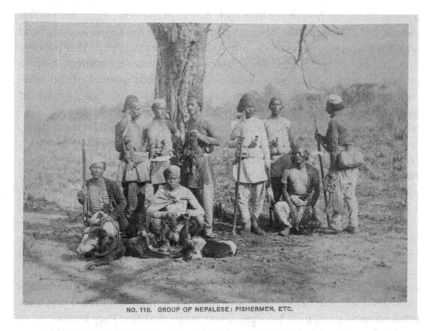

NO. 118. GROUP OF NEPALESE: FISHERMEN, ETC.

Figure 2.6 © British Library Board. 'Group of Nepalese: fishermen, etc.' Photographer: Bourne and Shepherd, 1876; Photo carries the following note: "The fishermen are Tharos, natives of the Terai, who have the peculiarity of being proof to its malaria (which in certain seasons is deadly to anyone else)...". (India Office Select Material, British Library. Shelfmark: Photo 992/1(118).

affected with black rust'.[288] By the mid-nineteenth century, malaria had emerged as predominantly a colonial concern. It is suggestive that by then malaria began to be associated more with brown and black than any other colour.

Figure 2.6 indicates that discussions about European vulnerability in the tropics coexisted with assertions of the immunity of the colonised 'primitives' from the effects of malaria. The 'tribes in the Terai and other forest districts of India', the 'negroes in some parts of the coast of Guinea'[289] and 'the deadly regions of Central America', the 'aborigines' inhabiting the 'virgin forests' of Java, the Malaya Peninsula, and ancient Mexico, were considered immune from the effects of malaria.[290] Various explanations were offered to explain such examples of 'racial immunity'

[288] E. A. Parkes, 'Report on Hygiene for 1867', *Army Medical Department Report for 1866*, Volume viii (London: Harrison and Sons, 1868), 316–317.
[289] Sternberg, *Malaria and Malarial Diseases*, 81.   [290] Wilson, *An Enquiry*, 106–107.

from malaria, such as the colour and texture of the skin. Thus wrote Oldham in 1871, 'One of the obvious peculiarities of the negro as compared with the European is his thick, oily, skin, rank to a degree . . . it is possible that the skin of the Negro does, from its thickness and oiliness, help to protect him from malarious disease'.[291] In the last quarter of the nineteenth century, such racial immunity from malaria was also explained by invoking the theory of natural selection.[292] Groups of people, who had inhabited tropical and therefore malarial regions from 'remote ages', it was suggested, tended to acquire 'collective acclimatisation'. In such regions, malaria, it was claimed, swept away from each generation individuals whose specific resistance was the feeblest; it spared only those who could offer strongest resistance. This, over generations, paved the way for a 'collective specific resistance in a race'.

Such perceived immunity amongst those who were collectively mentioned in various imperial narratives as primitives was attributed to their crude and uncivilised physical constitutions. Their compatibility with malaria was cited as corroboration of anthropological accounts, which described them as less-than-humans, whose unsophisticated existence resembled animals more than any form of human culture. They were referred to as primitives because it was suspected that they continued to be caught up in a 'state of nature'. 'Men in a state of nature', Thomas Wilson thought, 'seem to resist malaria'.[293] An anonymous article published in the *Medical Times and Gazette London* in May 1885 argued that such resistance could be observed amongst the 'savage men', 'the negro race' and the 'lower animals'.[294] A few decades later a senior medical bureaucrat in the British Indian government reflected similar prejudice when he wrote that malarial parasites were 'as natural amongst primitive races as flea infestation is to a dog'.[295]

Nonetheless, the so-called primitives were recommended subjection to colonial regimes of improvement and doses of quinine broadly for two reasons. It was suspected that although the 'primitive races' withstood malaria themselves having imbibed it across generations, they could infect the non-immune communities.[296] Commenting on colonial northern Australia at a later period Warwick Anderson has shown how the non-white population were projected in scientific texts as '"natural"

---

[291] Oldham, *What is Malaria?*, 173.   [292] Sternberg, *Malaria*, 80.
[293] Wilson, *An Enquiry*, 14.
[294] Anonymous, 'Special Correspondence: The Improvement of Malarious Countries', *The Medical Times and Gazette*, 1 (1885), 626.
[295] *Proceedings of the Third Meeting of the General Malaria Committee at Madras November 1912* (Simla: Government Central Branch Press, 1913), 13.
[296] Ibid.

careers of dangerous tropical pathogens'.[297] Moreover, such absolute immunity from malaria, nineteenth-century authors lamented, could hardly be witnessed any more. Exposure to European notions of civilisation and domesticity seemed to contaminate the pristine 'state of nature' inhabited by the 'aborigines' and the 'natives'.[298] It was argued, for instance, that the advent of specific remedies preserved the 'weakly resistant', and acted against the 'benefits' offered by 'natural selection'. It resulted in 'marked deterioration of race in malarious countries'.[299] The 'natives of Newfoundland and Canada'[300] and 'dark races'[301] including the 'negroes in Africa',[302] the Coles, Gonds and other 'tribes' inhabiting the jungle-regions in India,[303] 'the non-Aryan races of Assam'[304] began featuring in various reports as victims of malaria.

Thus, immunity of the so-called primitives from malaria in tropical locations could no longer be described as absolute. They began to appear as relatively more immune to malaria only when compared to the greater vulnerability of the Europeans. However, the propensity of such 'races' to malaria manifested itself whenever they were made to travel from one region to another. Immunity acquired by these 'primitives' was projected as not only relative, but also contextual.

In the moist and sultry climate of the West Indies, the negro thrives... more deadly the climate to the white race, the better does it suit the negro. Transferred to a cooler climate, however, the African loses his advantage over the white man; the liability to malarious disease become equalized and something more... the negro after a lengthened residence in a cooler climate, becomes more susceptible to the diseases of the tropics. The Negroes, who went out from England with the Niger expedition, suffered much less from fevers than the white men, but very much more than their countrymen who had never left the coast... [305]

Such impressions found wider currency from the 1870s, and were reflected in a range of sources. George M. Sternberg, an influential physician employed in the US army, for instance, wrote in 1884, 'Negroes born in Africa are much less susceptible to malaria than are their descendants born in more temperate and cooler climates'.[306]

Thus, by the mid-1870s, 'primitives' were incorporated amongst the potential victims of malaria. Oldham suggested in 1871: 'No race has yet

[297] W. Anderson, 'Geography, Race and the Nation: Remapping 'Tropical' Australia, 1890–1930', in Rupke (ed.), *Medical Geography*, 147.

[298] Wilson, *An Enquiry*, 14.

[299] Anonymous, 'Special Correspondence: The Improvement of Malarious Countries', *The Medical Times and Gazette*, 1 (1885), 626.

[300] Wilson, *An Enquiry*, 14.   [301] Oldham, *What is Malaria?*, 168.   [302] Ibid., 170.

[303] Ibid., 171.   [304] Sternberg, *Malaria*, 80–82.

[305] Oldham, *What is Malaria?*, 174–175.   [306] Sternberg, *Malaria*, 82.

been discovered, which is proof against malarious disease; though all do not suffer alike in the same climate',[307] Individuals belonging to every race, such statements suggested, were likely to benefit from regimes of improvement and the consumption of quinine. Such suggestions were revealing because, as I will show, the 1870s also witnessed the beginnings of attempts to define, manufacture and circulate pure quinine as an item of mass consumption in various British and Dutch colonies. Besides, with emphasis on British India in general and Bengal in particular, I will point out in what follows, how the intimate histories of malaria and quinine played out not only in the policies of the imperial state, but also in the vernacular markets in land, print and drugs.

Conclusion

In the half-century following 1827, when John MacCulloch's book about malaria was published, the category attracted the attention of various layers of commentators. The intellectual history of nineteenth-century malaria presents the curious case of a medical problem, which was addressed and shaped by, apart from medics, a range of geologists, chemists, meteorologists, natural historians, sanitary officials and colonial administrators. At the same time, writers about malaria, as I have suggested, were not only drawn from the Europeans. By the 1870s, for example, Bengalis employed in various capacities in the colonial bureaucracy had begun authoring articles and books on malaria in English as well as Bengali. It has been noted in existing histories that subordination and authority are relational and subjective positions.[308] In relation to their intended vernacular audience, writers of Bengali texts on malaria commanded a position of authority, even when they claimed to derive information from English textbooks. Their pedagogical tone was restricted within their spheres of ambition and influence set by the Bengali print market.

In contrast, Bengali writers in English found themselves at the bottom of the hierarchy of authors on malaria, pleading often with superior officials in the colonial bureaucracy or with European writers for their share of recognition. Gopaul Chandra Roy, for example, was the author of the most extensively cited English book on malaria written by a Bengali in the nineteenth century. Articles published by him later in his life vented

---

[307] Oldham, *What is Malaria?*, 172.
[308] F. Coronil, *The Magical State: Nature, Money and Modernity in Venezuela* (Chicago: University of Chicago Press, 1997), 16.

his desperation for recognition and patronage from European authorities and the state.[309] Such examples can be multiplied. In June 1882, the *Indian Medical Gazette* published a review of J. W. Moore's 'Malaria vs. Recognisable Climatic Influences', written by one K. D. Ghose, a Bengali trained in one of the medical colleges set up by the colonial government. Ghose began his article by proposing the following apology: 'Ten years residence and active practice in the most notoriously malarious district (Rungpore) in malarious Bengal is the only apology for coming out of this place of obscurity to take arms against such an authority as Dr Moore ... My hand trembles, when I hold my pen against the voice of one whose authority is well recognised ... '.[310] These authors projected themselves as marginal medical men who were deferential to their superiors in the world of knowledge about malaria. Thus, wrote a Hospital Assistant from Barishal in a letter to the editor of the *Indian Medical Gazette* in the same year: 'The Hospital Assistants have very limited knowledge either of book or practice ... they only follow the steps of higher medical authorities ... I being a man of same rank and position crave permission to state faithfully about my practical experience ... I feel shame for my inability to produce a paper ... '.[311]

Thus, malaria revealed various layers of authorities in the nineteenth century. Accordingly, many conceptions about the causes and cures of malarial diseases coexisted. By the third quarter of the century, for instance, an extensive range of plants was associated with malaria. These either figured as generative of malaria or were believed to neutralise its effects. In an article titled 'The Hygiene of Malaria' published in July 1874, Surgeon General C. A. Gordon summarised a catalogue of such plants. He mentioned the papaw in East Africa, the Manchineel tree of the West Indies, certain species of the *Rhus* encountered in America and China, and mangrove, tamarind, neem, oleander and narcissus as plants generative of malaria. Gordon included the sunflower, the eucalyptus, *Pistia Stratiotes*, 'several species of the natural order *Myrtaceae*' amongst plants with prophylactic influence. These plants, Gordon observed, were being planted in the Gold Coast, in Cuba, Algeria, Australian Colonies, in Corsica, Jamaica and India to stave off malaria.[312]

However, the relationships between various extracts of cinchona barks and malarial diseases appear to have been most invariable, consistent

---

[309] G. C. Roy, 'Vindication', *IMG*, 17 (1882), 24; Home, Medical, 1876, 1–5 A (NAI).

[310] Ghose, 'A Plea for Malaria', 150–151.

[311] Anonymous, 'Tincture of Iodine and Burnt Alum in Intermittent Fever', *IMG*, 17 (2 October 1882), 279.

[312] C. A. Gordon, 'The Hygiene of Malaria', *Indian Medical Gazette*, 9 (1 July 1874), 192–193.

and enduring in course of the century. In significant ways, as this book is in the process of highlighting, cinchona plants and their extracts could engender crucial transformations in the history of the diagnostic category, malaria. Although English writings on malaria did not begin in the 1820s, the discovery of quinine stoked an unprecedented gush of publications about malaria by the end of the decade. Besides, by the middle of the century, the cinchonas ceased to be confined within South American 'natural forests' and networks of circulation in Europe. Thousands of such plants and seeds were transported to the emerging colonial plantations in Dutch Java, French Algeria and British India. This coincided with a shift in the geographies of malaria: from a predominantly European disease to an almost exclusively colonial concern.

MacCulloch's comments and examples were predominantly associated with European locations, landscapes, beauty, grandeur and richness. Malaria, thought MacCulloch, was 'death knocking at the door of the opulent to spare the mean'.[313] His book was not initially intended for a colonial audience. However, in the decades that followed, it was received and reviewed extensively in colonial locations. By the mid-nineteenth century, malaria was defined in terms of colonial poverty, hunger, filth, insanitation, overpopulation and overcrowded ways of living. In the second half of the century, malaria was projected as almost exclusively associated with hot climates, tropical regions, torrid zones and the Indian Ocean belt. Such recurrent categories coalesced in a range of sources and almost revealed the map of European empires. The colonies, it was suggested, could be rescued only through intense regimes of improvement and extensive distribution of quinine.

Nonetheless, malaria did not absolutely disappear as a governmental concern within Europe.[314] Medical statistics, however, revealed sharply declining figures for malarial patients and victims within European states like Italy in the 1880s.[315] This could be sharply contrasted with statistics available for colonial locations like Bengal in the same decade. Quoting official annual mortality figures for Bengal between 1883 and 1887, the Bengali journal *Swasthya* (*Health*) suggested that 5,067,205 persons apparently died of diseases attributed to malaria within those five years.[316] In the next chapter, I will examine the production of a specific

---

[313] MacCulloch, *Malaria*, 293.
[314] For instance, see P. T. Volprignano, *The Future of the Port of London. A Provision Against the Malaria of the Metropolis, the Pollution of the Thames, the Collisions on the River Being The Outline of a Scheme for an Uninterrupted Navigation to and from the Port of London* (London: H Horne and Sons, 1890).
[315] Anonymous, 'Special Correspondence'.
[316] Anonymous, 'Malaria According to Various Physicians', *Swasthya*, 3, 1 (1897), 15.

malarial locality in the British Empire, and reveal how knowledge about a particular locality and an epidemic were simultaneously put together.

In this chapter I have hinted at how histories of nineteenth-century malaria can variously expose relationships between objects and imperial formations. First, malaria itself was an *object* of knowledge and governance re-inscribed by the exigencies and apparatuses of imperial rule. Malaria found itself intimately entangled in imperial conversations about colonial capital, migrant labour, cultures of intervention and compensation, and questions of race, regions, class and improvement. At the same time, malaria, in turn, consolidated Empire by reinforcing connections between a network of distant places, materials, professions and processes. Finally, in the imperial texts malaria was believed to personify in decaying vegetation, friable granite rocks, water casks, mouldy bed sheets, stale mushrooms, dusty old books, refuse of indigo factories and groups of humans pejoratively described as colonised tribes, aborigines, negroes and primitives. Although described as immune from the effects of malaria, these objects and groups of humans were perceived to signify and circulate malaria. Thus imperial embodiments of malaria transgressed the boundaries between humans and nonhumans; subjects and objects. Distinctions between wild animals and native robbers, primitives and parasites, lower animals and negroes were systematically blurred in the imperial narratives about malaria.

3   'A Cinchona Disease'
Making Burdwan Fever

The truth of the matter is that the terms "epidemic, "time", and "space" are the most general abstractions, which we can form and if we bring them together, the result must be something very vague and visionary... An abstract term "epidemic influence" is invented or utilized, and made to do as a substantive "theory" of a more occult or quasi-learned description... The whole process is a melancholy exhibition of false generalising.[1]

It is curious to note how mankind is led by watchwords. Be it religion, politics, or popular science, the commanding officer of the hour issues the countersign, and the sect, party, or society catches it up, and it is repeated, and echoed and re-echoed until the sound becomes faint, or the voice is deadened by the higher tone of new utterance. It is a strange phase of human life, this system of watchwords....[2]

In many ways Assam fever, Malta fever, Nagpur fever, Hong Kong fever, Amritsar fever, Peshawar fever, Niger fever, Mauritius fever, Bulam fever and Burdwan fever constituted disparate episodes within a shared history of colonial correspondence. In different moments of the nineteenth century, medical bureaucrats recognised them as epidemics attributable predominantly to malaria. Particular patterns of bureaucratic reporting recurrently identified maladies by referring to place-names. Such associations of place-names with maladies ended up circulating enduring impressions about lands, landscapes and people.

This chapter examines the making of Burdwan fever. Burdwan in the 1870s was a part of the Bengal presidency in British India. Burdwan was both the name of a division within the Bengal presidency as well as a district within the Burdwan division. Hooghly, Howrah and Midnapur were amongst the other districts within the Burdwan division.

[1] Anonymous, 'Prominent Fallacies in Epidemiology', *IMG*, 8 (1 July 1873), 188–189.
[2] Anonymous, 'Draining Bengal', *IMG*, 7 (September 1872), 209.

Divisions and districts represented geographical units for organising civil administration and revenue-extraction. In various official registers, the Burdwan fever featured as a malarial epidemic that hit the Burdwan division of the Bengal presidency in British India in the late 1860s and early 1870s. In these records, Burdwan fever, the malarial epidemic and 'Lower Bengal Epidemic fever' often tended to figure interchangeably as almost identical categories.[3] The making of Burdwan fever was inti-. mately connected to government discourses about malaria ostensibly prevailing in the Burdwan division and beyond.

Existing histories of Burdwan fever have explained this malarial epidemic as an event, characterised by the simultaneous manifestation of a single, fairly homogenous, monolithic malady in a million bodies.[4] Instead, expressions such as Burdwan fever and the malarial epidemic can also be understood as historically produced labels: shorthand expressions that provided convenient points of reference to a dispersed set of officials. Numerous bureaucratic reports in the second half of the century in Bengal presented the malarial epidemic as a flexible medical metaphor, which could be invoked to explain myriad expressions of physical unease, varying over time and across space.[5]

Historians have frequently defined epidemics as ontologically accessible phases of countless deaths and ceaseless sufferings. Critiques of colonial medicine have justifiably appropriated epidemics as excuses to highlight various historical processes ranging from government exploitation to mismanagement.[6] In the process, the category epidemic itself has often been inherited from the colonial archive at face value. Analysing the makings of such categories can reinforce critiques of colonial medicine. This chapter then refrains from probing into *why* there had been a malarial epidemic in Bengal in the nineteenth century. Nor is

[3] See, for example, L. Rogers, 'The Lower Bengal (Burdwan) Epidemic Fever Reviewed and Compared with the Present Assam Epidemic Malarial Fever (Kala-Azar)', *IMG* 32 (November 1897), 401–408; G. C. Roy, *The Causes, Symptoms and Treatment of Burdwan Fever. Or the Epidemic Fever of Lower Bengal* (Calcutta: Thacker, Spink and Co, 1876); J. H. French, *Endemic Fever in Lower Bengal, Commonly called Burdwan Fever* (Calcutta: Thacker, Spink 1875).

[4] For instance, A. Samanta, *Malarial Fever in Colonial Bengal, 1820–1939, Social History of an Epidemic* (Kolkata: Firma KLM, 2002); S. Sarma, *The Ecology and the Epidemic: A Study on the 19th-century Controversy* (Calcutta: India Book Exchange, 1999).

[5] For a study of the different meanings associated with 'malaria' in nineteenth-century British India and beyond, see R. Deb Roy, 'Mal-Areas of Health: Dispersed Histories of a Diagnostic Category', *Economic and Political Weekly*, 42, 2 (13 January 2007), 13–19.

[6] In relation to the history of Burdwan fever this is most evident in Samanta, *Malarial Fever*; and Sarma, *The Ecology and the Epidemic*.

it a study of the inadequate responses of the colonial government or the reactions of the local landed proprietors. Instead, it asks *how* a series of dispersed and dissimilar debilities could be put together as a single, continuous epidemic of malaria over a considerable period of time.

The biopolitical production of Burdwan fever needs to be located within the exigencies and apparatuses of imperial rule. Burdwan fever was occasioned by interactions between the overlapping worlds of pharmaceutical business, colonial governance, medical knowledge and vernacular markets (in land, prints and drugs). In these imperially enabled worlds, as the following pages will reveal, a drug could precede and delimit understandings about the malady it was meant to cure.

The production of Burdwan fever was also built upon ascribing active, lifelike, causal properties to inanimate nonhumans, particularly a range of plants. These processes were connected to the reinforcement of various layers of prejudices about colonised humans. Mark Harrison and David Arnold have shown already how official reports about Burdwan fever were deeply implicated in the discriminating discourses of race, class and civilisation.[7] Ultimately, the epidemic was not a passive and impotent biopolitical construct. While being occasioned by the Empire in British India, reports about the epidemic in turn reconstituted Burdwan as one of the many malarial localities in the colonial world. There was no 'local' that always and already existed as a natural geographical entity on the map of the British Empire. Locations like Burdwan were defined as the 'local' through conscious strategies of knowledge gathering initiated by the colonial state. Such strategies enabled cultural and medical stereotypes to proliferate. But, if at one level the making of Burdwan fever reveals the ways in which malaria emerged as a trope for colonial bureaucrats to make sense of localities in the interiors of British India; malaria itself did not merely remain a distant and unchanging medical jargon imported from Europe. Instead, the anecdotes, debilities, intellectuals, landscapes, landowners, markets, officials, peasants and plants encountered in the localities of Bengal in the late 1860s and especially in the 1870s, in turn, increasingly became accommodated within the existing global narratives about malaria.

---

[7] M. Harrison, '"Hot Beds of Disease": Malaria and Civilisation in Nineteenth-Century British India', *Parassitologia* 40 (1998), 11–18; D. Arnold, '"An Ancient Race Outworn": Malaria and Race in Colonial India', in W. Ernst and B. Harris (eds.), *Race, Society and Medicine: 1700–1960* (London: Routledge, 1999), 123–143; D. Arnold, *Science, Technology and Medicine in Colonial India* (Cambridge: Cambridge University Press, 2000), 78–80.

'Malarial Subjects'[8]

Contemporary sources described Burdwan fever as a spectacular disruption of the prevailing ways of life. It provided an occasion for dramatic lamentation for a world that was lost:

Its ravages have not yet been repaired, the ruined villages have not been yet rebuilt, jungle still flourishes where populous hamlets once stood, and many of those who fled before the fever have not returned . . . [9]

Rev Neale's school numbering 130 boys is now deserted . . . [10]

. . . the rich and the poor of all ages and castes have suffered alike; consequently, dwelling houses of all descriptions in equal proportions are to be seen in various stages of decay and ruin . . . many large '*barees*' [houses] in which there were formerly thirty and forty residents, have now been left with perhaps one solitary occupant; whole mohullahs and streets have been deserted, and large villages which formerly told their residents by thousands can now almost number them by hundreds . . . [11]

Ironically, reports about the epidemic also revealed a vocabulary which claimed to articulate and explain daily bodily niggles. These bureaucratic reports were couched in a language endorsed by institutional science, and seemed convincing, respectable and legitimate. In these reports, varieties of physical unease figured as necessary preconditions, symptoms, sequels or simulations of a collectively experienced malady.

The epidemic appeared to have unleashed itself at a time when there was no dearth of Bengali texts on malaria. Jodunath Mukhopadhyay, for instance, narrated detailed case-histories of individual patients suffering from malaria in successive medical texts published in Bengali through the 1870s.[12] He suggested that malaria expressed itself not necessarily by gifting fluctuating temperatures readable on the thermometric scale, or by assuming a contagious character inflicting innumerable mortalities. Instead, the impact of malaria on the body, Mukhopadhyay believed, could make one feel 'not sick, but out of sorts'. Malaria did not necessarily cause illness but rather 'a slight deviation from health'.[13]

---

[8] J. Fayrer, 'First Troonian lecture on Climate and the Fevers of India', *Lancet*, 119, 3055 (March 18, 1882), 423–426.

[9] Rogers, 'The lower Bengal (Burdwan) epidemic fever', 401.

[10] General, Medical, File 6, Prog-34–36, July 1873 (WBSA).

[11] Home, Public, 7 May 1870, 65–71 A (NAI).

[12] Jodunath Mukhopadhyay was a medical practitioner, who held a 'license for medicine and surgery' recognised by the colonial state. Between 1872 and 1880 he published at least eight medical manuals in Bengali. Mukhopadhyay and his works await more intense and detailed attention from historians.

[13] J. Mukhopadhyay, *Saral Jvar Chitiksa, Prothom Bhag (Curing Fevers, Part I)* (Calcutta: Sri Nityananda Ghosh, 1878), 39, 49, 50, 67. It would be misleading to suggest that

Malaria therefore figured as an onerous agent which could be invoked to explain a wide variety of maladies. Such maladies included diarrhoea, nausea, headache, infections on the eyeball, abscess on the female breast or in the ear, secretion of pus, or a general unlocatable malaise.[14] At the same time, malaria figured as a cause behind potentially fatal conditions like cardiovascular arrests. Mukhopadhyay identified experiences of unease such as general lassitude, repeated acts of yawning, the need to stretch oneself, pain in the ankle, wind, intense regular sluggishness, irritation and pain around the ear, as inevitable preconditions in a body which should anticipate another attack of malarial fever.[15]

It is hardly surprising then that the malarial epidemic figured as an occasion when medical practitioners could itemise these sensations as objects of medical knowledge. As items of medical knowledge, these appeared as predictable, manageable and curable categories. Dr Gopaul Chunder Roy's extensively cited account of the epidemic associated the frequent drying up of the tongue, accumulation of brown sores on the teeth and lips, bloated face, oedematous limbs, mouth ulcers, inflammation of the gum, loose teeth and swollen-bleeding gums as probable expressions of malaria in the body.[16]

Many commentators on malaria in the 1870s including Roy, Joseph Fayrer, C. F. Oldham and his anonymous reviewer in the *Indian Medical Gazette*,[17] had classified malarial diseases in terms of their predictable rhythms of recurrence. However, careful analysis of the caveats and qualifications accompanying discussions about such expected rhythms of malarial diseases suggests that categories like intermittent, remittent and malarial fever were flexible and commodious. Such labels were inscribed upon different forms of debilities, which manifested in the body with various symptoms and in diverse rhythms.[18]

---

such trends were unique to Bengal or to Burdwan fever. Mukhopadhyay's understandings were shared across a variety of contexts. See A. Christie, 'On Latent Malarial Disease', *Medical Times and Gazette London*, 1 (11 May 1872), 550; Home, Medical Board, 21 October 1858, 14 (NAI); Home, Medical, January 1877, 47–48 B (NAI); Note the categories 'masked' and 'pernicious malaria' and 'malarial cachexia' in Fayrer, 'First Troonian lecture', 426 and 467–470.

[14] J. Mukhopadhyay, *Quinine* (Calcutta, 1893), 57–90.

[15] Mukhopadhyay, *Saral Jvara Chitiksa*, 39, 49, 50, 67.

[16] Roy, *The Causes, Symptoms and Treatment of Burdwan Fever*, 84, 98–100. Roy's work was widely circulated and reviewed. For a brief overview of the ways it was received in the *Lancet, Medical Times and Gazette, Medical Press and Circular* and *The Doctor* see Home, Medical, June 1879, 1–5 A (NAI).

[17] Anonymous, 'Review of C. F. Oldham, *What is Malaria? And Why Is It Most Intense in Hot Climates?*' *IMG*, 6 (1 May 1871), 99 and 100.

[18] For instance, see W. Hensman, 'Remarks on Malaria', Appendix no. L, in *Army Medical Department Report For the Year 1866*, Volume viii, 1868, 505–511; Fayrer, 'First Troonian lecture', 467–470.

Who then could be defined as a 'malarial subject' in the 1870s in Burdwan? Roy suggested that unexceptional attacks of malaria seldom deterred their victims from eating, drinking and bathing as usual.[19] The unhappy effects of malaria became a natural phenomenon, part and parcel of the necessary constituents of their body. Most would remain without fever for months or years and yet the slightest cause could upset the balance of health. Thus malarial subjects could be someone suffering from pigmentation of the skin, bleeding from the nose or from the rectum, mental inaptitude, rheumatism, night-blindness, impotence or pregnant women weakened by the embolism of the heart and women suffering from menstrual flux.[20]

'Cinchona Disease'

Surgeon Major Albert M. Vercherie inspected several cases reported as malarial in the Burdwan town in September 1873. In his diary, he referred to the case of a dhobi's daughter, who happened to be a patient of one Dina Bondhu Dutt, a local physician. She was recorded in the official registers as suffering from malaria. In the fourteen days Vercherie kept track of her it was found that she was gradually diagnosed with the following maladies successively: typhus, enteric fever, cholera, relapsing fever. 'I heard from Dr French that the case became complicated by pleuro-pneumonia about thirteen or fourteen day of disease'.[21] Thus, individual case histories reveal that those who were labelled as suffering from malaria could be diagnosed with different diseases in different phases of the same course of illness. This example also specifies some of the numerous designations, apart from malaria, which were available to medical science for explaining a similar set of clinical symptoms.

How could such confusion, presented by an overabundance of closely related diagnostic tropes, be resolved? Jodunath Mukhopadhyay narrated a similar experience of attending to a little girl, eight to ten years of age. She was initially diagnosed to suffer from cholera. When the relevant fever mixtures and stimulants failed, and the physician was about to give up the 'case', he decided to gamble with quinine. Subsequently, the girl recovered. Mukhopadhyay narrated this experience to suggest that the malarial identity of a particular form of physical unease could be

---

[19] Roy, *The Causes, Symptoms and Treatment of Burdwan Fever*, 75.
[20] Ibid., 84 and 94–105.
[21] A. M. Vercherie, 'Extracts From a Diary Kept During a Visit to Burdwan', *IMG*, 8 (1 November 1873), 287–289.

determined by how a body reacted to quinine.[22] He hinted at how quinine was often invoked as a diagnostic tool in quick-fix pharmacological tests. Such examples can be multiplied.[23]

In many more ways, the malarial epidemic owed itself to quinine. Decades before dispersed expressions of quotidian debilities in various parts of Bengal began being projected as diverse articulations of single, continuous malarial epidemic, quinine had already been convincingly advertised as the quintessential remedy of every form of malarial disease. Such advertisements were vigorously reiterated in the official registers at various moments in the 1850s.[24] Quinine was confidently acknowledged not only as a febrifuge, but also as a prophylactic. This is evident, for example, in the military files of the government. In various military regiments in British India, specific doses of quinine formed a part of the mandatory breakfast.[25] Even when officials like Lieutenant G. S. Hills doubted the labelling of an epidemic as malarial, they nonetheless consumed daily preventive doses of quinine.[26]

As late as 1874, many colonial officials sounded unsure about the malarial character of Burdwan fever. For instance, Dr Albert Vercherie, a member of the Indian Medical Service, was convinced that it was typhus.[27] Lieutenant Governor Sir Richard Temple, writing a decade after Hills, was equally hesitant to attribute the series of maladies in contemporary Bengal to 'any particular cause'.[28] Such doubts amongst some of the senior officials about the precise cause of fever, ill health and death, and whether they could be collectively

---

[22] Mukhopadhyay, *Saral Jvara Chitiksa*, 103–106.

[23] Quinine acted as an agent in similar diagnostic tests. See for instance, W. A. Green, Inspector General of Hospitals, Lower Provinces, to Secretary, Government of Bengal, – No. 40, dated Fort William, 15 April 1868. Municipal, Sanitation, Prog 14–15, June 1868 (WBSA). See also R. T. Lyons, 'The Burdwan Fever', *IMG*, 7 (1 August 1872), 204–205. Such tests were arranged to confirm the malarial identity of 'epidemics' in other instances as well. For instance, see, Home, Sanitary, August 1882, 97–103 A (NAI). See also G. Bernard, 'Was it Malarious Fever or Sun Stroke Cured by Quinine?', *IMG*, (March 1), 1870; P. Sanyal, 'Remittent Fever e Quinine' (Quinine in Remittent Fever), *Chikitsa Sammilani*, 4, 1 (1887), 243.

[24] For instance, A. Bryson, 'Navy Medical Report Number XV on the Prophylactic Influence of Quinine', Medical Times and Gazette *of* London, viii (New Series, 1854), 6–7; D. Blair, 'On the Employment of Quinine in West India Fevers', *Lancet*, 52, 1308, (23 September 1848), 344.

[25] Home, Medical Board, 21 October 1858, File no. 14; 28 October 1858, File no. 52, 2 December 1858. File no. 58, (NAI).

[26] G. S. Hills, Executive Engineer, Shillong Division, to H. L. Dampier, Commissioner of the Nuddea Division, dated 31 December 1864. Home, Public, 7 March 1868, 140–143 A (NAI).

[27] Vercherie, 'Extracts from a Diary', 8–12.

[28] Richard Temple, 'The Causes of, and Remedies for the Burdwan Fever', dated 25 August 1875. Home, Medical, November 1875, 53–55A (NAI).

considered as expressions of a single general outbreak, persisted in the 1870s.

However, there seemed to circulate a consensus that quinine could be its unquestionable remedy. Years before doubts over the malarial character of the epidemic could be conclusively resolved, quinine had made its way into the interiors of Bengal.[29] The indiscriminate use of quinine was being condemned even in government correspondences in the early 1870s.[30] Official files in Bengal reveal, through most of the late 1860s and the early 1870s, organised efforts to procure additional quinine from the Madras and Bombay presidencies to combat the outbreak.[31] They also reveal efforts to requisition quinine from England,[32] tracking the details of its journey from England,[33] measuring its stock in the rapidly exhausting medical stores,[34] and requesting the military department to spare some for the civil department.[35] There was correspondence between officials placed at different levels in the subdivision, districts and divisions towards supervising the distribution of quinine. Such distributions were carried out in the villages through panchayats and dispensaries.[36] These suggest how the units of revenue-extraction began to be projected as units for affording relief.

From the 1850s, the careers of malarial diseases and quinine were repeatedly written about as inseparable parts of a single, shared history. Widely circulating publications in medical journals,[37] stories narrating past glories of the Jesuit Bark,[38] reports of adventures into the interiors of the Peruvian forests,[39] the foundational programmatic statements written by the early managers of cinchona plantations in India[40] informed official understandings. This resulted in impressions that quinine and malarial diseases were invariably associated. The presence of one seemed to imply the presence of another. At a time when official characterisation of dispersed debilities and deaths in Bengal suffered from imprecision,

[29] Home, Public, April 1872, 508 A (NAI).
[30] General, Medical, May 1872, 92–93 B (WBSA).
[31] Home, Public, September 1872, 441–444A (NAI).
[32] Home, Public, December 1872, 344–353 A (NAI).
[33] Home, Public, September 1872, 441–444A (NAI).
[34] Home, Public, August 1872, 574–577 A (NAI).
[35] Home, Public, December 1872, 344–353 A (NAI).
[36] See General, Sanitation, July 1870, Prog. 8–10 (WBSA).
[37] Bryson, 'Navy Medical Report', 607; Blair, 'On the Employment of Quinine', 344.
[38] For instance, C. R. Markham, *A Memoir of the Lady Ana de Osorio, Countess of Cinchon and Vice Queen of Peru (A.D. 1629–1639) With a Plea for the Correct Spelling of the Cinchona Genus*, (London: Trübner & Co, 1874).
[39] C. R. Markham, *Travels in Peru and India* (London: John Murray, 1862).
[40] As quoted, for instance, in Home, Medical, January 1884, 9–11 A (NAI).

governmental alacrity in distributing quinine contributed to the reinforcement of the malarial identity of the epidemic.

An understanding that the introduction of quinine into Bengal immediately preceded the outbreak of the epidemic was reflected in various publications in the late nineteenth century. In an anonymous editorial entitled 'Burdwan Fever', the homoeopathic journal, *Calcutta Journal of Medicine,* described the epidemic as a consequence of the introduction of quinine in Bengal. The editorial characterised the epidemic as a 'Cinchona disease' that resulted from the side effects of consuming regular doses of quinine to stave off intermittent fever. It argued that while quinine relieved the body from milder and temporary forms of intermittent fever, it plagued the body with a worse and enduring form of disease (i.e., Cinchona disease).

It is not intermittent fever ... on the contrary, it is another and worse disease than intermittent fever; it is a Cinchona-disease worse than intermittent fever ... [41]

Such impressions survived well into the last decade of the nineteenth century. The Bengali journal *Chikitsa Sammilani* in 1893 blasted the government policy of distributing quinine at cheap rates from the post offices for causing general sickness and fever in rural Bengal.[42]

'... Opportunity of the Epidemic ... '

The careers of malarial epidemic and quinine in Bengal were caught up in a symbiotic relation. The figure of quinine was invoked to provide precision to the malarial identity of the epidemic. The epidemic was conceived to have unleashed itself at a time when the credibility of quinine itself was being called into question. Contemporary files quoted extensively from bureaucratic reports that were published earlier in the 1860s which expressed doubts about quinine's potential as either a febrifuge or a prophylactic. The epidemic proved to be an occasion when the usefulness of quinine as an effective drug could be tested once again.[43]

---

[41] Anonymous, 'Burdwan fever', *Calcutta Journal of Medicine,* 6, 6 (June 1873), 198.

[42] Anonymous, 'Quinine i malaria' (Quinine is malaria), *Chikitsa Sammilani,* 9, 10 (1893), 402–405. Such trends of attributing malarial fever to the intake of quinine have been witnessed in other contexts. For instance, see, W. B. Cohen, 'Malaria and French Imperialism', *Journal of African History,* 24 (1983), 29; A. S. Mackinnon, 'Of Oxford Bags and Twirling Canes: The State, Popular Responses, and Zulu Antimalaria Assistants in the Early-Twentieth Century Zululand Malaria Campaigns', *Radical History Review,* 80 (Spring, 2001), 76–100.

[43] J. Elliot, *Report on Epidemic Remittent and Intermittent Fever Occurring in Parts of Burdwan and Nuddea Divisions* (Calcutta: Bengal Secretariat Office, 1863), quoted in Home, Public, 7 May 1870, 65–71 A (NAI). Similar impressions were subsequently elaborated in Bengali medical texts. Anonymous, 'Bhati', *Anubikshan,* 1, 6 (1875), 185–188.

Scepticisms involving quinine acquired at least two forms. There were suspicions about the usefulness of quinine as a drug itself. Some authors argued that the merits of administering quinine had been exaggerated.[44] Another set of complaints was concerned with the rapid depletion of pure quinine from the market. The distribution of quinine, it was alleged, fell into the hands of 'unqualified imposters' and 'mischievous quacks' who frequently tampered with its purity, producing adulterated versions. Quinine gave them access to quick, easy money despite its weak curative functions. Writing in June 1869, the Sanitary Commissioner of Bengal expressed concern about the rapidly depleting faith in quinine in a context when different corrupt versions circulated in the market under the same name.

Under the existing circumstances, when a villager himself, or a member of his family, is weakened by fever in a malarious district, it is customary for him to purchase *what is called quinine* from some village Apothecary who deals in medicines, which he sends for to Calcutta. In many instances I have examined and tasted the *so called quinine mixture* of the Bengal villages, and often found it be an altogether spurious and useless remedy; and yet for a small quantity of this and similar preparations, it is common for a villager to give two or three rupees at a time; – the consequence being that the poor man remains uncured, whilst at the same time he is being beggared.[45]

How could the distribution of state-endorsed pure quinine be ensured? It was suggested that the government could depend on 'reliable agents' at the village level. Such agents included 'headmasters of village schools' and gurus at the pathshalas.[46]

What constituted this quinine, which the state in India was keen on marketing as 'pure'? Government factories had repeatedly failed to produce pure quinine in India till then. These factories managed to yield instead several substitutes of quinine: quinovium, quinidine, cinchonidine, cinchonine, etc. The government appeared keen on endorsing these substitutes as acceptable variations of pure quinine. These substitutes were often regarded as adulterated quinine, while the state contested such allegations. Quinine continued to be advertised as an exotic drug which was very difficult to produce, and could not be procured

[44] W. J. Moore, 'The Value of Quinine', *IMG* (1 August 1870), 160–163.

[45] D. B. Smith, Sanitary Commissioner of Bengal, to A. Mackenzie, Officiating Junior Secretary to the Government of Bengal, dated Darjeeling 5 June 1869. Home, Public, January 1870, 15–29 A (NAI). See also, J. M. Tagore, Honorary Secretary to the British Indian Association to S. C. Bayley, Junior Secretary to the Government of Bengal dated 18 March 1864. General, General, April 1864, Prog 23–25 (WBSA).

[46] General, Medical, July 1873, Prog 192, 1–4 A (WBSA).

easily, but its virtue could only be sensed from the healing qualities of its substitutes.

I had frequently been told that sulphate of quinine sold by native druggists in Calcutta and mofussil was largely adulterated by mixing it with flour, magnesia, arrowroot and other articles. I was therefore agreeably surprised to find that after analysis... were not adulterated by any foreign substances, but were either pure cinchonidine, or contained cinchonine, which are alkaloids found in the Cinchona bark, and which cannot be distinguished from quinine by the naked eye or unless by analysis... [47]

The epidemic confirmed the supply of bodies affected by malaria. The epidemic provided an 'opportunity' to verify the purities of different drugs circulating as quinine in the medical market. These tests also aimed to enquire whether the extracts of raw unprocessed cinchona barks or the substitutes could cure malarial patients. If confirmed, the government could give up its tedious projects of manufacturing pure quinine in India. In a correspondence drafted in July 1872, the Lieutenant Governor instructed the Inspector General of Civil Hospitals to 'take *opportunity of the epidemic* to test the capabilities of the cinchona bark':

The Lieutenant Governor desires that opportunity may be taken of the epidemic fever in Burdwan to test the use there of the cinchona bark which has already been ordered to be sent, in order to ascertain the capabilities of the bark when used as a simple infusion with boiling water. His Honor would like to find out whether a simple infusion of the bark is a really reliable febrifuge. [48]

I have noted in the earlier section how quinine acted as a diagnostic tool in determining the malarial identity of various maladies. Here, it appears that bodies identified as malarial were, in turn, employed to verify the quality of quinine in circulation. The epidemic became thus an occasion to test the medical efficacy of different extracts of cinchona barks or the raw bark itself.

'Local'

The configuration and ordering of myriad sensations of physical unease into a particular epidemic in nineteenth-century Bengal was conditioned

---

[47] S. Wauchope, Officiating Commissioner of Police, Calcutta, to the Officiating Secretary, Government of Bengal, Judicial Department. No.1238 dated Calcutta, 16 October 1872. General, Medical, October 1872, Prog 6–8 (WBSA). See also, Anonymous, 'Adulterated Sulphate of Quinine', *IMG*, 7 (1 August 1872), 187.

[48] J. Ware Edgage, Officiating Junior Secretary to the Government of Bengal to Inspector General of Hospitals, Lower Provinces. Dated Calcutta, 6 July 1872. General, Industry-Science, 5, July 1872 (WBSA).

by an emergent culture of bureaucratic correspondence. The colonial medical bureaucracy and the intricate network of correspondences sustained by it shaped the acts of reporting, recording and recapitulating the epidemic.[49] These converged in different moments with commentaries in the vernacular press and in the medical journals, deliberations solicited from the perceived experts of local/subdivisional knowledge, retrospective literary works and postcolonial histories to provide credibility to the projected story of the malarial epidemic.

The bureaucratic correspondences reveal an intimate engagement with the geography of interior localities. Almost coinciding with the first Census Report presented in 1871, the demand for aetiology of a coherent epidemic converged with an aggravated desire for knowledge of the locality. The causes of the epidemic, it was argued, were inherent in 'the numbers and the classes of the population, of tenures and rents, rates of wages and prices of food'. A series of twelve questions were circulated from the office of the Governor General in Council and the 'local officers' were 'specially desired to give in their periodical reports all they know...'.[50]

The locality had to be known in credible ways. Such knowledge found expression in the languages of science, governance and improvement. Some of the correspondents appeared aware that, in the process, they were correcting or adding to some of the limitations of the census returns of 1871 or the statements of the Registrar General.[51] These questionnaires were not merely circulated to the 'local officers' within the Burdwan division. To avoid similar epidemics in the near future, accumulation of detailed information about the interior of neighbouring divisions was solicited. The Commissioners of Chotanagpur, Chittagong, Orissa divisions, for instance, had to summarise the responses of district officers placed under them.[52]

Most of these questions enquired about the living conditions of 'the people'.

---

[49] Besides, these reports recognised the units of revenue extraction as the geographical frames of reference, i.e., the presidency, subdivisions, thanas, districts, etc. These reports show how these categories were being naturalised as rigid boundaries. Any transgression beyond the borders of one district was taken note of, and accounted for. It seemed commonsensical that the diseases should be confined to one particular division or district. Diseases reported to spread beyond one district into another were considered to flout some natural principle and taken note of. For instance, Roy, *Burdwan Fever*, 57; Rogers, 'The lower Bengal (Burdwan) epidemic fever', 402–403.

[50] R. Temple, 'The Causes of, and Remedies for the Burdwan Fever' dated 25 August 1875. Home, Medical, November 1875, 53–55A (NAI).

[51] G. Campbell, 'Minute: Hooghly Fever and Conditions of the Ryots', Ibid.

[52] Ibid.

What is the usual food of the mass of the people? What is estimated to be the weight of rice eaten ordinarily by each man, woman and child? And how many meals are eaten daily?... Is there any ground for thinking that the people stint themselves in such necessaries as rice, salt etc?... Have daily labourers any difficulty in procuring the means of subsistence? Are beggars or paupers common?... Are the people clothed more poorly than twenty years ago?[53]

Responses to these questions varied. Predictably, prevalence of poverty and hunger amongst 'the people' was denied in most official responses. The Magistrate of Hooghly, Mr Pellew considered paupers and beggars almost as figures of the past. 'The practice of the lower classes congregating uninvited at feasts and picking up scraps has almost died out', he thought. However, another set of officials led by Colonel Haig and Dr Saunders argued in their reports that the epidemic could be convincingly explained in terms of poverty and inadequate access to food. They suggested that the poorer classes in Hooghly and Burdwan districts were 'under-fed and ill-nourished'. This made them 'predisposed' to the miasmatic poison.[54] It is difficult to ascertain whether a humanitarian instinct inspired the reports of Haig and Saunders. However, quite clearly, hunger and chronic dearth provided these authors with a credible language in which to describe the epidemic. Hunger seemed to have figured as a probable cause behind fever epidemics in other parts of the contemporary world. The reports of Colonel Haig and Dr Saunders referred to the 'hunger theory of fever', which was apparently invoked to explain events in distant Germany and Great Britain. It was claimed that this theory was established in Ireland in the post-famine literature of the 1840s.[55] The reports of Colonel Haig and Dr Saunders portrayed Burdwan fever as a reenactment of that proven medical understanding. Thus, 'insufficiency of food' seemed to provide one of the commensurate and convincing explanations for the epidemic. In the process, it reinforced the assumption that the epidemic could be narrated as a homogenous and monolithic event.

That these explanations had currency is evident from brief attempts during these years at organising food relief camps for the sick poor. Such charitable camps followed the rules usually in place concerning relief to famine victims.[56] It is not clear from available sources how effectively these food relief camps for the sick poor really functioned.

[53] H. S. Cotton, Officiating Junior Secretary to the Government of Bengal to the Secretary, Government of India, Department of Revenue, Agriculture and Commerce. Ibid.

[54] Ibid.   [55] Temple, 'The Causes of, and Remedies for the Burdwan Fever'.

[56] W. E. Ward, Magistrate and Chairman to the Municipality, Burdwan to C. T. Buckland, Commissioner of Burdwan, No.180, dated Burdwan, 29 December 1869. Political, Medical, January 1870, Prog 8–13 (WBSA).

It has already been indicated that hunger and dearth did not consistently figure as a cause behind Burdwan fever. Instead, an editorial published by the *Indian Medical Gazette* in June 1873 entitled 'The Cause of Burdwan fever' ascribed it to excessive eating. It recalled how elders from within the Muslim community in a village called Munglecote had discovered that eating too much beef caused Burdwan fever. It quoted from a report submitted by the local civil surgeon:

The village of Munglecote recently suffered and is suffering very severely. The population consists chiefly of Musalmans, who consume beef so largely that a movement was set on foot by the head men and Maulavis to put a stop to it, as they thought the stimulating character of the meat produced the fever. Here we see that something besides starvation and low fat must act as a cause.

The editorial went on to ridicule the impression of these villagers. It observed that even if the 'beef eating Mussulmans' and the 'vegetarian Hindoo' occupied different 'mohullas' of the same village the epidemic did 'attack' both groups equally. The editorial concluded sarcastically 'the Munglecote theory is probably as correct as that would connect the fever with rice and greens'.[57]

Search for an aetiology of the epidemic also led to a series of questions involving land and land tenures. 'Are there any symptoms of pressure upon the land? Are rents rising, and are there many applicants for any vacant lands?' Summarising the responses from local officers the Lieutenant Governor of Bengal Sir George Campbell admitted that the mass of figures received was 'very wide and vague'. The answers supplied from Howrah, Burdwan, Midnapore, Hooghly, Chotanagpore, Chittagong and Orissa often differed from each other. However, this wide range of responses revealed certain strategic options that the state could adopt in relation to governance of land. In areas marked by increasing pressure on land and rise in rents, the government recommended rackrenting. Campbell argued that if the ryots had fixity of rent as the zamindars had fixity of revenue then the condition of ryots in Bengal would be more comfortable. Campbell believed that these concerns underlay 'the theory of the regulations of 1793'. However, he added that 'the practical working of the Permanent Settlement' failed to live up to the originally intended visions. The districts that had been hit by the epidemic 'do not imply that rents are more racked there than elsewhere, but that the people have not yet submitted to rack-renting to the same extent as elsewhere ... the degree to which rent have been racked in different districts is a great degree the measure of the comfort or discomfort of the

[57] Anonymous, 'The Cause of Burdwan Fever', *IMG*, 8 (2 June 1873), 159–160.

people'. On the other hand localities characterised by considerable margin of wasteland were earmarked for reclamation. Once reclaimed, such areas could be made available to the land market.[58]

The official responses often tended to relate the epidemic to immobile labour. 'Would the people be willing to immigrate to other parts of India, or to Burma, or Assam, if assisted by the government to do so?... Whether the people of the fever-stricken tracts go largely to Calcutta and Howrah for work?'[59] These reports celebrated mobile labour by characterising it as more healthy. Chotanagpore supplied cheapest labour available in India. Labourers were recruited in the industrial regions around Calcutta and Howrah or in the plantations as far as Burma, Assam, Mauritius and Trinidad. Campbell detailed in his minute how Chotanagpore as the home of cheap, mobile, tribal labour escaped the ravages of the fever-epidemic. 'This facility of immigrating or going out for labour extends wherever *the aboriginal blood* predominates; e.g. into the Raneegunge portion of Burdwan, Bancoorah, Beerbhoom and upper Midnapore. But the fever tract is to the *east of this in an Aryan country*.'[60] This he contrasted with localities in Bengal affected by the epidemic. Such localities were marked by sedentary labour.

People of this part of Bengal do not emigrate... so long as they are not killed down by disease they go on increasing at home... they won't go out and work and prefer to stay at home on their patches of ground and starve.[61]

Such apparent concern for rescuing the people from starvation should be read with caution. It seems that official priorities predominantly lay in enabling the recruitment of cheap and mobile labour.

'Undergrowths'

Many contemporary official correspondences about the epidemic quoted widely from earlier reports that systematically advocated destruction of unkempt vegetation while encouraging cultivation of agricultural crops. Unlike most agricultural products, these usually uncombed vegetation failed to circulate extensively as profitable commodities in distant markets. However, those who inhabited the interiors of the fever-tracts considered some of these as cheapest sources of food. These reports suggest that most 'local officials' tended to discredit such rural vegetation, other than agricultural crops, as unwanted, rank and malarial.

Thus, the desire for acquiring knowledge about the locality was not confined to ascertaining the living conditions of the people. It extended

[58] Campbell, 'Minute'.   [59] Ibid.   [60] Ibid.   [61] Ibid.

to consolidating information about the landscape and the vegetation it bred. In the context of Burdwan fever, an official file in 1870 carried a report originally written in 1863 in English by Sunjeeb Chunder Chatterjee, a prominent figure in Bengali literature, who intermittently occupied various colonial administrative positions in the region in the 1860s and 1870s.[62] In this letter Chatterjee drew attention to the difficulties in authentic gathering of knowledge in the localities. The magistrate was expected to carry out 'detailed and careful inspection of each of the infected villages' in person. This being impossible, he often distributed his responsibilities amongst the police *darogahs* under him. Overburdened with assignments themselves, the police *darogahs* in turn ended up assigning responsibility to the *fareedars* and *barkundauzes* to execute the orders transmitted to them by the magistrates. Chatterjee added that the *fareedars* and *barkundauzes* would inevitably prove incapable of exercising the discretion that was required in judging how far certain trees and plants, by their proximity to human habitations, affected public health. Besides, he doubted their ability to determine whether the entire rooting out of such vegetation secured greater benefit to the public than loss to their owners.

The mass of people on the one hand, are ignorant of the malarious influence of the jungles, and on the other hand regard them as particularly useful in screening their zenanas from exposure to the public gaze, and especially in supplying their kitchen with vegetables, fruits and fuel. Therefore they would not miss an opportunity to induce the fareedars to pass over unnoticed such portions of the jungles as lie behind their houses, and have on that account little chance of being discovered from the principal road of the village if ever the magistrate should happen to pass along it.[63]

To prevent these, Chatterjee recommended the appointment of three special officers with sufficient penal authority, whose 'local presence' might keep the fareedars and the villagers 'under control'. It is not clear from the records whether his recommendations were implemented.

From the mid-1860s, however, special engineers were assigned to the 'affected districts'. They were entrusted to 'examine and collect information' on any specific 'local works' that might be required for the 'sanitary

---

[62] B. Mukhopadhyay, *Sanjibchandra: Jibon o Sahitya (Sanjibchandra: His Life and Works)* (Calcutta: Pustak Biponi, 1988), 24–27; B. Chattopadhyay, 'Sanjibchandra Chattopadhyayer Jiboni (The Life of Sanjibchandra Chattopadhyay', in J. C. Bagal (ed.), *Bankim Rachanabali Volume 2* (Calcutta: Sahitya Samsad, 1954/1890), 790–795.

[63] S. C. Chatterjee, Cantalpara, to A. Eden, Secretary to the Government of Bengal, dated 1 May 1863. Home, Public, 7 May 1870, 65–71 A (NAI).

improvement' of particular villages.[64] In 1868, in the wake of Burdwan fever, an official file reprinted the diary of one such special engineer in the Burdwan division. C. Ducas' diary was originally written in 1864, and was part of his assignment to report the causes and remedies of the extensive ill-health prevailing in the Burdwan division during that time. He reported after having visited villages Tribeni and Mugrah:

The *Kutchoo* and *ole*, both bulbous plants, thickly cover the village land, so much so that village roads have disappeared under them, and the ditches have been choked with them. The slopes of tanks are also covered with the *Kutchoo*. The bulbs of these plants are much used by the natives in daily food. The *Kutchoo* is used in place of potatoes and the *Ole* makes nice *chutney*, which is prepared in mustard oil, much in the same way mango chutney is prepared in the United Provinces...There is not a single village road to be traced, except by the foot tracks...[65]

After having narrated his visits to other localities including Balagore, Kanchrapara and Goopteepara, Jerat the engineer suggested his recommendations:

Where foot tracks exist, regular village roads must be of necessity constructed...So long as rank vegetation will be promoted, no engineering work can be carried out so as to ensure permanent advances...nothing can be done to assist...these *localities* when the surface of the country is scarcely visible from the covering of undergrowth, and when village paths have disappeared under them in most places...[66]

How could 'improvement' be guaranteed? Ducas' solution was simple: denudation of excess and rank vegetation followed by the introduction of agricultural cultivation. Similarly, Sunjeeb Chunder Chatterjee provided a list of thirty-three shrubs, creepers and plants out of which twenty-seven required to be burnt down and completely destroyed as a preventive against malaria; six of them had to be uprooted. Amongst them, Chatterjee argued, plants like *Kuchoo*, *Mankuchoo*, *Laoo*, *Shim*, *Koomra*, when methodically cultivated in the fields could be spared, while *Monsha* had to be preserved for worship.[67]

Such details, otherwise quotidian and mundane, emerged as credible inputs informing the bureaucrat's and the engineer's analysis of the locality. Officials preoccupied with the Burdwan fever, who circulated Chatterjee's and Ducas' narratives amongst their colleagues in the late 1860s

---

[64] H. L. Dampier, Commissioner of the Nuddea Division, to Lieutenant G. S. Hills on Special Duty, No. 127 dated 1 September 1864. Home Public, 7 March 1868, 140–143 A (NAI).

[65] 'Journal of the Occupation and Duties of Mr C. Ducas,' Ibid. (NAI).   [66] Ibid.

[67] Chatterjee to Eden. Home, Public, 7 May 1870, 65–71 A (NAI).

were convinced that such detailed engagement with certain aspects of local vegetation could provide them with a clue to understand the causes behind the epidemic.

Similar tales about perceived shifts in subtle aspects within an elaborate landscape: the drying up of many rivers, excessive deposition of silt, shifting levels in the adjacent subsoil, inconsistent rainfall,[68] state initiatives at the subdivisional level that had backfired,[69] gossips circulating out of rural gatherings resurfaced in government reports as reliable causes behind another malarial outbreak.[70]

These various explanations could speak to each other in a shared vocabulary as the authors of these reports rearranged these stories by invoking some branch of science. Thus the idea of malarial Bengal as a landscape undergoing myriad range of mutations was articulated in a language endorsed by varieties of sciences. These local tales were rewritten as physical changes in the landscape,[71] engineering debacles,[72] meteorological inconsistencies,[73] debates concerning contagion[74] and so on. The epidemic was reified in these reliable and credible ways.[75]

The Meteorological-Malthusian theory propounded by Colonel Haig is yet another example of how current scientific knowledge was invoked in providing authentic explanations of Burdwan fever.

Chiefly due to an increase in population having outstripped the means of production, to an impoverished and under-fed condition of the great mass of the people; in fact that we now witness the last sad stage of that process by which over population, in the absence of any special counteracting or remedial measures, works its own cure... [76]

Each 'local' act of explaining the cause or course of the epidemic required ratification by the distant and dominant codes of respectable knowledge. One Babu Thakur Dass Chuckerbutty argued in a letter written to the Lieutenant Governor of Bengal in January 1871 that the epidemic was caused by the importation of a hitherto unknown plant

---

[68] E. H. Whinfield, Officiating Magistrate of Burdwan to the Commissioner of the Burdwan division. No. 129 P, dated Burdwan, 24 June, 1873. General, Medical, July 1873, File 6, Prog-34–36 (WBSA).

[69] Rogers, 'The Lower Bengal (Burdwan) Epidemic Fever', 401–408.

[70] R. Mookherjee, Deputy Magistrate of Kishaghur, to E. Grey, Magistrate of Nuddea, dated 30 November 1863. Home, Public, 7 May 1870, 65–71 A (NAI).

[71] Rogers, 'The Lower Bengal (Burdwan) Epidemic Fever', 407.

[72] 'Journal of the occupation and duties of Mr C. Ducas'.

[73] Mookherjee to Grey, Home, Public, 7 May 1870, 65–71 A (NAI).   [74] Ibid.

[75] The previously mentioned trends in medical reporting were elaborately witnessed in contemporary Mauritius. See, C. Meldrum, *Weather, Health, and Forests* (Port Louis: Mercantile Record Co. Printing Establishment, 1881).

[76] Anonymous, 'Burdwan fever', *IMG*, 8 (1 May 1873), 126.

in Bengal. He identified this plant as *Bellaty Bharandah*. 'Its progress is simultaneous with that of the disease. Wherever this plant was propagated, the disease has arisen'. He added that if sunflower could be attributed to neutralise the effects of malaria, it was reasonable to suppose that some other plant could possess the qualities of malaria. In response C. B. Clarke, the Officiating Superintendent of the botanic garden, identified *Bellaty Bharandah* as Iatropha glandulifera, an American weed. He suggested that the plant had indeed somehow made its way into Bengal and formed 'a particularly obnoxious and *useless* low shrubby jungle'. However, Clarke believed that in designating this plant as the sole cause behind the epidemic Chuckerbutty was ignoring the fundamental rules of inductive logic. He added that the projected equation with sunflower was a flawed exercise of 'reversed analogy'. He suggested that Chuckerbutty's association of the introduction of sunflower with the disappearance of malarial fever was merely based on the logical method of coincidence. Sunflower caused abatement of malarial fever by enhancing ozone in the surrounding air. Clarke argued that to make his point Chuckerbutty had to show that *Belatty Bherandah* caused depletion of ozone from the air. Clarke maintained that the fallacies in Chuckerbutty's arguments surfaced as he had 'not thoroughly mastered J. S. Mill's chapter on the Method of Differences'.[77]

The officials deputed in the interiors of Bengal to furnish knowledge concerning the 'local' were thus uniquely placed. They could at least peep into the professional world of natural and engineering sciences while claiming to provide exotic local details. In their claim of knowing this locality and its inhabitants they provided coherence to different experiences of unease in distant regions as local variations of one commensurate malady: malaria. They were agents, however unaware or unintended, in a 'larger pathologisation of space'; a trend reflected in medical writings across local, regional and national contexts.[78] Thus the beginnings of revelation of the interior of the body through dissection and postmortem converged with trends of framing knowledge about the 'local' in British India that deepened possibilities towards construing medical and geographical stereotypes.

'Agriculture'

Lack of tolerance towards rural, unkempt, 'useless' vegetation was paralleled by encouragement of agricultural cultivation. It was argued that

[77] Municipal, Medical, February 1871, Prog 34–35 B (WBSA).
[78] Harish Naraindas, 'Poisons, Putrescence and the Weather: A Genealogy of the Advent of Tropical Medicine', *Contributions to Indian Sociology*, 30, 1 (1996), 1–35.

fallow wastelands otherwise considered malarial became harmless when reclaimed for agriculture. As a colonial official posted in a neighbouring division observed in the early 1860s: 'The germination of malaria lessened, if not prevented, by cultivating the soil...'.[79]

English newspapers expressed consistent concern whether the epidemic had an adverse effect on agriculture. They enquired whether the epidemic in Burdwan would cause the prices of agricultural goods to fluctuate. An editorial in the *Englishman* dated 23 October 1867 alleged that cultivation in the interiors had suffered adversely following the epidemic. The issue was considered serious enough to necessitate an immediate response. Quoting from reports of the local officials placed in Bood Bood, Cutwa, Culna, Mymaree, Serampore, Jehanabad, Oolooberiah, Shanpore, F Montresor, the Commissioner of the Burdwan division dismissed such apprehensions.[80]

However, it might seem simplistic to explain the projected geography of Burdwan fever in terms of the exigencies of colonial capital. In the 1860s, bamboo jungles had often been suspected to generate malaria. Mr M. J. Shaw Stewart, Collector of Canara in Western India, for instance, speculated whether prevalence of malarial fever in Soopa talook could be attributed to the great increase of bamboo jungles. To bolster further his understandings associating wild bamboo seeds with malarial fever he solicited information from Bengal. In his response Thomas Anderson, Superintendent of the Botanic Gardens in Calcutta was not very clear. He pointed out that unlike western India extensive tracts of land were not covered with wild bamboo plants in Bengal. However, Anderson noted that organised plantation of bamboo was practiced in certain villages in lower Bengal since 1857–1858. He was ambiguous whether such plantations were as liable in generating malaria as the wild bamboo plants in Western India.[81]

In March 1868 Dr H. T. Thompson, Civil Assistant Surgeon of Hooghly, asserted the need to preserve carefully planted bamboo trees around the villages of lower Bengal. He recognised bamboo as indispensable for protecting the inhabitants from the ill effects of malaria. Official reports suggested that 'in all rice-producing countries like Burmah,

[79] J. C. Snow, Civil Assistant Surgeon of Jessore, to the Magistrate of Jessore, No. 5, dated 15 January 1864. General, General, March 1864, Prog 84–85 (WBSA).

[80] C. F. Montresor, Commissioner of the Burdwan divison, to the Officiating Secretary to the Government of Bengal No. 148, dated Burdwan, 23 October 1867. General, General, December 1867, Prog 6 (WBSA).

[81] M. J. Shaw Stewart, Collector of Canara to Mr W. Hart, Revenue Commissioner, Southern Division, No. 874, dated 16 April 1864. General, General, August 1864, Prog 25–28 (WBSA).

China and other malarious localities (sic)' a preventive custom of rais-
ing the houses on piles was observed. This was to allow free passage
of underneath air and avoiding damp and rot. In Burma, these reports
argued, abundant supply of woods of superior quality assured reasonably
priced piles. Alternatively, people in the *mofussils* of Bengal followed a
contrivance of their own. They erected what they called bamboo *machans*
for sleeping purposes. 'By this cheap and simple arrangement, the people are protected from the damp floors and influence of malaria during
the night, when the system is relaxed and more predisposed to receive
it after the toil, fatigue, hunger and anxiety of the day...'.[82] Earlier,
the uprooting of bamboo plants was also severely condemned by the
British Indian Association, an influential collective of Bengali landown-
ing interests. Its Honorary Secretary, Baboo Joteendro Mohun Tagore,
underplayed suppositions that bamboo plants generated disease. He concluded by insisting, 'There is not in the country another substitute for
bamboo'. The destruction of bamboo plants had to be prevented, as they
required 'nourishment of years to grow into maturity'.[83]

In course of the 1860s, the possibility that malaria could have its origin in planting bamboo trees or rice cultivation[84] or in the process of
maceration of jute was seriously considered in Bengal. However, unlike
in the case of a range of rural uncombed vegetations, local officers could
not afford to instruct the uprooting of such practices which were integral
to the proliferation of the colonial economy. The harshness and alacrity
of anti-malarial measures were deliberately relaxed to enable the con-
tinuation of these practices. For instance, the Lieutenant Governor of
Bengal had authorised the Commissioner of Nuddea to take relevant
steps under Section 62 of the Code of Criminal Procedure for preventing
the maceration of jute in the immediate proximity of towns and villages.
Maceration of jute was considered to affect the purity of air and cause ill
health. Conveying the writ of the Lieutenant Governor, S. C. Bayley the
Junior Secretary to the Government of Bengal added:

...but I am to impress upon you on the necessity of making careful provision that the preparation of Jute is not interfered with more than is absolutely
necessary for sanitary purposes. I am to request the Magistrate of the district in which this process is carried on many be directed to try to induce the

---

[82] J. Sutherland, Deputy Inspector-General of Hospitals, Presidency Circle, to H. M.
Macpherson, Secretary, Inspector-General of Hospitals, Lower Provinces, No. 51,
dated Fort William, 13 April 1868. Municipal, Sanitation, June 1868, Prog 14–15
(WBSA).

[83] J. M. Tagore, Honorary Secretary to the British Indian Association to S. C. Bayley,
Junior Secretary to then Government of Bengal, dated 16 July 1863. General, General,
October 1863, Prog 92 (WBSA).

[84] General, Medical, March 1869, Prog 75–76 (WBSA).

inhabitants of large villages to fix upon some particular piece of water for this purpose...[85]

'Draining Bengal'

Official efforts towards dealing with the epidemic, in turn, sustained and reinforced the identity of Burdwan division as a malarial locality. Existing histories have commented on the elaborate pamphlets published serially in the *Hindu Patriot* by Digambar Mitra.[86] In such histories the pamphlet-savvy elite in Bengal appear locked in a polemical dialogue with the colonial state. These works consistently empathise with Mitra. It is suggested that powerful men in the colonial establishment ignored his suggestions towards improving stagnating drainage networks in the interiors of Bengal. Careful revision reveals that both Digambar Mitra and the representatives of the colonial state considered it necessary to reclaim stagnant swamps and to facilitate the flow of dying rivers and other drainage channels. However, they were indeed engaged in a debate while explaining the main cause behind the stagnation of waterways. Mitra considered newly constructed roads and railways under colonial supervision responsible. On the contrary, superintending engineers employed by the government blamed unprofessional construction and handling of private zamindari embankments.[87]

Different groups from the late 1860s proposed the 'improvement' of drainage networks in Bengal. Such groups harboured different interests and represented varying investments. Studying them reveal numerous habitations of power in the interiors of Bengal in the third quarter of the nineteenth century. In an aggressive and sustained way the government had advocated the need to 'improve' drainage networks, reclaim wastelands, promote agriculture and navigability and clear jungles. These, the government consistently maintained, were credible ways of dealing with the threat of the malarial epidemic. These measures enabled detailed and legitimate intervention of the colonial state into the interiors of Bengal. It was argued that 'such an apathetic race can only be preserved from the consequences of their own ignorance and folly by constant supervision...'[88] Colonial intervention in the late 1860s often took the form of 'constant supervision' of public works geared towards 'agricultural improvement'.

---

[85] S. C. Bayley, Junior Secretary to the Government of Bengal, to the Commissioner of the Nuddea Division, No. 6064, dated 28 December 1864. General, General, December 1864, Prog 53–54, File 1–3 (WBSA).

[86] Sarma, *Ecology and the Epidemic*; D. Mitter, *The Epidemic Fever in Bengal* (Calcutta: Hindu Patriot Press, 1873).

[87] Home, Sanitary, April 1884, 112–116 A (NAI).

[88] Sutherland to Macpherson, Municipal, Sanitation, June 1868, Prog 14–15 (WBSA).

In June 1872, the *Indian Medical Gazette* conveyed the admiration drainage projects had begun commanding in contemporary Bengal. It ridiculed the 'mushroom crop' of theories which had so far been furnished to explain the Burdwan fever. The journal provided an 'exhaustive catalogue of theory mongers', and ridiculed them as: supernaturalists, transcendentalists, pseudo-inductionists, hobby-riders, intuitionists and plagiarists. In contrast, the editorial privileged 'modest, laborious and cautious ... genuine workers-men ... ' over such seekers of futile knowledge. Such 'genuine workers-men', it argued, included those who were actually fighting the epidemic by taking part in the drainage works.[89]

The colonial state systematically pursued the question of drainage from the late 1860s. A mammoth memorandum submitted by C. C. Adley, Executive Engineer on Special Duty in June 1869, bore a detailed programme of draining three huge swamps (i.e. at Danconee, Kathlia and Roypore) in the Hooghly district of the Burdwan division. Adley recalled how *khalls* or natural drainage channels once led from these swamps to the River Hooghly and were formerly navigable for small crafts round the year. Referring to contemporary texts on malaria available in French, Italian and English, he reinforced the understanding that Burdwan fever might have been caused by filth generating around declining rivers, stagnating channels and proliferating swamps. He located improvement schemes being initiated to resist Burdwan fever as part of a larger history. He pointed out how successful works of drainage had effectively reduced malarial fevers in Lincolnshire, Holland, Mauritius, Burgundy, Jessore and Serampore.[90]

Public projects of improvement would require considerable intervention into lands held by numerous proprietors. Adley initiated detailed negotiations with the 'principal proprietors' in the region relevant to the project. It was discovered that the bulk of land belonged to the Seorapooly Rajas and their co-heirs. On the behalf of the government, Adley and his colleagues interacted with other influential proprietors in the region (i.e., Baboo Joykrishna Mukherjee and Bamapada Chaudhuri). In the process crucial assurances were extracted. An elaborate list of every 'minor proprietor' in that region was solicited and collected. However, there is barely any evidence suggesting that the government bothered to engage with most of them. In course of their conversations with the principal proprietors the government revealed the commercial profits,

---

[89] Anonymous, 'The Epidemic Fever in Bengal', *IMG*, 7 (2 June 1872), 164; Anonymous, 'Draining Bengal', 209.

[90] C. C. Adley, Executive Engineer on special duty, to Major J. J. Hume, Officiating Superintending Engineer, Western Circle, No. 109, dated 25 June 1869. Home, Public, 12 March 1870, 167–170 A (NAI).

which were likely to result from the drainage works. It surfaced that drainage works on Dancoonee, Kathlia and Roypore would enable reclamation of 19000 bighas of cultivated and 24000 bighas of uncultivated land.

...the average present value of the cultivated land under the most favorable circumstances is 8 annas per bigha per annum; when drained, its minimum mean value would be Rs. 3 per bigha per annum; thus showing a clear additional profit to the landlords of Rs. 2–8 per bigha per annum. The value of the uncultivated land would be raised from nil to Rs. 3 per bigha per annum.[91]

As a consequence of reclamation of land by drainage, it was suggested, relevant landholders would reap an 'additional profit' of Rs. 47500 from cultivated land and Rs. 72000 from uncultivated land (i.e., a total additional profit of Rs. 1,19,500). Besides, it was pointed out that drainage would inevitably promote navigation and irrigation. Apart from befitting the cultivation of sugarcane, rice and vegetables, it was expected to guarantee easier access to the Calcutta market.[92]

The projected economics of profit seems to have convinced Baboo Joykrishna Mookerjee as well as Raja Poorno Chunder Roy of Seorapooly. Mookerjee proposed that the initial financial burden of the project should be borne by the government. The cost was to be repaid by the landowners in instalments, spread over several years. Each landlord had to pay in proportion to the holding. Mookerjee agreed that a law had to be passed compelling landowners to join any scheme convened towards 'public good'. To these suggestions the Raja added that once the amount advanced by the government had been refunded, the drainage works and canals should become the property of the zamindars. However, the zamindars were expected to pay the government a fixed sum annually for maintenance and repairs. The Raja wished the works to remain 'under government supervision.'[93]

These ideas found expression in the document that made up the Hooghly and Burdwan Drainage Bill. This bill was eventually endorsed by the Lieutenant Governor and passed into an Act on 18 March 1871. Passed with the intention of facilitating drainage in the concerned districts, this bill opened up tricky questions about landownership. For the execution of this act the Lieutenant Governor had to appoint Drainage Commissioners. These commissioners had to be at least seven in number. Amongst them the majority had to be constituted of proprietors of lands which would be affected by the drainage works. Within fifteen days of notifying a proposed scheme to concerned proprietors, the commissioners had to ascertain their responses. If half amongst the

[91] Ibid.   [92] Ibid.   [93] Ibid.

affected proprietors assented to the proposed scheme the commissioners could proceed with it irrespective of what the other proprietors thought. If more than half amongst the relevant proprietors objected, the commissioners had to reconsider the proposed scheme. Thereafter, the commissioners as a collective could reject the scheme, modify it or proceed with it unaltered. The commissioners were thus under no compulsion to respect the objections raised by the proprietors to the schemes proposed. Once the Lieutenant Governor had sanctioned a scheme he could acquire the relevant pieces of land for public purpose. Within one month after any scheme had been completed the commissioners had to determine the sums payable by each of the proprietors of land reclaimed or improved. If the proprietor failed to pay up within one month from the day the sum was payable the commissioners could recover that sum by the sale of such lands. Where the ownership of a piece of land was in dispute or if there was more than one claimant to proprietorship the commissioners were empowered to determine the proprietor as it applied to this Act.[94]

Unsurprisingly, such provisions did not leave every landholder elated. Responses from these unhappy petty landholders often revealed shades of enmity between them. The following case suggests how the question of drainage revealed conflicts amongst different layers of proprietors. In a petition addressed to Adley, a 'petty zemindar' named Showdaminy Debi objected to the construction of a channel of water through the cultivated low grounds of the village she owned. Showdaminy Debi happened to be the zamindar of the village called Gobra under the Thannah Hurripal in the district of Hooghly. She wrote:

The revenue of the village (Gobra) is very poor; if the Government take the canal through the cultivated parts of the place then it will be too injurious for so petty a zemindar as I am . . . there is only one Government Khas Mehal which gives small revenue therefore it is unnecessary to have such expensive and useless canal . . . The place which your honour has selected as a site for the canal is not at all fit for the purpose, as there was no canal at any time before . . . [95]

The last section of the petition was most revealing:

The people who applied for cutting a canal are my enemies, and thinking me to be a helpless woman, they are merely trying to injure me by cutting a canal through the fertile grounds of my zemindary and the rent-free lands of other holders; their principal object is not to make general good, but to put their enemies into trouble . . . [96]

---

[94] Home, Public, 22 April 1871, 57–59 A (NAI).
[95] Adley to Hume, Appendix D. Home, Public, 12 March 1870, 167–170 A (NAI).
[96] Ibid.

Thus, efforts to prevent malaria often merged into projects of improvement. As indicated, such projects advocated clearance of wastelands and jungles. Once cleared these lands could be reclaimed for agriculture. The British Indian Association was a voluntary association of absentee landlords settled in Calcutta. Its members often possessed property in the form of orchards, gardens and other tracts of lands in the interiors of rural Bengal. Since the early 1860s, excessive emphasis by government representatives on the reclamation of rural land for agriculture often clashed with the interests of the members of the Association. A letter written by its Secretary, Joteendro Mohun Tagore, objected to the following observation by Dr Elliot, a senior medical bureaucrat.

> ...Patches of land in the centre of villages held rent-free produce only jungles. Land occupied by mangrove, plantain, and other fruit trees generally belong to people of high castes, who do not cultivate themselves, and are unwilling to let it out to others for that purpose. Until these and similar tracts are brought under cultivation and until the soil is exposed to the sun's rays at least twice in the year, I am of opinion that such places can never be healthy or habitable.

Tagore considered Elliot's recommendation of bringing under cultivation all village lands not occupied by homesteads as considerable infringement on private property. Tagore disputed the labelling of land occupied by orchards consisting of plantain, mango and other fruit trees as 'wastelands'. He urged the government against imposing sanitary improvements on villages by any means that might have semblance of force or compulsion or by any legislation, which would interfere with private property. Tagore suggested that 'reciprocation of sentiments' between 'local officers' and 'private proprietors' worked better than any form of coercion. In communicating such views to the government, Tagore functioned as an efficient spokesman of the interests of his colleagues in the British Indian Association.[97]

Alliances struck with influential zamindars over the issue of drainage and improvement enabled the colonial state to explore new opportunities of trade. C. T. Buckland, the Commissioner of Burdwan proposed in April 1872 the cultivation of sunflower in Burdwan and Hooghly. He referred to cases in Sonmaar, Belgium, France and Northern America where sunflower had been cultivated to 'neutralize the deleterious effects of marshy exhalations'. Buckland's message referred to a detailed report from R. T. Thompson, the civil surgeon of Hooghly. Thompson wrote about the remunerative aspects of sunflower cultivation on account of the valuable oil, which was produced in it. He suggested

---

[97] Tagore to Bayley, General, General, October 1863, Prog 92 (WBSA).

that sunflower yielded 'a beautiful clear oil' that could be cultivated all the year round in Bengal and North Western Provinces. He believed that sunflower oil tasted sweet, was nearly inodorous and that 50 per cent of its seeds contained this oil. Although sunflower oil was well adapted for machinery soaps, cerates, liniments and plasters, its chief use was thought to be as an aliment suited for culinary purposes. As an ingredient in cooking, Thomson thought that it was better than the costly olive oil. He hoped that sunflower oil, once produced in Bengal, could compete with the costly imported Spanish olive oil if not quite throw it out of the market. Once again the lure of commerce converged with the obligation to deal with the epidemic. Buckland promised that the preliminary cost of procuring sunflower seeds from Agra might be charged from the epidemic fever-fund. Joykrishna Mookerjee was again requested, along with Mr Pellew, the Magistrate of Hooghly, to arrange for these experiments in four different villages: Kolora, Kinkurbutty, Madhabpur and Ooterparah. Buckland mentioned that all these villages lay on the edge of the Dancoonee, Kathlia and Roypore swamps that formed the core of the drainage scheme in the Hooghly district. Mookerjee found it very difficult to induce the ryots to displace a known crop for an experimental one. Sources suddenly go silent on what happened next.[98]

Certain practices of agricultural improvement and drainage in Bengal in the 1870s stoked a series of discussions. Such discussions, quite predictably, revealed the colonial state, the influential zamindars, absentee landlords and the petty zamindars as overlapping and conflicting layers of propertied authority in the interiors of the Hooghly and Burdwan districts of Bengal. At the same time, in different narratives Burdwan and its vicinities began to appear as one of the many malarial localities in the world. Burdwan in particular or more generally Bengal, figured as one of the many regions in the world, which were in need of improving their networks of drainage. It was suggested how the British bureaucrats in Burdwan could take lessons from the French in Algeria or medics in Massachusetts or sanitary officials in Natal. The experience of drainage initiated in the Burdwan division could then be compared with other regions.

In reference to the vexed question of the Burdwan fever in Bengal, the following account by Dr Derby of Massachusetts will be found of interest . . . [99]

---

[98] Memorandum by C. T. Buckland, Commissioner of the Burdwan division No. 178, dated Burdwan, the 8 April 1872. Municipal, Sanitation, March 1873, Prog 16–23, File 7 (WBSA).

[99] Anonymous, 'Marsh Fever Produced by Obstruction of the Outlets of Subsoil Water', *IMG*, 8 (1 October 1873), 279.

It is scarcely necessary to say that what has been accomplished in the way of water supply, drainage and agricultural improvements, in Algeria can be done in India.[100]

John Sutherland of the Indian Medical Service wrote a report on the applicability of methods of preserving the health of troops in Algeria to reducing the mortality of troops in India.[101] He insisted on the introduction of the Algerian mode of drainage to deal with the epidemic in lower Bengal. The *Indian Medical Gazette* quoted from the works of Colonel Mundy and Mr Hudgkinson emphasising the similarity of the 'swamps of Australia' to those of Bengal.[102]

'Travelling Epidemic'

Did such discussions and practices inevitably converge into yet another condescending colonial statement against the poor levels of native sanitation? Was the geography of Burdwan fever explained necessarily in terms of defective networks of drainage and heinous standards of sanitation? Bureaucratic commentators like Campbell or Haig seldom associated Burdwan fever with unsanitary localities alone. Campbell concluded his minute by observing: 'all sanitary science notwithstanding... Colonel Haig truly observes that up to this time there has been much less fever in these reeking swamps than in the higher parts of Burdwan and Hooghly, where there is a sensible natural drainage...'.[103]

Some amongst the prevalent histories on the subject have tended to organise different contending explanations of the epidemic into a debate between two opposite positions. It has been suggested that while the emergent vernacular Bengali press, keen on resisting policies of improvement conceived by the colonial state, were explaining the epidemic in relation to the new channels of communication, construction of railway tracks, embankments, renovated roads, the colonial officials attributed the epidemic to 'indigenous' sanitary practices.[104]

However the fragmented nature of the official explanation to the epidemic is revealed in statements like this emanating from within the files of the colonial medical bureaucracy:

[100] J. Sutherland, R. S. Ellis, Joshua Paynter and C. B. Ewart, 'Report on the Causes of Reduced Mortality in the French Army Serving in Algeria', *IMG*, 8 (1 May 1873), 139.

[101] J. Sutherland, 'On the Causes of Endemic Fever in Lower Bengal, the Influence of Canal Irrigation in their Production in Upper India, and the Means of Prevention to be Employed', *Edinburgh Medical Journal*, 15 (June 1870), 1086–1091.

[102] Anonymous, 'Malaria', *IMG*, 7 (1 September 1873), 241.

[103] Campbell, 'Minute: Hooghly Fever and Conditions of the Ryots'.

[104] Samanta, *Malarial Fever in Colonial Bengal*; Sarma, *The Ecology and the Epidemic*.

The history of the epidemic itself is equally strange. It is shown to have been unaccountably capricious and fitful in its incidence, seizing indiscriminately on towns whose sanitary arrangements were the best, and others where sanitation was quite neglected, and entirely over leaping tracts which there was every reason to suppose most liable to its attacks.[105]

Reports published in the 1870s often suggested that the malarial epidemic was not confined to localities characterised by low lands, insufficient drainage or stagnation of water. The epidemic appeared to reveal itself in apparently contradictory geographical surfaces. Confuting some of the theories advanced to explain the epidemic, the magistrate of Hooghly wrote in 1872:

The country round Jehanabad and Myapore is high; the country round Gohaut is high also. In neither of these tracts are there any railroads, nor is there any interference with drainage. The country around Singboor is high also; round Kishtonagore is low; yet all these places have this year been remarkable for the amount of fever. The soil around Bally is sandy; at Jehanabad, clay and sand; at Myapore sand with a little clay; at Krishtonagore black clay. In all these places there are good tanks and bad tanks. The Jehanabad people have beautiful river water as well. The prisoners in the lock up there always drink river water. Yet these circumstances make no difference whatever.[106]

Colonial medical bureaucrats frequently explained such 'eccentric geography' of the epidemic by invoking the logic of communication. In the process they often distinguished between communication and contagion. Such distinctions figured in an extensive range of official reports.[107] Thus wrote Leonard Rogers:

... it progresses steadily although slowly, it has followed, like a rolling wave, the chief roads or means of communication and there was no evidence that sanitary conditions had changed to any extent during or shortly before the epidemic.[108]

In contemporary bureaucratic reports, malaria surfaced as a sinister entity that could communicate itself across distant regions. However, the use of the expression 'communication' in these medical bureaucratic reports might have referred to a different set of connotations than what figured in vernacular commentaries written by the Bengalis. In medical bureaucratic imagination malaria could travel even when agents

---

[105] E. C. Bayley, Secretary to the Government of India, to H. L. Dampier, Officiating Secretary to the Government of Bengal, No. 867, dated 21st February 1868. Home, Public, 7 March 1868, 140–143 A (NAI); General, Miscellaneous, August 1872, Prog 1–2 (WBSA) See also, General, Miscellaneous, August 1872, Prog 1–2 (WBSA.)

[106] Anonymous, 'Burdwan fever', *IMG*, 7 (August 1, 1872), 188.

[107] Elliot, *Report on Epidemic*; French, *Endemic Fever in Lower Bengal*; Sutherland, 'On the Causes of Endemic Fever', 1086–1091.

[108] Rogers, 'The Lower Bengal (Burdwan) Epidemic Fever', 404.

of development like renovated roads, extensive railway tracks, embankments were not communicating it. As wrote one Dr Jackson, 'I regard the supposition that a line of railway embankment could, under any circumstances, originate a *travelling epidemic* like that in Burdwan as ridiculous and unworthy of serious consideration' [emphasis mine].[109]

What communicated malaria was in dispute, but there existed a belief across different sections of the medical bureaucracy that malaria was indeed travelling and was carrying the epidemic along with it. Thus, when these medical bureaucrats were referring to the 'lines of communication' they were not necessarily subscribing to the anti-government positions profoundly articulated by the likes of Digambar Mitra.[110] On the contrary, they were implicitly referring to and drawing from extensive imaginings of malaria as an elusive yet mobile category, represented in medical journals, published and circulated across and beyond local contexts. In these correspondences malaria itself was imagined as a substantially mobile entity that could travel like invisible waves across districts and provinces; which could remain latent in the body and travel with it across continents,[111] 'could drift up the ravines',[112] or 'it moves like mist and rolls up the hill sides, and may travel with the wind for miles...'.[113] The transit of malarial particles, Dr Massy of the Army Medical Department in Jaffna believed, was hampered by certain trees the leaves of which were eventually stained with black rust.[114]

It is in light of such imaginings one has to read the characterisation of the 'malaria fever epidemic' as a 'travelling epidemic'.

That the fever did travel is no matter for doubt. Like the waves of a flowing tide it touched a place one year and receded, reached it again next year with greater force and again receded, repeating this process until the country was wholly submerged and tide passed further on...[115]

...Its main feature is, as we have shown already, that it is travelling, slowly indeed, but, as some have remarked, yet travelling.[116]

Unlike the sweeping but uncertain marches of cholera and small pox, its progress has been slow but sure...[117]

[109] Ibid., 405.
[110] D. Mitra, *The Epidemic Fever in Bengal* (Calcutta: The Hindu Patriot Press), 1873.
[111] Christie, 'On Latent Malarial Disease', 550.
[112] Anonymous, 'Review of C. F. Oldham, *What is Malaria?*', 102.
[113] Fayrer, 'First Troonian Lecture', 423–426.
[114] E. A. Parkes, 'Report on Hygiene for 1867', *Army Medical Department Report for the Year 1866*, Appendix xxxvi, Volume viii, 1868, 316–317.
[115] Rogers, 'The Lower Bengal (Burdwan) Epidemic Fever', 402.
[116] Vercherie, 'Extracts From a Diary', 287.   [117] Roy, *Burdwan Fever*, 57–58.

Such widely circulating stories on travel fed into the idea of malaria as an ordering principle. These imaginings bound diverse symptoms of physical unease dispersed across time and space into the radar of a coherent, continuous, single malarial epidemic. This explains how as late as 1899 Leonard Rogers could suggest a biography of Burdwan fever that boasted a lifeline spanning half a century. He extended the life of Burdwan fever back and forth and wove 'outbreaks' in Jessore in 1824, Nuddea in 1862, Mauritius in 1869, Burdwan particularly in the 1870s, Assam and Rangpur in the late 1890s as different expressions of the same unending epidemic.[118]

A close reading of contemporary bureaucratic correspondences reveal how the distances covered by the epidemic were represented in quantifiable terms. 'We have found it in our time to have travelled in thirteen years from Nuddea to Hughly'.[119] 'From Jessore it spread slowly (from 5 to 10 miles per year) from one district to another for a period of over 20 years.'[120] Leonard Rogers quoted the Sanitary Commissioner for Burdwan in 1874, who suggested that the epidemic followed this repetitive pattern until it left one locality for another:

During the fourth, fifth and sixth years – six years being the average duration of the fever in any place, – there was a general and slow recovery, the fever in each successive year attacked fewer persons, was of a less fatal type, and prevailed for a shorter period, finally disappearing altogether in the seventh year.[121]

The literature on Burdwan fever tended to bind not only distant places, but also stoked memories of different times. John Sutherland, for instance, disputed impressions that epidemic malarial fevers in Bengal were of recent origin. Bengal had known such epidemics since the sixteenth century, he argued. He attributed the destruction of the 'ancient and prosperous' city of Gour as early as 1574 to a similar epidemic. Sutherland informs us that the epidemic killed an entire Mughal contingent under Monaim Khan, a Lieutenant of Akbar, which had then held the city under siege.[122] Bureaucratic reports on the epidemic could also speak to similar correspondences in other parts of the contemporary world. The epidemic began to be compared with similar events in history. Thus the malarial epidemic in Burdwan in the late 1860s and 1870s was made to appear as an unexceptional phase in the history of epidemics. It fitted into a larger pattern of such epidemics in different parts of the world and in other moments in history.

---

[118] Rogers, 'The Lower Bengal (Burdwan) Epidemic Fever', 401–408.
[119] Roy, *Burdwan Fever*, 57–58.
[120] Rogers, 'The Lower Bengal (Burdwan) Epidemic Fever', 404.   [121] Ibid., 402.
[122] Sutherland to Macpherson, Municipal, Sanitation, June 1868, Prog 14–15 (WBSA).

Conclusion

'Native' expert opinions about the causes and remedies of Burdwan fever were solicited. However the medical establishments of the government closely monitored such opinions. Thus 'indigenous' impressions about the epidemic often reflected the understandings and biases of the colonial state. A prize of Rs. 1000 for the best essay by a 'native' on the epidemic declared by Lord Northbrook in August 1872 provides an interesting case. The Viceroy and Governor General of India encouraged all sub-assistant surgeons to submit essays on 'The nature and causes of the fever which now prevails in and near Burdwan, and best means of preventing its continuance'. The competitors were warned that they had to adduce to facts and could not indulge in 'speculation and theorising'. All papers sent in were supposed to be examined and the prize adjudged by the Principal of the Medical College and the Officiating Sanitary Commissioner for Bengal.[123]

A gleaning of contemporary advertisements and medical manuals in Bengali enables us to locate 'others' operating in the medical marketplace alongside those who were configuring diverse expressions of physical unease into a continuous epidemic. This alternative archive suggests how dissimilar ordering principles could be employed to frame quotidian little debilities that were being explained and expressed through the metaphor of malaria in certain other contexts. Practitioners who were contributing to this 'other' archive were often, with some exceptions, subjected to vigorous condescension. Gopaul Chunder Roy for example spoke of 'a band of lawless resolute...whose prototypes we observe in quacks and empirics. These infest the country like locusts, and cause more devastation amongst humanity than the diseases which they pretend to combat'.[124]

Karal Chandra Chattopadhyay, for instance, attributed his healing skills to divine benevolence and his collection of medical recipes to his extensive travels across a geographical space he identified as Bharatvarsha. In a booklet entitled *Bibidha Mahaushadh*[125] he does not acknowledge his debt to any other individual or medical tradition. He barely met his patients in person, but interacted with them through the post, rarely finding the scope for diagnosing his patients. His patients wrote to him about their precise complaints: expressions of pain and

---

[123] General, Medical, August 1872, 147–148 B (WBSA).
[124] Roy, *Burdwan Fever*, 151–152.
[125] K. C. Chattopadhyay, *Bibidha Mahaushadh (Specifics discovered and experimented by K. C. Chatterjee)*. (Calcutta: Iswar Chandra Basu and Company and K. C. Chattopadhyay, 1876).

physical unease ranging across bleeding from the rectum, impotency, physical infirmity, gonorrhoea, ulcers, fever, mercurial disorders etc. Such complaints, as I have already noted, were co-opted otherwise within the vortex of the epidemic: as preconditions, sequels, or simulations of a single malarial malady. Chattopadhyay, in return, responded by writing back to his patients, packing the required medicines in an envelope without forgetting to mention the exact dosage and of course, the price with postage that varied with every ailment. Through advertisements in the Calcutta and Bombay newspapers his patients got to know of him and wrote testimonials acknowledging his abilities in local newspapers published from places as distant as Dinajpur, Benaras and Lahore. Advertisements published in Bengali newspapers towards the end of the 1870s suggests that Chattopadhyay was not alone in the medical market in his silence on the malarial epidemic. Nor was he the only self-proclaimed healer in Bengal to prescribe generic medicines other than quinine, or to exploit the emergent networks of postal communication to extend his trade.[126]

The Burdwan fever malarial epidemic in the 1870s was an epistemological and administrative configuration. There were many 'indigenous' medical actors like Chattopadhyay who represented other modes of framing diseases, alternate cosmologies and patterns of cure, and did not seem to bother or have any clue whether an epidemic had unleashed itself.

Such indifference to and disinterest in the language of the malarial epidemic, its aetiology and its management, were paralleled by sustained contemporary critiques on the idea of epidemics from within 'medical science' itself. The *Indian Medical Gazette* published a series of editorials in instalments in different volumes through the course of 1873 on a common topic entitled 'prominent fallacies in epidemiology'. These editorials described epidemics as a fallacy within medical understanding. It was argued that 'present-day epidemiology' would not qualify as an inductive science and should be considered instead as a 'pseudo-science'. These editorials placed epidemiology amongst a 'species of mild speculation with a spicing of mystery', which could merely amuse the idle and satisfy the curious. Epidemiology, it was alleged, appeared as a source of 'amusement of children, not the work of grown up men'. These editorials urged readers to rethink some of the basic assumptions associated with 'general epidemics'. General epidemics were understood as

---

[126] For instance see these advertisements. 'Morrison's Tonic', *Sambad Purna Chandroday* (30 August 1862), 1–2; 'New Apothecaries' Hall', *Somprakash* (15 April 1867) [CSSSC].

a widespread disease phenomenon spreading over time and across an extended space.[127]

The human mind is, moreover incessantly hankering after causes...An abstract term "climate" or "epidemic influence" is invented or utilized, and made to do as a substantive 'theory' of a more occult or quasi learned description...The whole process is a melancholy exhibition of false generalising.[128]

This questioning of the projection of epidemics as a general, widely dispersed, homogenous phenomenon was followed by considerable doubts articulated in some contemporary medical texts about the existence of malaria itself. An official correspondence drafted by Surgeon Major Moore, Superintendent-General of Dispensaries and Vaccination, Rajputana in January 1877 suggested, for instance:

...it is probably the uncertainty and difficulty in accepting seemingly opposed facts which have caused a minority amongst eminent medical observers both in this country and in other parts of the world, to doubt, or altogether deny the existence of any such poisonous agent as malaria. In France and Algeria Dr Burdel regards marsh poison as 'a myth'; Armam entirely rejects it as a figment of the brain. Amongst Anglo-Indian officers, Renine writing of China says: 'Let mud and malaria alone, it will give no one the ague'...Hutchinson thinks malaria will be 'only an old friend: Carbonic acid'; Dr Knapp, the President of the Iowa University, regards malaria as a 'hypothetical cause' that could never be empirically verified, which some practitioners were using as 'cloaks for ignorance' that would eventually 'hinder the progress of medical science'.[129]

It was in such an overall context of suspicion and doubt about the integrity of both the epistemological categories malaria and epidemic that the Burdwan fever, in predominant records, was identified as a malarial epidemic – a credibly describable and sustained phase in the history of Bengal. The making of Burdwan fever epidemic can hardly be ascribed to conveniently locatable intentions or a straightforward series of causes. The history of unfolding of the epidemic hints at a 'game of relationships': between diagnostic protocols and pharmaceutical interests; codes of bureaucratic reporting and information gathering; medical relief, land control and commercial priorities; indenture labour market and medical geography; between the colonial government and different layers of landed proprietors. Burdwan fever reveals an intimate interplay

---

[127] Anonymous, 'Prominent Fallacies in Epidemiology', *IMG*, 8 (1 July 1873), 188–189.
[128] Ibid., 217.
[129] Home, Medical, January 1877, 47–48 (NAI) Dr Moore elaborated his views harbouring doubts about the existence of malaria in another article. W. J. Moore, 'An Enquiry into the Truth of the Opinions Generally Entertained Regarding Malaria', *Indian Annals of Medical Science*, 20 (1866), 375–404.

between the histories of epidemics, empire, modernity, capitalism, environment and locality.

Consolidation of knowledge about the epidemic and colonial extraction of information about the locality happened simultaneously. While shaping these overlapping processes colonial bureaucrats in Burdwan were uniquely placed. They had access to a prolific mass of details concerning Burdwan. Further, they were entrusted with the task of repackaging them in accordance with the commensurate and cosmopolitan codes of imperial correspondence. Knowledge of the locality and the epidemic converged to stereotype the Burdwan division as a malarial landscape. Once identified as such, Burdwan began being projected along with Massachusetts, Natal, Australia, Mauritius, Assam and Algeria as one amongst many unexceptional malarial localities on the map of British Empire and beyond.

The case of Burdwan fever reveals specific historical processes through which categories like malaria, which proliferated in post-Enlightenment Europe in general and Edwardian and Victorian England in particular were made to appear as commonplace in the wider colonial world through much of the nineteenth century. Burdwan fever also provided an occasion when categories like malaria began to acquire a thicker Indian accent: Bengali names of places, peoples and plants were incorporated within the expanding vocabularies of malaria. Therefore, whilst malaria began to be described in official discourses as an intrinsic feature of the locality, 'local' debilities, landscapes, landowners, markets, personnel and vegetation were in turn inscribed as inalienable components in the global narratives about malaria.

The making of Burdwan fever witnessed the bureaucratic attribution of significant causative properties to animate and inanimate nonhumans, particularly a variety of plants, for instance, sunflower, paddy, bamboo, jute and a myriad range of unspecified vegetations referred collectively as 'undergrowths'. Such activation of plants in the bureaucratic imagination, in turn, was linked to the entrenchment of exclusionary discourses about colonised humans. Mark Harrison and David Arnold have shown how Burdwan fever was cited in administrative reports as an example of racial degeneration, effeminacy and poor attainments of civilisation in lower Bengal.[130] Even projected collective immunity from malaria could be perceived as an indicator of racial inferiority. The santhals recruited from Chotanagpore as indentured labourers in the distant colonial plantations, for example, were described as free from the effects of malaria. It

---

[130] Harrison, 'Hot Beds of Disease', 11–18; Arnold, 'An Ancient Race Outworn', 123–143.

was conjectured later that the so-called primitive people like the santhals were compatible with malaria because of their crude and laborious racial constitutions. Burdwan fever thus constituted yet another phase in the history of imperial biopolitics in which the ascription of *active* properties to various nonhumans coalesced with processes of dehumanisation.

In different moments of this chapter I have argued that quinine often acted as a pharmacological agent in quick-fix diagnostic tests. The malarial identity of a malady could be retrospectively established by how the relevant body responded to quinine. Thus Burdwan fever owed its identity to quinine in different ways. Malaria in the 1860s and 1870s could be associated with a range of maladies. Quinine, it appears, could determine the limits to which the category malaria could be flexed. In the next chapter I ask whether quinine itself referred to a rigid, inflexible and homogenous category. These decades were also significant in the history of manufacturing quinine in British India.

4 'Beating About the Bush'
Manufacturing Quinine in a Colonial Factory

> ...Quinine is an article of which a great value travels within a small weight...[1]

Quinine has attracted the attention of a range of scholars pursuing the histories of medicine, warfare, environment and empire. It has been pointed out that the chemical isolation of quinine in the Parisian laboratories in the 1820s led to its subsequent recognition in the European markets as the most valuable extract of cinchona barks.[2] The beginning of commercial manufacture of quinine by private firms in Europe was followed by the establishment of cinchona plantations in the 1860s by the colonial governments in Dutch Java, British India, Ceylon and Jamaica, and French Algeria. Many historians have justifiably situated quinine as an essential component in imperial economic botany.[3] While they have located quinine as a bridge between imperial commerce and ideology, Daniel Headrick has characterised it as one of the 'tools of empire', which ensured the military expansion of European imperial rule in the nineteenth century.[4]

Such sustained interest in the history of quinine is understandable. Quinine was arguably the drug circulating most extensively in the

---

[1] C. B. Clarke to the Secretary, Government of Bengal, No. 202, 1 July 1870 Rungbee Home, Public, 17 December 1870, 123–125 A (NAI).

[2] J. L. A. Webb Jr., *Humanity's Burden: A Global History of Malaria* (Cambridge: Cambridge Universty Press, 2008), 92–126; M. Honigsbaum, *The Fever Trail: The Hunt for the Cure for Malaria* (London: Macmillan, 2001), 6–7; F. Rocco, *Quinine: Malaria and the Quest for a Cure that Changed the World* (London: HarperCollins, 2003).

[3] K. Philip, *Civilising Natures: Race, Resources and Modernity in South Asia* (Hyderabad: Orient Longman, 2004), 238–272; L. H. Brockway, *Science and Colonial Expansion: The Role of the British Royal Botanic Gardens* (New Haven: Yale University Press, 2002); A. Mukherjee, 'The Peruvian Bark Revisited: A Critique of British Cinchona Policy in Colonial India', *Bengal Past and Present*, 117 (1998), 81–102; R. Drayton, *Nature's Government: Science, Imperial Britain, and the 'Improvement' of the World* (New Haven: Yale University Press, 2000).

[4] D. R. Headrick, *The Tools of Empire: Technology and European Imperialism in the Nineteenth Century* (Oxford: Oxford University Press, 1981).

second half of the century, within the distant corners of the British
Empire and beyond. Talk about quinine figured in a variety of sites: business letters,[5] advertisements,[6] published governmental reports,[7] transit
insurance documents,[8] medical and pharmaceutical journals.[9] Such discussions involved various distant places which had been identified as
malarial in myriad colonial correspondences. Quinine was considered a necessary constituent of a traveller's kit. It was recommended,
for instance, while journeying through the rivers in the West Africa,
the Black Sea and 'all hot, moist and unhealthy districts of South
America.'[10] Quinine was prescribed 'wherever malaria was generated'.[11]
Dispersed localities in the interiors of Ceylon, West Indies, Hong Kong,
British India, Malta and North America were regularly supplied with
quinine. Quinine could be served in the form of wine,[12] biscuits,[13]
tea,[14] or administered as pills,[15] tonics,[16] and hypodermic subcuta-
neous injections.[17] Quinine was believed to cure or act as a prophylactic for an elaborate range of malarious diseases including malarial fever.
Quinine was also prescribed as a cardiac sedative in arresting internal
haemorrhage,[18] as a solution for curing diphtheritic ophthalmia,[19] as a

[5] J. Low to A. Low, 2 June 1828, Calcutta. File ACC 1037/853/2D (LMA.); Anonymous,
'Note about Import of Quinine', 20 December 1848, New York, ACC/1037/659, 1–7
(LMA).

[6] Anonymous, 'On Quinine Wine', *The Chemist and Druggist: A Monthly Trade Circular*
(15 September, 1859), 4. B/WHF/243 (LMA).

[7] The Committee appointed to examine the properties of the cinchona alkaloids other
than quinine to Secretary, Government of India, Home department. 29 October 1868.
ACC/1037/699/3 (LMA).

[8] See for instance, Howard to The London and Oriental Steam Transit Insurance Office,
London. ACC/ 1037/ 690 (LMA).

[9] G. Barnard, 'Was it Malarial Fever or Sun Stroke Cured by Quinine?', *IMG*, 5 (1870),
50.

[10] Anonymous, 'On Quinine Wine'.   [11] Ibid.

[12] Ibid; A. Bryson (ed.), 'Practice of Giving Quinine or Quinine Wine on Distant Expeditions on the West Coast of Africa', *Statistical Report of Health Navy 1857* (London:
House of Commons, 1859), 82–85.

[13] W. Purvis, *Specification of William Purvis: Medicinal Biscuit* (London: Great Seal Printing
Office, 1871) (WL).

[14] I. Smith and Company to Howard, 8 November 1860, Birmingham. ACC/1037/
649/135 (LMA).

[15] Home, Medical, March 1879, 58–60 A (NAI).

[16] L. J. Jordan, *Specification of Lewis Jacob Jordan: Tonic* (London: Great Seal Printing
Office, 1861) (WL).

[17] W. J. Moore, 'On the Treatment of Malarious Fever by the Sub-Cutaneous Injection of
Quinine', *Lancet*, 82, 2083 (1 August 1863), 126.

[18] C. Salvatore, 'The Action of Quinine as a Cardiac Sedative in Arresting Internal Haemorrhage', *Medical Records*, 9 (1874), 285–287.

[19] J. Tweedy, 'On the Treatment of Diptheritic Ophthalmia by Local Application of Solution of Quinine', *Lancet*, 115, 2943 (24 January 1880), 125–126.

gargle in sore throat,[20] aphrodisiac,[21] anti-pyretic,[22] to relieve 'alarming head symptoms after violent exercise in hot weather,'[23] dental pain[24] and suppuration.[25]

I have indicated how quinine acted as a pharmacological agent in quick-fix diagnostic tests. As a diagnostic category, malaria was associated with a plethora of maladies. Malaria was defined in different ways. Quinine was often administered to retrospectively determine whether an ailing body had been exposed to malaria.

Yet, quinine itself did not figure as a definite, homogenous, inflexible and rigid category. Rather than internalising the imperial projections of quinine as a generally stable and consensual category, I aim to pierce through this veneer of stability and consensus, and to explore the ways in which quinine was 'black-boxed' as a preordained, commonsensical, scientifically endorsed, homogenous entity. Empire produced and maintained the image of pure quinine in British India through a set of mundane processes, strategies and assemblages.[26] Particularly, attempts to manufacture cheapest possible pure quinine in government factories in British India between late 1860s and 1889 is in need of detailed analysis.

I have already noted that the first bag of cinchona seeds to be sown in the government plantations reached British India from South America in 1860. By the mid-1860s, government factories at Rungbee (which expanded in the early 1880s to nearby Mungpoo) in British Sikkim and at Ootacamund in the Nilgiris had been set up in the vicinities of experimental cinchona plantations. It is noteworthy that Rungbee and Mungpoo occupied contiguous sites and particularly from the early 1880s they were referred to almost interchangeably in the official sources. The Bengal government claimed to have invented the process of manufacturing cheapest possible pure quinine in a factory owned by it in Mungpoo

---

[20] D. J. Brackenridge, 'On the Use of Quinine as a Gargle in Diptheritic Scarlatinal and other Forms of Sore Throat', *Practitioner*, 15, 86 (August 1875), 110–114.

[21] Jordan, *Specification*.

[22] C. Allbutt, 'On the Antipyretic Action of Quinine', *Practitioner*, 12, 67 (January 1874), 29–37.

[23] R. L. Bowles, 'Alarming Head Symptoms after Violent Exercise in Hot Weather Relieved by Quinine', *BMJ*, 1, 34 (1857), 711.

[24] M. A. F. Mannons, *Specification of Marc Antoine Francois Mannons: Elixir* (London: Great Seal Patent Office 1862) (WL).

[25] D. Morton, 'Quinine and Suppuration', *Practitioner*, 13, 77 (November 1874), 348–351.

[26] For repair and maintenance, see B. Latour, 'Whose Cosmos, Which Cosmopolitics? Comments on the Peace Terms of Ulrich Beck', *Common Knowledge* 10, 3 (2004), 459; E. C. Spary, 'Of Nutmegs and Botanists: The Colonial Cultivation of Botanical Identity', in L. Schiebinger and C. Swan (eds.), *Colonial Botany: Science, Commerce and Politics in the Early Modern World* (Philadelphia: University of Pennsylvania Press, 2005), 187–203.

in British Sikkim in 1889. A micro-history of attempts to manufacture 'cheapest possible pure-quinine' in the British Indian government factories would reveal how pure quinine was constructed and sustained as a credible scientific fact. This reveals the history of how it was possible for the factory at Mungpoo to manufacture cheapest possible pure quinine in 1889. In other words, under what circumstances could such claims made by the cinchona factory at Mungpoo in British Sikkim appear credible and sustainable in the late 1880s?

This question, in turn, is closely connected to these following set of questions: What could be the range of attributes associated with the word quinine in factories in British India in the nineteenth century? Who could be trusted with the manufacture of pure quinine? What was referred to by purity in quinine? Who had the power to define and judge pure quinine? Who or what were considered as legitimate custodians of pure quinine? What role did ideas about race and place play in all this? Answers to these questions will be revealed when the intricate networks of correspondence between travelling geographer-botanists, European drug manufacturing families, the office of the Secretary of State for India, British Indian chemical examiners, Dutch experts on cinchona plants in Java, private investors in cinchona trade and managers of government plantations in Jamaica, Ceylon, Java, Nilgiris and British Sikkim are examined. This would expose shifting configurations of authority in the overlapping imperial worlds of medical knowledge, colonial governance and pharmaceutical business. Authority over pure quinine in these decades was not monopolised by any specific institutional edifice, but fluctuated asymmetrically amongst intricately entangled actors. Here I map the imbrications of commerce, science and politics to analyse how contending claims to authority over quinine were asserted and resisted: paving the way for the emergence of newer nodes of expertise and tutelage.

The history of quinine manufacture also reasserts scholarly insights about the relevance of substitutes in the colonial medical marketplace in British India.[27] Not only was pure quinine defined in relation to its substitutes, the prestige of the producers of pure quinine was delimited and contested by those who claimed to manufacture its substitutes. Mapping the political economy of substitutes is necessary to understand the shifting epistemologies of pure quinine.

Finally, the history of quinine manufacture opens up the opportunity to examine the material configurations of pure quinine in

---

[27] P. Chakrabarti, 'Empire and Alternatives: Swietenia Febrifuga and Cinchona Substitutes', *Medical History*, 54 (2010), 75–94.

nineteenth-century British India: its colour, taste, smell and appearance. The imperial assemblage which constructed pure quinine constituted not only of pharmaceuticals, botanists, geographers, chemical examiners, planters, bureaucrats, workmen, but also material ingredients like alcohol, colouring substances, cinchona barks, alkalis, oil, paraffine and protective devises like carmine, sealing wax, officially endorsed bottles and glass cases with patent locks. Even when these indispensible materials (that is, ingredients and protective mechanisms) converged, products manufactured in each factory were not necessarily ascribed the identity of quinine. Products were recognised as 'pure quinine', or retained as 'substitutes', or discarded as 'wastes'. These varying labels were contingent upon the shifting locations of their manufacturers in the hierarchies of imperial commerce and politics. The material, the social and the scientific were not self-sufficient, autonomous domains, but were instead intimately symbiotic.[28]

At the same time, quinine tells us a lot about Empire. Despite being a product of Empire, pure quinine as a commodity-in-the-making in turn reinforced Empire. Quinine exposes various expanses, depths, tensions, prejudices as well as human and material constituents of Empire.

An Exclusive Drug

In December 1875, a report drafted by the Government of Bombay alarmed the office of the Secretary of State for India in London. It said that quinine was being sold in the bazaars of Poona and Bombay 'in the original bottles, full as issued from the medical stores, with the government mark on the sealing wax'. The Secretary of State for India promptly responded. He requested the Governor General to enquire whether government quinine was similarly in circulation in bazaars in other parts of British India as well. He specifically solicited information about 'Calcutta or other bazaars in the Bengal Presidency'.[29] Earlier in September, certain measures were proposed to 'prevent robbery' of quinine from the medical stores and depots owned by the British Indian government. Messrs Howard and Sons of London were by then the most celebrated family of British druggists. They suggested, for instance, that quinine

---

[28] On the theme of co-constitution, see F. Trentmann, 'Materiality in the Future of History: Things, Practices and Politics', *The Journal of British Studies*, 48, 2 (April 2009), 297, 300; A. Pickering, 'The Mangle of Practice: Agency and Emergence in the Sociology of Science', *American Journal of Sociology*, 99, 3 (November, 1993), 559, 567, 576.

[29] Secretary of State for India to the Governor General, No. 305, 9 December 1875, India Office London. Home, Medical, May 1876, 45–48 A (NAI).

requisitioned for British India could be coloured in England by 'some harmless substance'. Dyed quinine, it was believed, would be an indicator of pure quinine imported from England and endorsed by the British Indian Government.[30] It was argued that once coloured, it would be convenient to distinguish pure quinine from objects of fraud; quinine that had 'legitimately found its way into the Indian market' from objects of 'theft, robbery'. Such deliberate convergence of the identity, colour and purity of quinine indicated a recurrent pattern. The Surgeon General of the Bombay Presidency appeared convinced by the suggestion from the Howards. He found it 'necessary to *arrange* with Messrs Howard and Sons' to tint quinine exported to British India with 1 per cent carmine.[31] It was suspected that this *arrangement* could be an excuse for ensuring the effective monopoly of the supply of quinine to Messrs Howard and Sons. On behalf of the Medical Board, Bombay Presidency, Dr J. L. Paul emphatically denied such allegations. The denial, however, was not justified by sufficient explanations.[32]

In the perception of most government officials in British India, production and circulation of pure quinine appeared restricted along certain predictable, legitimate and exclusive routes. The scientific laboratory was believed to represent one such sacrosanct site.[33] However, the translation of laboratory knowledge into commercial manufacture of pure quinine was considered rare and difficult. C. B. Clarke, the Officiating Superintendent of the Botanical Gardens, Calcutta and In-charge of Cinchona cultivations in Bengal wrote in December 1870: 'Now, any good text book of chemistry will give, not only a laboratory process to produce sulphate quinine, but will also give an account of the process pursued by manufactures. The real secret is to *perform* this process with reasonable economy...'.[34]

The products manufactured by very few firms were recognised as pure quinine by the British Indian government in the 1870s. Those firms were mostly based in Europe, particularly, England, France and Germany.[35] The London-based pharmaceutical family associated with Thomas Whiffen claimed to manufacture and sell commercial sulphates

[30] Secretary of State for India, 'Paragraph 16 of Military Letter', No. 227, 22 August 1876. General, Medical, October 1877, File 294, Prog. 83–85 B (WBSA).
[31] J. L. Paul to the Director General of Stores, 23 September 1875. Home, Medical, May 1876, 45–48 A (NAI).
[32] Ibid. Dated London, 28 September 1875.
[33] Anderson to Secretary, Government of Bengal, No. 49, 7 August 1863. Home, Public, 19 August 1863, 85–87 A (NAI).
[34] Clarke to Secretary, Bengal. Home, Public, 17 December 1870, 123–125 A (NAI).
[35] G. E. Shaw, *Quinine Manufacture in India, Seventeenth Streatfield Lecture* (London: Institute of Chemistry of Great Britain and Ireland, 1934).

of quinine since the 1850s.[36] In the 1870s and 1880s, the Whiffens began to feature regularly in the official correspondences of the British Indian governments. But, as I have noted in Chapter 1, the Howards of Tottenham represented the most influential pharmaceutical interest in quinine in the nineteenth century.[37] By the 1870s, the Howards had been investing in the manufacture of pure quinine over three generations. The successes of the Howards were based on their ability to coordinate amongst extensive networks of collaborators. Collaborators ranged from traveller-botanists specialising in the cinchonas and 'cinchona forests' of South America,[38] senior officials at the Kew gardens[39] and the British government in India. Even before his two books on the cinchonas were published, J. E. Howard was recognised as an expert on the different varieties of the plant.[40] He had been functioning as an advisor to the government of India in questions involving the cinchonas since the early 1860s.[41]

By the late 1860s, following the footsteps of the Howards, two government factories were set up in British India near cinchona plantations at Ootacamund in the Nilgiris and at Rungbee in Sikkim. It may be recalled that the declared purpose of introducing cinchonas in British India was humanitarian. The advertised intention was to manufacture and circulate the cheapest possible pure quinine in British India. The possibility of commercial profit was, nonetheless, mentioned as a 'secondary consideration'. Till the late 1880s, however, the products of these government-owned factories were denied the status of quinine. In this situation, the Howards were certainly amongst the most substantial suppliers of pure quinine to the governmental medical stores and depots in British India. They had considerable business investments in British India, and were considered as well amongst the leading intellectual authorities on quinine in the British Empire. They were frequently requested to judge the claims of the managers of the quinine factories owned by the British Indian governments. The Howards, then, enjoyed a unique position. They were conferred with the authority to examine products

[36] 'Process for Manufacturing Sulphate of Quinine', 1840. B/WHF/145 (LMA).

[37] For detailed information on the background of the Howards, please see Chapter 1.

[38] For correspondences between Clements Markham and the Howards see, ACC/1037/693/1–3 (LMA). See the introduction of the two books on cinchona written by J. E. Howard. Howard, *The Quinology of the East Indian Plantations* (London: L Reeve, 1869) and Howard, *Illustrations of the Nueva Quinologia of Pavon* (London: L Reeve, 1862).

[39] Two of J. E. Howard's books were dedicated to the Hookers, father and son.

[40] He had become a member of the Linnean society in 1857. See, J. H. Kirkwood et al. (ed.), *John Eliot Howard, A Budget of Papers on his Life and Work* (Oxford: Crewsdson Howard Lloyd, 1995), 2.

[41] Ibid., 7.

manufactured by their prospective competitors.[42] Later in this chapter, I shall follow the story of how the Howards performed this twin role as judge and competitor simultaneously.

Thus, the attempts of certain specific agents towards manufacturing quinine were recognised by the British Indian government as legitimate. Such agents were conferred different degrees of authority in judging, identifying and defining quinine. Similarly, governmental efforts to circulate and distribute pure quinine were confined to an exclusive network of institutions, individuals and positions. On receiving indents ratified by the office of the Secretary of State for India, a limited group of manufacturers (most notably the Howards) supplied quinine to the medical stores in different British Indian Presidencies. Under the careful vigil of the provincial medical boards or the medical department, pure quinine was distributed amongst the military hospitals and the civil dispensaries. The acts of distribution in the *mofussil* or the interiors were conducted through official agents: medical officers at the *sudder* and subdivisional stations,[43] police stations[44] and patrol boats.[45] In the military-medical stores, quinine was considered amongst the valuables and preserved with extra protection. 'Strong case required for storing quinines and valuables for military stores ... glass cases to be made extra strong with patent locks for the special storage of quinine and other valuables at the military stores'.[46]

The circulation of quinine from the medical stores was strictly monitored. In the wake of proposals that quinine supplied for India should be coloured with some 'harmless substance', the Secretary of State for India wrote in August 1876: 'Of course the adoption of this step should not in any way relax the vigilance of those in charge of medical stores to guard against the pilfering of valuable drugs by subordinates or others'.[47]

However, the government did not necessarily ban drugs that circulated as quinine, beyond this insular network of exclusive institutions and personnel. Such forms of quinine were not always attributed to belong to the clandestine market. However, the legitimacies of private druggists dealing in quinine were often called into question by the state. They were often blamed for selling adulterated or fraudulent versions of quinine. The most landmark judgment against 'acts of fraudulent' business

---

[42] C. R. Markham to J. E. Howard, 17 October 1873, India Office. Home, Medical, May 1874, 54–62 B (NAI).

[43] Home, Public. April 1872. 508 A (NAI).

[44] General, Medical, July 1876, File 290, Prog. 92–93 B (WBSA).   [45] Ibid.

[46] IOR/L/SUR/2/7/f.193, September 1868 (BL).

[47] 'Paragraph 16 of military letter' General, Medical, October 1877, File. 294, Prog. 83–85 B (WBSA).

in quinine in the 1870s and 1880s came from outside the British Empire. In 1887, Alexander Boehringer and Christian Boehringer, Directors of Milan Quinine Works, Fabbrica Lombarda de Prodotti Chimici, were sentenced to fifteen and ten years in prison, respectively.[48] It is difficult to locate such harsh measures in British India in the 1870s and 1880s. Nonetheless, private druggists were often accused of selling impure quinine. Such accusations were followed up variously by investigations, punitive measures and even justifications.[49] Allegations against private dealers in quinine, however, could take other forms. Private druggists were often believed to sell pure quinine. These druggists could, in such cases, be suspected of having benefitted from daring acts of stealing and robbing pure quinine from carefully guarded government medical stores.[50]

Such suspicions were premised on the understanding that pure quinine was a precious commodity. In the perceptions of the British Indian governments, the manufacture of pure quinine was rare and difficult. The chemistry textbooks outlined the laboratory methods of procuring pure quinine. However, the commercially viable process of manufacturing quinine was considered a 'zealously guarded secret'.[51] Such impressions were conveyed by C. B. Clarke, the Officiating Superintendent of the Botanical Gardens and in-charge of cinchona cultivation in Bengal to the Secretary to the Government of Bengal in July 1870.[52] It was believed that this secret was confined to an exclusive network, which constituted a handful of institutions and individuals based in Europe and Dutch Java. The Dutch expert on cinchonas Dr J. E. de Vrij, for instance, claimed to have been aware of a process of manufacture, which he was 'unhappily... not at liberty to divulge'.[53] The British Indian governments claimed to be in immediate correspondence with such experts.

Small wonder, then, that the indiscriminate circulation of pure quinine, beyond the earmarked routes made the governments in British India suspicious. Acts of 'robbery' from the medical stores of the government, it was argued, resulted in the selling of bottled quinine in the

---

[48] Newspaper clipping from page 335 of *The Chemist and Druggist*, 17 September 1887, preserved in ACC/1037/711/4/3 (LMA) mentions this.

[49] Anonymous, 'Adulterated Sulphate of Quinine', *IMG*, 7 (1 August 1872), 187–188 and 7 (2 September 1872), 211–212; 7 (1 October 1872), 239.

[50] Secretary of State for India to the Governor General. Home, Medical, May 1876. 45–48 A (NAI).

[51] Shaw, *Quinine Manufacture in India*.

[52] Clarke to Secretary, Bengal. Home, Public, 17 December 1870, 123–125 A (NAI).

[53] J. E. de Vrij, to the Under Secretary of State for India, 21 October 1881, Hague. Home, Medical, 1882 November, 67B (NAI).

bazaars of Bombay and Poona in September 1875. Such lines of reasoning, in turn, revealed certain prejudices of senior officials in the colonial medical bureaucracy. It was suggested, it may be recalled, that quinine ordered from England into British India should henceforth be coloured with 1 per cent carmine. It would introduce, it was hoped, 'a further protection to the Government property'. However, Dr J. D. Paul on behalf of the Medical board, Bombay Presidency, advocated the following words of caution:

I should question the advisability of colouring the stocks already in the stores and depots in India, as the persons who would carry out the process of imparting a colour to quinine in the different medical stores in India are amongst those *generally implicated of robberies* of the drug; and it seems to me undesirable that they, of all persons, should be made acquainted with the means of colouring the drug by the very mode that will be applied by the manufacturer for future supplies [Emphasis mine].[54]

Further Paul noted that quinine was stolen in small quantities by native hospital assistants who sold it to the customers. 'The government drug is employed to cure disease, but it *enriches the Native doctor,* which was not intended...'.[55] Other suspects included patients and their representatives who were selling those drugs, it was alleged, at a much higher price in the bazaars. As a preventive measure, the Surgeon General of Bombay Presidency suggested that the supply of medicines from dispensaries be restricted to genuine patients who could collect them in person.[56]

Foolproof protection of quinine from acts of adulteration and robbery was acknowledged as difficult. It was predicted, however, that this could be achieved with the introduction of 'mixed cinchona alkaloids" in the drug market of British India: '...When the mixed cinchona alkaloids come into general use, dispensaries will practically *have a quinine* which can be distinguished as a government preparation, for in appearance it differs essentially from any other form of cinchona manufacture' [Emphasis mine].[57]

The description of mixed cinchona alkaloids as 'a quinine' is revealing. It indicates that in official correspondences, quinine did not necessarily mean the name of a single, inflexible drug. Quinine was a label that could be attached to drugs. Till the late 1880s, manufacture of quinine remained the unattained goal of the British Indian government factories. In government correspondences, quinine most frequently figured as a point of reference; it was a pharmaceutical designation. More tangibly

---

[54] Paul to the Director General of Stores. Home, Medical, May 1876, 45–48 A (NAI).
[55] Ibid.
[56] Ibid. 'Note from the Military Department', No. 594, 13 March 1876.   [57] Ibid.

circulating drugs in British India often derived their names, identities and legitimacies in relation to quinine. Officials in the government factories struggled to unravel the 'secret' behind commercial manufacture of pure quinine. Meanwhile, various products of the government factories began circulating as inferior, incomplete versions of quinine (e.g., cheaper quinine,[58] amorphous quinine,[59] and rough hospital quinine).[60]

Moreover, quinine also appeared as a relational category. The identities of drugs labelled as quinine could be volatile. Such identities could be asserted and erased; labels could be ascribed to drugs and later withdrawn. For instance, F. Odevaine, a Surgeon Major in the medical bureaucracy, spoke of 'one advantage of the mixed cinchona alkaloids': '... Its solution is perfectly clear, and in dispensary practices the patients, concluding that they are getting pure quinine, will, with greater confidence, have recourse to those institutions'.[61]

Similarly, there are evidences to suggest that the tag of quinine could be deliberately withdrawn from drugs. In March 1882, Chetan Shah, Officiating Civil Surgeon at Jhang, narrated this revealing story.

I particularly observed a lady relation of mine who could never take quinine under its proper name without suffering from severe vomiting and intense depression... Once, one of my dispensers administered to her pills made of quinine under the name of 'sat gilo', which she believed was cooling in its effects as well as a cure for fever. On this occasion she had none of the symptoms that she used to ascribe to Quinine. Since then it became a custom in the family to administer quinine to this lady – whenever occasion required it – under the guise of 'sat gilo', and then the terrible symptoms of the fancied quininism never returned. Occasionally, when by mistake quinine was given to her as Quinine, the old symptoms appeared with the usual severity.[62]

These examples constitute different physicians' narratives about their encounters with patients. In such narrations, the patients hardly figure as obedient recipients of prescriptions from doctors. They are represented as active agents who could make choices between restricted options. Nonetheless, on each occasion, the identity of quinine appears to have been defined and negotiated by the imposing authority of manipulative physicians.

[58] Clarke to Secretary, Government of Bengal. Home, Public, 17 December 1870, 123–125 A (NAI).
[59] Clarke to the Secretary, Government of Bengal, No. 223, 24 October 1870 Rungbee. Home, Public, 24 December 1870, 128–132 A (NAI).
[60] Clarke, to the Secretary, Government of Bengal, No. 165, 10 February 1870 Botanic Gardens. Home, Public, 12 March 1870, 157 A (NAI).
[61] J. F. Beatson to the Officiating Secretary, Government of India, No. 548, 15 May 1879 Fort William. Home, Medical, 1879 October, 64–80 A (NAI).
[62] C. Shah, 'Uncomfortable Effects of Quinine', *IMG*, 17 (1 March 1882), 75.

Quinine in nineteenth-century British India thus did not only refer to an exclusive drug – legitimised and identified by a range of protective mechanisms – but was also indicative of a flexible label which could be attached to or withdrawn from various drugs. Identities and definitions of quinine in British India in the second half of the century were shaped by contending assertions of authority. This trend was certainly not confined to narratives of interactions between cunning physicians and their vulnerable patients. Identities of pure quinine produced in British Indian factories, as I will elaborate in the following sections, were established or repudiated by biased judgments from individuals or institutions in command of particular situations. The history of manufacturing quinine in these government factories exposes the shifting equations of authority amongst contending actors within British India and beyond.

'The Authority to Judge'

Cinchona plants and seeds extracted from forests in South America started arriving in British India in the late 1850s. Within a decade, attempts to produce cheapest possible pure quinine began in factories set up in the immediate vicinities of government cinchona plantations in the Nilgiris and British Sikkim. Meanwhile, various pharmaceutical firms, phytochemists, botanists in Germany, France, Italy, England, North America and Dutch colonial officials had credibly asserted themselves as experts in the manufacture of pure quinine. Quinine factories in British India began by soliciting ratification from some of these established authorities. Seeking recognition for such projects in British India as viable and legitimate appeared as the necessary first step.

It has been indicated already that in the 1860s and 1870s the office of the Secretary of State for India repeatedly approached Howard and Sons for such endorsements, reinforcing the claims of the Howards as the most predominant authorities on quinine.[63] The Howards manipulated this position of superiority variously. They could exercise the prerogative of refusing to judge, and they often delegated such authority to agents of their choice. For instance, John Eliot Howard wrote in April 1868 to the Undersecretary of State for India refusing to analyse extracts of cinchona barks from Darjeeling: 'It would require more time and labour than I am prepared to give to the subject'. Instead, the Howards submitted those samples to the inspection of drug brokers Messrs Phillips and Jenkins.[64]

---

[63] Secretary of State for India to the Government of India, No. 34, 27 April 1871 India Office. Home, Public, 3 June 1871, 69–70 A (NAI).

[64] General, General, January 1868, Prog. 70 B. (WBSA).

It would be fair to add, however, that in the 1860s the Howards derived much of their authority in relation to such projects initiated by the British Indian governments by offering precise judgments.

Drugs manufactured commercially in the government factories in British India in the 1860s and much of the 1870s were consistently denied the status of pure quinine by the Howards. In October 1866, Mr John Broughton had been appointed as the Quinologist to the Madras government. In successive reports, the Howards suggested that Mr Broughton's efforts could, at best, be considered to yield amorphous versions of quinine. The Howards deemed the barks of certain varieties of cinchona trees grown in the Nilgiris rich in quinine content, and there-fore valuable. They considered the investment of those barks towards the preparation of 'half manufactured products' in the Madras Presidency redundant. Instead, they recommended that these barks be shipped to England for sale in the London market. Quite predictably, such judg-ments would enable the Howards to conveniently access the barks from Madras in London as sources of cheap raw material.

Experience has hitherto shown, . . . that the collectors and importers in the end reap *more profit* from sending in to the European market the *raw material* than the *half-manufactured product*. The latter would command no price worth mentioning as a febrifuge per se. It would simply come into competition with the refuse product of the bark operation.[65]

In the early 1870s, it was reported that 'amorphous quinine' was being manufactured at a 'very serious loss to the public revenue . . . its commer-cial value is less than one-half the value of the raw material and manufac-turing charges'.[66] The 'local manufacture of amorphous quinine' in the Madras Presidency was discontinued thereafter. Broughton resigned his appointment. The post of the Government Quinologist in Madras Pres-idency had not been filled up for more than a decade. The entire crop of bark from the Madras Government plantations had since the mid-1870s been sent to England for auction in the London market.[67]

Unlike their counterparts in the Nilgiris, cinchona barks grown in British Sikkim featured in reports from the Howards as 'quite unsaleable', and never shipped to London. The Howards suggested that certain varieties of cinchona barks suffered from 'extreme poverty in alkaloids'.[68] In April 1871, commenting on 'preparations from cinchona barks, manufactured at the Sikkim plantation', J. E. Howard suggested

[65] A note from Howard dated 15 June 1864. Home, Medical, 9–11 A, January 1884. (NAI).
[66] Ibid.   [67] Ibid.   [68] Ibid.

that 'the preparation contains a very large percentage of copper, and that it is consequently inadmissible as a medicine'.[69]

The particular variety of cinchona plants that was believed to thrive most extensively in British Sikkim was recognised as cinchona succirubra. The bark of the succirubra species of the cinchonas was considered particularly weak in quinine content whereas cinchona officinalis and calisaya were amongst the varieties regarded as rich in quinine. However, it was reported that such quinine-rich varieties were not suited to the climate and landscape of British Sikkim.[70] By contrast, cinchonas growing in the Nilgiris were reported as relatively rich in quinine. This explains why the Howards preferred such barks being shipped to England for sale in the London market. The Howards appeared keen to resist the misuse of those valuable barks in the manufacture of incomplete versions of quinine in Madras. The Howards' activities suggested that government factories in Ootacamund in the Nilgiris or Rungbee in British Sikkim were inadequately equipped to produce pure quinine. Such impressions appeared firmly entrenched in cumulative reports from the Howards by the 1870s. However, acts of defining and identifying pure quinine in British India were not solely restricted to unilateral judgments from the Howards. As it unfolded, the story accommodated many diverse voices. Some of those set limits to the authority asserted by the Howards.

Contesting 'Pure Quinine'

Official correspondences in British India in the 1860s and 1870s rarely commented on the physical appearance of pure quinine. Sporadically surviving sources describe it as a 'white crystalline substance'.[71] In the laboratory, quinine was believed to crystallise into comparatively 'short crystals', in the shape of 'beautiful, long needles'.[72] By the 1870s, officials in British India appeared aware of the method 'in general use' of manufacturing crystallised sulphates of quinine.[73]

---

[69] Secretary of State for India to the Government of India. Home, Public, 3 June 1871, 69–70 A (NAI).

[70] Ibid.

[71] H. A. Cockerell, to Secretary, Government of India, Home, Revenue, and Agricultural departments, 22 August 1879, Darjeeling. Home, Medical, October 1879, 64–80 A (NAI).

[72] Clarke to the Secretary, Government of Bengal. Home, Public, 17 December 1870, 123–125 A (NAI).

[73] Clarke, to the Secretary, Government of Bengal. Home, Public, 12 March 1870, 157 A (NAI).

Replication of closely similar methods at government factories in Rungbee and Ootacamund, however, produced different results. Efforts of Thomas Anderson, Superintendent of the Botanical Gardens, Calcutta, and in charge of cinchona cultivation in Bengal, failed to yield desired versions of white pure quinine. Instead, he ended up preparing two substances from the cinchona barks grown in Darjeeling. Those substances contained 'alkaloids mixed with some extraneous matter'. He called one of those quinium. It was described as a 'brown viscid substance'. The other figured as a grey powder that consisted of alkaloids in an 'impure and non-crystalline condition'. From bark grown in the Nilgiris, Broughton, the Government Quinologist, prepared a 'closely resembling yellowish grey powder'.[74] However, neither Broughton nor Anderson considered their inability to manufacture pure quinine in the form of a 'white crystalline substance', a failure.

On the contrary, it was claimed that the preparation of these different substances was deliberate. They were projected as attempts at 'experimenting' with alternative methods of manufacturing pure quinine. The 'usual, alcoholic process', it was suggested, was unsuitable to the conditions at the factories in Ootacamund or Rungbee. Instead, Broughton claimed to have been 'engaged in devising a new, unusual process'. Anderson's successor in the Botanic Gardens in Calcutta, C. B. Clarke, endorsed such attempts: ' ... The impression which I have gained from my protracted experiments is that the successful manufacture of quinine is not any particular secret or the adoption of any particular route ... '.[75]

While the received methods of preparing pure quinine were being regarded with suspicion, the figure of pure quinine itself was subjected to considerable scrutiny. The laboratory definition of pure quinine was increasingly seen as ever changing. Since the early nineteenth century, it may be recalled, the chemical constitution of cinchona barks had been characterised by the presence of different alkaloids. The healing qualities associated with these barks were believed to result from such alkaloids, particularly quinine. Pure quinine was understood as a residual category which could be derived by chemically isolating the other alkaloids inherent in the cinchona barks. The definition of pure quinine, then, was intimately tied to the identities of 'other alkaloids' present in the cinchona barks. Pure quinine could be defined by what remained after the elimination of 'other alkaloids' from the extracts of the cinchona barks. Cinchonine was the only alkaloid other than quinine that Pelletier and

---

[74] T. Anderson, to the Secretary, Government of Bengal, 14 January 1869. Ibid.
[75] Clarke to the Secretary, Government of Bengal. Home, Public, 12 March 1870, 157 A (NAI).

Caventeau claimed to have detected in the cinchona barks in 1820. Ever since, the presence of several 'other alkaloids' had been claimed by the phytochemists. These implied corresponding changes in the laboratory definitions of pure quinine. Pelletier suggested the presence of a third alkaloid (i.e., Aricine) in 1829. In the mid-nineteenth century, Pasteur added to the list two more alkaloids, quinidine and cinchonidine. By the 1880s, phytochemists A. C. Oudemans and O. Hesse claimed to have discovered three 'new alkaloids' – quinamine, conquinamine and cinchonamine. In the laboratory sense, therefore, pure quinine could hardly be considered as an unchanging reality since the 1820s. Phytochemical understandings of pure quinine kept altering with the discovery of each 'new alkaloid'.[76]

The Howards often judged efforts pursued in the factories in British India towards manufacturing pure quinine. These provided them with numerous occasions to assert their superiority over the officials located in such factories. Since the late 1860s, officials at the receiving end of dismissive judgments from the Howards often questioned the sanctity of the category of pure quinine itself. In such official statements purity of quinine figured as a subject of sarcasm, ridicule or shocking revelation. Pure quinine was most recurrently alleged as 'deeply adulterated with cinchonidine'. Officials found it difficult to distinguish between pure quinine and some of the 'other alkaloids'. C. B. Clarke wrote thus in February 1870:

... Cinchonidine is about one-third the value of quinine, and the crystals of Cinchonidine are exceedingly like those of quinine. There is really very little quinine in general use that is not at present deeply adulterated with Cinchonidine, and I doubt whether any amount of chemical knowledge will enable the medical officer to detect the percentage of Cinchonidine present, unless he were provided with quite a different laboratory apparatus from that generally at his command.[77]

In a similar correspondence drafted a few months later, Clarke doubted the received understandings concerning the physical appearance of pure quinine: 'I may remark in passing that quinine itself crystallizes in comparatively short crystals, and that the beautiful, long needles which are regarded as almost a test of quinine are generally Cinchonidine'.[78] Such

---

[76] 'Enclosure no. 6: Report on the Bengal Cinchona febrifuge, called for by the Secretary of State for India, in Letters dated 6 April and 6 September 1878, and 11 January 1879'. Home, Medical, November 1882, 67 B (NAI).

[77] Clarke to the Secretary, Government of Bengal. Home, Public, 12 March 1870, 157 A (NAI).

[78] Clarke to the Secretary, Government of Bengal. Home, Public, 17 December 1870, 123–125 A (NAI).

impressions seem to have had extensive currency. In September 1878, G. Smith the then Surgeon General of the Indian Medical Department, Madras Presidency, suggested that 'impure quinine of the shops' constituted a combination of sulphates of quinine and cinchonidine.[79]

Suggestions that impure quinine was circulating extensively in the shops did not necessarily indicate a scandalous fraud in British India in the 1870s. Rather certain influential officials employed in the cinchona factories had begun questioning the integrity of the phytochemical category of pure quinine itself. These officials tended to suspect the distinctness of quinine as an alkaloid, suggesting that specific alkaloids supposedly inherent in the cinchona barks were not exceptional, distinguishable and autonomous entities. The identities of such alkaloids were often fluid, overlapping and seldom mutually exclusive. In 1871, Broughton showed how, once exposed to certain conditions, alkaloids changed identities. He suggested that quinine and cinchonidine shared 'chemical similarity',[80] 'a natural connection.'[81] He argued that quinine could convert into cinchonidine and vice versa when exposed to sunshine and heat. He claimed that this hypothesis was not 'contradicted by a single fact' and was 'in harmony with observations made with very diverse species of cinchona'. These alkaloids, Broughton asserted, were 'especially sensitive to light'. Whiteness, according to Broughton, had been an indicator of the purity of alkaloids, but whiteness faded, Broughton believed, on exposure to Indian sunshine: 'The purest and whitest alkaloids I have been able to prepare become coloured brown when exposed to the Indian sunshine...'.[82]

The authority of the Howards was based on their claim as experts in the manufacture of pure quinine. By contrast, British Indian officials like Broughton and Clarke tended to question the chemical viability of pure quinine itself. Circulation of impure quinine, then, could not necessarily be attributed to inefficient manufacturers or clandestine traders. The purity of alkaloids, these officials suggested, was often compromised by 'idiosyncrasies'[83] inherent in the 'living cinchona plants'. Purity of alkaloids could wane, it was argued, once exposed to adverse colonial conditions. Thus, quinine could lose its purity prior to moments of manufacture and circulation. Corruption of quinine was often seen to be beyond

[79] G. Smith to Acting Chief Secretary, Government of Madras, No. 527, 25 September 1878, Fort St George. Home, Medical, March 1879, 55–57 A (NAI).
[80] J. Broughton, 'Chemical and Physiological Experiments on Living Cinchonaey', *Philosophical Transactions of the Royal Society of London*, 161 (1871), 8.
[81] Ibid., 1.   [82] Ibid., 8.
[83] G. E. Shaw, *Quinine Manufacture in India* (London: Institute of Chemistry of Great Britain and Ireland, 1935), 3.

the control of commercial manufacturers. Clarke argued that this made the manufacture of pure quinine often 'speculative and uncertain', and that this was why John Eliot Howard, in his books, had never elaborated on the process of manufacturing quinine with clarity and precision.[84] The volatile identities of 'pure alkaloids', in turn, reshaped understandings of 'adulterated versions of pure quinine'. In October 1872, the Officiating Commissioner of Police, Calcutta, S. Wauchope, refused to consider the circulation of cinchonidine or cinchonine under the name of pure quinine, a particularly unacceptable act.[85]

Even in distant contexts, chemical definitions of pure quinine acquired similar flexible forms. French botanist Gustave Planchon defined 'raw quinine' in 1866 as an 'admixture of quinine, chinchonine, unctuous matter, and colouring parts . . .'.[86] Having questioned the viability of the category pure quinine, successive Superintendents of the Botanic Gardens in Calcutta began advocating deliberate manufacture of 'impure forms of quinine'. Thus in February 1870, Clarke wrote thus: 'Dr T. Anderson now advocates the manufacture of a rough hospital quinine at Rungbee, by which he means the production of the precipitated alkaloids in a more or less *impure* form'.[87]

An Economy of 'Substitutes'

Managers of the cinchona factories in British India set limits to the authority of the Howards in certain other ways. A four-member committee, including John Broughton, was appointed in March 1866 to examine the relative therapeutic value of cinchona alkaloids other than quinine. The committee reported to the Secretary to the Government of India, Home Department on October 1868 that there was no longer doubt that alkaloids 'other than quinine' were capable of being generally used with best results in India: 'Compared with quinine . . . [they] have been found, by more than one observer, to supplement this sovereign remedy in some of its points of deficiency'.[88]

---

[84] Clarke to the Secretary, Government of Bengal. Home, Public, 17 December 1870, 123–125 A (NAI).

[85] S. Wauchope, to the Officiating Secretary, Government of Bengal, Judicial Department, No.1238, 16 October 1872 Calcutta. General, Medical, October 1872, Prog. 6–8 (WBSA).

[86] G. Planchon, *Peruvian Barks* (Bangalore: Mysore Government Press, 1867), 34.

[87] Clarke to the Secretary, Government of Bengal. Home, Public, 12 March 1870, 157 A (NAI).

[88] The Committee appointed to examine the properties of the cinchona alkaloids other than quinine to the Secretary, Government of India, Home, 29 October 1868. Howard

Amongst these different alkaloids, only quinine had hitherto been accepted into the British pharmacopeia, and the committee suggested that this position was untenable.[89] Recognitions of the medical values of alkaloids other than quinine were reflected elsewhere. Commercial manufacture of pure quinine ceased to be the sole declared goal of the cinchona plantations. Nor is it entirely coincidental that the Annual Report of the cinchona plantations at Darjeeling removed the word 'Quiniferous' from its title since October 1866.[90]

In January 1870, the office of the Secretary of State for India forwarded copies of the Medical Committee report to the Howards. This implied a break with the prevailing equations of authority. In relation to the cinchona factories in British India, this, for the first time, placed the Howards at the receiving end of instruction. The Howards were informed that the value of febrifuge other than quinine, should be generally known both in England and in India, and that the Duke of Argyll 'will not have any objection to you making any use you may seem fit of the information contained in the report'.[91] Already in 1869 official correspondences in British India began recognising the cinchona alkaloids other than quinine as not only effective, but also desirable. It was suggested that the extensive circulation of such 'cheaper' alkaloids would be compatible with the declared ethical intentions of the government, since they would represent considerable saving.[92]

Official opinion in British India as well as Burma encouraged a variety of medical preparations, often different combinations of cinchona alkaloids, other than quinine. The Secretary to the Chief Commissioner of British Burma wrote in October 1870: 'General Fytche understands that the plant can be prepared in a rough way and used as a febrifuge by those growing it, without having to send it away for chemical manipulation and conversion into the form in which it is generally used'.[93] Such 'rough preparations' enjoyed considerable legitimacy in British India. Managers of cinchona plantations and factories tended to invest such preparations with respectability and pedigree. Clarke suggested that such 'rough',

Private Papers. ACC/1037/699/3 (LMA); See also, Home, Public, 26 February 1866, 58A (NAI).

[89] J. A. Gammie, 'Manufacture of Quinine in India', *Bulletin of Miscellaneous Information* (Royal Gardens: Kew), 18 (1888), 139–144.

[90] T. Anderson, 'Report on the Cultivation of Cinchona at Darjeeling from 1 April 1865 to 31 March 1866', Home, Public, October 1866, 21–22 (NAI).

[91] Secretary of State for India to Howard, dated January 1870, India Office. Howard Private Papers. ACC 1037/699/1 (LMA).

[92] Home, Public, 17 April 1869, 31 B (NAI).

[93] A. Fraser to Secretary, Government of India, PWD, No. 612–15F, 10 October 1870. Home, Public, 17 December 1870, 43–44 A (NAI).

'amorphous' preparations of alkaloids conformed to the 'original recommendations' of Pelletier, 'the great medical authority on quinine'.[94]
Pelletier had preferred these alkaloids to quinine, argued Clarke. Poster-
ity chose to ignore such insight, reasoned Clarke, as 'making the amorphous alkaloid contained some details which the manufacturers found
especially troublesome to work in practice'.[95]

The 1870s and the early 1880s witnessed a plethora of such preparations in British India. These bore a variety of names and claims. In
November 1876, Rai Bahadur Kanai Lall Dey, the Deputy Surgeon
General of Bengal hinted at the various 'colloquial names' of cinchona-
related drugs in use in Bengal: cinchona khar, cinchona yaraghana, cinchona alkaloids, Indian cinchona alkaloid, Indian febrifuge cinchona
alkaloid, desaja cinchona khar and bharatta yaraghana cinchona khar.[96]
The celebrated Dutch expert on the cinchonas and their alkaloids Dr J.
E. de Vrij argued that quinetum, cinchona febrifuge, quinium, quinine
brute and rough quinine indicated different names for almost identical
preparations.[97] John Eliot Howard, in contrast, emphasised difference.
He suggested that four different varieties of drugs were circulating in the
name of quinetum.

Quinetum No. 1 is that prepared in British India, and sold by the Government
there at Rs. 20 per English pound. It is of a fine white colour, and has a peculiar
sweet smell. It is packed in tin boxes holding half an English pound, which are
provided with direction for use in English and Hindustani. No. 2 was prepared
at Wettevreden. It has the same appearance and smell as the Bengal, but is a little
darker coloured. No. 3 is a sample of the first quinetum prepared by Broughton
in Madras, and called amorphous quinine. It is a yellow stuff, sticky like resin,
and looking like rhubarb powder, on the whole a very impure preparation. No.
4 is quinetum of the manufacturer Whiffen, in London. This had a grey-brown
tint, smell or meth.[98]

Comments from J. E. de Vrij and Howard can hardly be read as disinterested assessments. These experts had begun investing in such preparations themselves. Their products were locked in relations of comparison and competition with preparations they were judging. Physical
appearance and chemical compositions were not the only indices for

[94] Clarke to the Secretary, Government of Bengal. Home, Public, 17 December 1870,
123–125 A (NAI).
[95] Ibid.
[96] K. L. Dey to Superintendent, Campbell Medical School, No. 76, 30 November 1876
Calcutta. General, Medical, December 1876, File 365, Prog. 25–27 A (WBSA).
[97] de Vrij to the Under Secretary of State for India. Home, Medical, November 1882, 67
B (NAI).
[98] J. E. Howard to the Under Secretary of State for India, 21 June 1881, Lord's Meade,
Tottenham, Ibid.

comparison. Given the ethical pretentions of the British Indian government, inexpensiveness emerged as a measure of the worth of a product.[99]

By the late 1860s, quinine was no longer considered the only efficacious alkaloid inherent in the cinchona barks. Quinine was shown to share its curative properties with 'other alkaloids' believed to be present in the cinchona barks and these extended also to the 'waste products' derived from the cinchona factories in British India. Clarke wrote in December 1870: 'The waste in practice is not so great as appears, because the uncrystallizable alkaloid is not thrown away, but forms the basis of many well known medicines, and is also purchased as an amorphous powder...'.[100]

Judging the Howards

Contesting the indispensability of quinine implied setting limits to the authority of those groups of men who claimed expertise in the manufacture of pure quinine. Ironically, however, such experts located in The Hague or London, found in these statements promising business prospects. In successive letters written from Hague to Clements Robert Markham in April 1871, de Vrij pointed out the therapeutic virtues of one of the 'waste products of the Cinchona plants'. Referring to 'experience and information' from hospitals and dispensaries in Java, Sumatra, Samaran, Dr de Vrij suggested that quinovin could be considered as an 'excellent cure' for dysentery, diarrhoea, cholera and ague.[101]

By October 1873, the Howards had themselves begun advertising the virtues of the cheaper alkaloids.[102] They began by offering 'the refuse of the quinine factory' under the name of quinoidine at about five shillings per pound.[103] However, in these years, the most emphatic claims of the Howards were for cinchonidine. J. E. Howard suggested that he found cinchonidine 'in most cases not inferior to quinine', and went on to claim that on certain occasions he considered the 'therapeutic action of cinchonidine preferable to that of quinine'.[104] Howard retold the story

---

[99] A Note from Surgeon General, Indian Medical Department, No. 1418, 17 February 1876. Home, Medical, March 1876, 53–57 B (NAI).

[100] Clarke to Secretary, Government of Bengal. Home, Public, 17 December 1870, 123–125 A (NAI).

[101] J. E. de Vrij to C. R. Markham, 17 April 1871, Hague. Home, Public, 1 July 1871, 34–35 A (NAI).

[102] J. E. Howard to C. R. Markham, 21 October 1873, Tottenham. Home, Medical, May 1874, 54–62 B (NAI).

[103] C. H. Wood, to C. J. Lyall, 13 July 1874, Rungbee. Home, Medical, August 1874, 44–49 A (NAI).

[104] Howard to Markham. Home, Medical, May 1874, 54–62 B (NAI).

of the recovery of the Countess of Cinchon in the seventeenth century. The Countess had apparently recuperated from a fatal ailment after consuming extracts of cinchona bark. Howard retrospectively attributed her recovery to the richness of cinchonidine in that particular variety of cinchona bark.[105] Howard suggested that an extensive supply of cinchonidine to British India would be absolutely necessary in the wake of the Burdwan fever.[106] In February 1874, Howard proposed to furnish 3000 pounds of cinchonidine in six months at 45 shillings per pound.[107] The Howards seem to have had the backing of the office of the Secretary of State for India at this stage. A note from the latter preceded the proposal. 'I hope your Government will take the suggestions contained in Mr Howard's letter into consideration ...'.[108]

The newly appointed Quinologist in Bengal, Mr C. H. Wood, responded to the Howards' proposals with considerable scepticism. He suggested that the Howards were desperately trying to foist accumulated cinchonidine on the Government of India: 'by hook or by crook', a position that A. O. Hume, on behalf of the India Office, endorsed. 'Howard has enormous stock in hand and wants to get rid of it', it was noted, with the cynical aside that a large sale to the Indian government could enhance the legitimacy of the same product in Europe.[109]

Wood's response was suggestive. I have already shown that the Howards were often requested to judge the identities and qualities of drugs manufactured in the factories at Rungbee and Ootacamund since the mid-1860s. Wood's response suggested, yet again, that the authority asserted by the Howards had limits. While the Howards continued to judge the efforts of the Government Quinologists employed in Madras and Bengal Presidencies, the Quinologists had themselves by the mid-1870s begun scrutinising and even contesting assertive judgments from the Howards. From 1875, such reciprocal judgments were often witnessed between Wood and the Howards. Wood continued to hold the position of Quinologist of Bengal until he resigned in April 1879, but from the mid-1870s, the office of the Quinologist of Bengal acquired more relevance than ever before.

Several reports on the value of cinchonas grown in the emerging plantations in British India were presented after 1860. These reports, it may be recalled, revealed considerable regional variation. The cinchonas

---

[105] Ibid.   [106] Ibid.

[107] Secretary of State for India to Government of India, No. 33, 4 June 1874, India Office. Home, Medical, August 1874, 44–49 A (NAI).

[108] Secretary of State for India to Governor General of India in Council, 16 December 1873 India Office. Home, Medical, May 1874, 54–62 B (NAI).

[109] Note from A. O. Hume. Ibid.

thriving in plantations on the Nilgiris were identified as predominantly belonging to the officinalis and succirubra varieties. The barks of the officinalis plants were considered rich in quinine. In contrast, it was suggested that succirubra represented the most extensively proliferating species of cinchonas in British Sikkim, but their barks were considered poor in quinine. J. E. Howard kept denying the products manufactured in the factories at Rungbee in British Sikkim and Ootacamund in the Nilgiris the status of quinine. Following his recommendations, efforts at manufacturing quinine at Ootacamund were finally discontinued in March 1875. The entire crop of cinchona barks grown in the Nilgiris had been thereafter regularly sent to England as sources of cheap raw materials. As a result Broughton resigned as Government Quinologist in the Madras Presidency, and this post remained vacant ever since.

This made C. H. Wood the only Government Quinologist employed in British India in the later 1870s. Government efforts towards manufacturing quinine, however inchoate, were now solely confined to the factory at Rungbee in British Sikkim. This coincided with the ascription of new meanings to the succirubra species of the cinchonas. With the therapeutic virtues of alkaloids other than quinine being variously asserted, succirubra began to acquire the reputation of a valuable species. In December 1873, the Secretary of State for India suggested that the extensive use of the febrifuge in the form of cinchonidine would have the advantage of extending the cultivation and increasing the value of succirubra, 'the species which, while producing that particular alkaloid in very considerable quantities also grows more readily and over a wide range than any other in the hill districts of the (Bengal) presidency'.[110]

The barks of the succirubra species of the cinchonas, it was suggested by officials in British Sikkim, were enormously rich in alkaloids other than quinine. Figure 4.1 and Figure 4.2 suggest that photographs were circulated within official circles to bolster the claim that the cinchona plantations in British Sikkim were abound in succirubra plants. Such impressions conferred considerable prestige on these cinchona plantations. C. H. Wood and his colleagues appeared to assert intimate knowledge on these plantations, claiming expertise on the extraction of alkaloids inherent in the succirubra barks. The Howards had, by then, found new enticing business prospects in 'other alkaloids' besides quinine.

In relation to these newly found interests of the Howards, then, Wood and his colleagues in British India were placed in a position of comparative advantage and authority. In a revealing reversal of roles, for instance, samples of quinoidine and 'amorphous quinine' prepared

[110] Markham to Howard. Home, Medical, May 1874, 54–62 B (NAI).

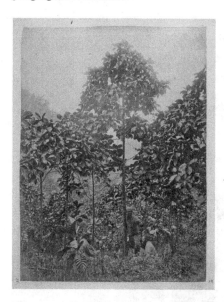

Figure 4.1 © British Library Board. Photograph of 'A cinchona tree (succirubra) at the Government Plantation at Rungbee.' Photographer: Robert Phillips; Photo contains the note: 'View of three European men sitting beneath cinchona trees. 1870s.' (India Office Select Material, British Library. Shelfmark: Photo 637/(28).

by Messrs Howard and Sons and Dr de Vrij, respectively, were sent out between November and December 1875 to British India for trial. Reports on the efficacies of these preparations were presented by a range of medical bureaucrats, including H. Cayley (Surgeon Superintendent, Mayo Native Hospital), Norman Chevers (Principal, Medical College Calcutta), Robert Bird (Civil Surgeon, Howrah General Hospital) and S. C. Mackenzie (Second Resident Surgeon, Presidency General Hospital). The preparations manufactured by the Howards and de Vrij were found to produce 'troublesome nausea, frequent vomiting, vertigo and anorexia', and were denied the status of efficacious drugs.[111] This represented a trend that would often be repeated.[112]

It appears from the foregoing narrative that officials located in the government cinchona factories in British India were hardly passive recipients of dismissive judgments. Between the late 1860s and mid-1870s, they had recurrently questioned the basic foundation of the claims to

[111] Note from Surgeon General, Indian Medical Department. Home, Medical, March 1876, 53–57 B (NAI).
[112] Home, Medical, July 1882, 44–46 A (NAI).

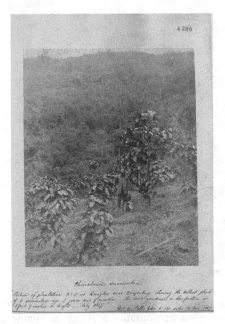

Figure 4.2 © British Library Board. Photograph carrying the following note: 'Chinchona succirubra. Portion of Plantation No. 5 at Rungbee near Darjeeling showing the tallest plant of C. succirubra age 2 years and 9 months. The head gardener in the picture is 5 feet 9 inches in height.' Photographer: Sir Benjamin Simpson; July 1867. (India Office Select Materials, British Library. Shelfmark: Photo 1000/40 (4200).

authority asserted by de Vrij or the Howards. This was achieved, as I have suggested, in two different ways. At one level, the viability of pure quinine as a phytochemical category was subjected to vigorous scrutiny. At another, the indispensability of quinine as a febrifuge was questioned. It was recognised that other alkaloids besides quinine inherent in the cinchona barks were considerably endowed with curative properties. Such recognitions led to newer and disparate claims to knowledge on the cinchonas. Most regularly, these claims were manifested in correspondences drafted by various British Indian officials: the Quinologist of Bengal and his subordinates in the factory at Rungbee, Superintendents of Botanic Gardens, medical bureaucrats and physicians located in dispensaries, military and civil hospitals.[113] Pharmaceutical business and medical relief in British India, since the early 1860s, involved a shared set of individuals, institutions and interests. In these overlapping worlds,

[113] Ibid.

the 'authority to judge' did not signify an inflexible, unchanging status. It referred to relations that could vary with shifts in contexts. The 'authority to judge' has to be understood with reference to these shifting terms of hierarchical relation between concerned parties; and not as a universally agreed upon designation. Besides, 'the authority to judge' could have its limits. The judge in a particular situation could be on the receiving end of judgment in another. From the previously mentioned context, it is clear that the Howards and the Quinologist in Bengal judged the products manufactured by one another. Thus, 'authority to judge' should be understood as shifting, relational and even reciprocal positions.

The Return of Quinine

Excessive emphasis on the medical virtues of alkaloids other than quinine did not necessarily erase the relevance of quinine. The difficulties and often the impossibility of manufacturing pure quinine in British India were mentioned in official correspondence. However, quinine remained relevant as an agreed point of reference. A wide range of preparations supposedly manufactured from alkaloids other than quinine, from the late 1860s, were often collectively referred to as substitutes of quinine.[114] Whether quinine could be identified as a tangible drug remained a matter of dispute. Nonetheless, quinine frequently figured as an index, a yardstick for comparison. The virtues of newly prepared drugs manufactured from 'other alkaloids' inherent in cinchona barks were asserted by claiming their similarities with quinine. Similarly, the credibility of some preparations was contested by indicating their differences from quinine. For instance, Robert Bird, Civil Surgeon, Howrah General Hospital, labelled a drug prepared by de Vrij as an amorphous version of quinine. He found it more 'akin to quinidine in its power. It creates irritability of the stomach and brings on vertigo and anorexia'.[115] Thus, quinine was invoked to assert or deny the relative worth of different products prepared from the cinchonas.

Seventeen medical officers located in British India were requested to test the value of two such preparations manufactured in England, namely cinchonine alkaloids and quinetum tartrates. They responded in a variety of ways. Most responses were articulated in reference to quinine.[116] Relations between 'other minor alkaloids' and quinine were

---

[114] Home, Public, 17 April 1869, 31 B (NAI).
[115] R. Bird, to the Deputy Surgeon General, Presidency Circle, Calcutta. No 131, 14 December 1875 Howrah. Home, Medical, March 1876, 53–57 B (NAI).
[116] Home, Medical, July 1882, 44–46 A (NAI).

often expressed in quantifiable terms. C. B. Clarke, the Superintendent of Botanic Gardens, Calcutta, wrote thus: 'Roughly it may be
said that two grains of cinchonidine are equal in all respects to one
grain of quinine... cinchonidine is about one-third the value of quinine...'.[117] These correspondents very rarely spoke of the attributes
of quinine itself. Quinine seldom appeared to figure as a commodity
on its own. Quinine and its substitutes were mentioned in relation to
each other. The credibility of these substitutes was claimed with reference to quinine. Such claims, in turn, hinted at the qualities of quinine.
Writing in defence of one such substitute, mixed triple sulphate, Surgeon Major R. W. Cunningham, XV Sikh's regiment, Sealkot suggested:
'The taste is less intensely bitter than quinine...'.[118] Explaining why the
mixed triple sulphate could emerge as a more satisfactory substitute for
quinine, a memorandum suggested that the triple sulphate 'is a white
crystalline substance, closely resembling pure quinine in appearance'.[119]
Thus, descriptions of the substitutes not only hinted at the curative
properties of quinine, they indicated the taste and the colour of pure
quinine as well. Even texts emphasising the 'desirability' of the substitutes retained the manufacture of pure quinine as the ultimate aim of
introducing cinchona into British India.[120] Small wonder, then, that the
managers of the cinchona factory at Mungpoo would gradually invest
their newfound prestige in claiming expertise on manufacturing quinine.
Already in 1872, the caption of an anonymous sketch published in *The
Graphic* (see Figure 4.3) contained the claim that all the various activities
undertaken in the cinchona plantations in the region were connected to
the ultimate goal of 'the production of quinine in India'.

In March 1888, James Alexander Gammie, then Resident Manager
of the government cinchona cultivation at Darjeeling, filed an application for patent. It involved a process of extracting quinine, pure and
cheap, which he claimed to have invented.[121] George King, the Superintendent of the Royal Botanic Gardens in Calcutta and the cinchona
cultivation of Bengal, endorsed Gammie's claim. King suggested that
the process could enable the extraction of the whole quinine inherent
in cinchona barks. Such quinine, he claimed, would be 'undistinguishable, either chemically or physically, from the best brands of European

---

[117] Clarke, to the Secretary, Government of Bengal. Home, Public, 12 March 1870, 157
A (NAI).
[118] Beatson, to the Officiating Secretary, the Government of India. Home, Medical, October 1879, 64–80 A (NAI).
[119] G. King and C. H. Wood, 'Memorandum on the Desirability of Manufacturing Pure
Alkaloids from Succirubra Bark', Ibid.
[120] Ibid.   [121] Home, Patents, June 1888, 166–169 A (NAI).

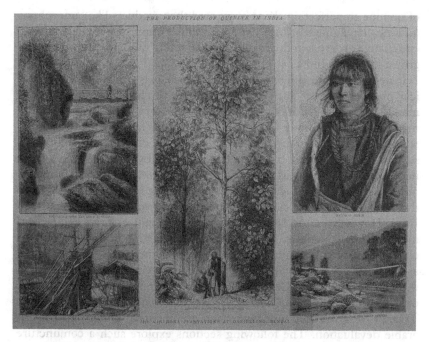

Figure 4.3 Artist unknown. 'The production of quinine in India, the cinchona plantations at Darjeeling Bengal; Cinchona succirubra 30 feet high'. *The Graphic* (October 26, 1872), 385, Author's collection.

quinine'.[122] In recognition of this, Gammie and C. H. Wood, the ex-Government Quinologist in Bengal, received monetary awards from Viscount Cross, the then Secretary of State for India, in October 1889.[123] It might be tempting to place such detail as a happy ending to a teleological success story: 'The efforts of the Governments of Great Britain and Holland, to secure for their tropical subjects a cheap remedy for the commonest of all tropical diseases, have thus culminated in a more triumphant success than was ever anticipated.'[124] The official history of this accomplishment acquired the form of an uncomplicated linear narrative. King narrated the careers of J. Broughton, C. H. Wood and J. A. Gammie in British India, as part of a single, continuous story. The story constituted a journey from confusion in the art of chemical manufacture

---

[122] G. King to the Secretary, Government of Bengal, Financial Department, No. 28 Q, 18 February 1888, Calcutta. Finance, Miscellaneous, August 1888, File M Q/1, Pros 1–13 (WBSA).
[123] Home, Medical, December 1889, 12 A (NAI).
[124] Rev-Agriculture, Agriculture, November 1891, 29 B (NAI).

of quinine to perfection. King suggested that products like 'amorphous quinine, 'cinchona febrifuge', and 'Gammie's quinine' were indicative of cumulative progress in the method of extracting quinine from cinchonas grown in British India.[125]

Instead, it is possible to read these as labels attached onto medical products. Such labels signified the hierarchical location of their manufacturers in relation to contending actors. The history of the manufacture of quinine in British India in the latter half of the nineteenth century was largely shaped by the ability of the manufacturers to sustain credible claims. It was no less informed by the abilities of others in contesting them. It was claimed, for instance, that samples of pure quinine were being manufactured 'in a remote place like Mungpoo'[126] from the early 1880s. Such claims had been faintly voiced earlier in British India. However, in the 1880s, these carried weight as never before, and indicated that Gammie, King and their colleagues in the government cinchona plantations and factory in British Sikkim had by then emerged as a collective force to reckon with. This converged with a situation when the superiorities of the Howards, the Whiffens and the office of Secretary of State for India were variously questioned in matters related to quinine. This, in turn, initiated a decade when quinine itself underwent considerable devaluation. The following sections explore such a conjuncture to explain how a convincing process of manufacturing cheap and pure quinine was 'invented' at Mungpoo in the late 1880s.

Cinchona Febrifuge: The 'Impure' as 'Desirable'

I have mentioned that C. H. Wood, the Government Quinologist in Bengal, began attempts to produce cheaper substitutes of quinine in the factory at Rungbee (Mungpoo) from his appointment in 1873. He worked very closely with George King, the then Superintendent of the Botanic Gardens, Calcutta, who was entrusted with the additional responsibility of the Superintendent of the Cinchona plantations in Bengal soon after Wood's resignation in 1879. King discharged these twin functions for more than a decade. In June 1875, Wood claimed to manufacture a 'mixture in the precipitated form of all the alkaloids present in the succirubra bark in the following combination: quinine (15.5 per cent), cinchonidine (29 per cent), cinchonine (33.5 per cent), amorphous

---

[125] King to Secretary, Government of Bengal. Finance, Miscellaneous, August 1888, File M Q/1, Pros 1–13 (WBSA).
[126] Ibid.

alkaloid (17 per cent), colouring matter (5 per cent)'.[127] Over the next three years, the preparation came to be widely circulated in Bengal.

In May–June 1878, elaborate correspondence ensued between Sir Richard Temple, the then Lieutenant Governor, J. F. Beatson, the Surgeon General, Indian Medical Department and senior medical bureaucrats including J. M. Cunningham regarding an official name for this 'substance' manufactured by Wood. Probable names discussed included quinetum, cinchona febrifuge, Darjeeling quinine and cinchona mixed alkaloids.[128] Such detailed discussions indicate that the 'substance' attributed to Wood had by then attracted considerable attention and interest amongst high-ranking officials in the bureaucracy. It was predictably suggested that the official name should not sound like a quack remedy. At the same time, it was proposed that the name should emphasise its differences from quinine. The medical bureaucrats wished to underscore its autonomous identity. 'Any pseudo-scientific name for it should be avoided... an appearance of scientific structure would lead many persons to regard it as denoting a compound of quinine, or some definite chemical body. The 'febrifuge' in reality is neither of these...'.[129] Despite significant reservations, the name cinchona febrifuge was adopted. The decision appears to have been motivated by the concern of appealing to the people and 'to the natives' and reveals an official ambition extensively to circulate and distribute the medicines manufactured in Rungbee under this specific name. Officials considered the term quinetum as 'a purely fanciful name, which would be unintelligible to the natives of the country'. Besides, as the preparation was already known as cinchona febrifuge in various parts of Bengal, it was felt that any change of name would affect 'public' trust in the drug.[130]

Since its introduction into the market in March 1875, the drug circulating as cinchona febrifuge had been variously compared with quinine. Cinchona febrifuge derived considerable legitimacy through numerous such acts of comparison. It gradually emerged as a respectable substitute for quinine: '...Somewhat less powerful than *pure quinine*...The taste appears to be nearly that of quinine...it is a very good *substitute* for quinine...[emphasis mine]'.[131] A collage of reports complied by J. F. Beatson, Surgeon General, Indian Medical Department in October 1879 suggests extensive use of cinchona febrifuge in all native

---

[127] R. Cockburn, to A. P. Howell, No. 307, 5 June 1875, Fort William. Home, Medical, August 1875, 49–58 A (NAI).
[128] Beatson, to The Officiating Secretary, Government of India. Home, Medical, September 1878, 126–128 A (NAI).
[129] Ibid.   [130] Ibid.
[131] Cockburn to Howell. Home, Medical, August 1875, 49–58 A (NAI).

hospitals, military and civil.[132] Official physicians associated with the military regiments tended to prefer cinchona febrifuge to quinine. Reports submitted by Surgeon Major W. E. Allen of the Bhopal battalion, Surgeon General R. W. Cunningham of XV Sikhs, Sealkot and Surgeon Major F. Odevaine, for instance, revealed a bias in favour of cinchona febrifuge. Odevaine claimed to have treated 600 cases of malarious fever in a regimental hospital exclusively with the drug; 593 were discharged 'cured', while the rest survived. Beatson, was doubtful if quinine would achieve better results: 'When nausea, headache, etc are attributed to the "cinchona" febrifuge by the opponents to its use, it is left to be inferred that quinine is free from all such noxious qualities; but what practical physician is not aware how often it is contra-indicated...?'[133]

Cinchona febrifuge was also projected as cheaper and more affordable, and its use instead of quinine was upheld as an effective cost-cutting measure. In view of the ever-mounting price of quinine in the late 1870s, more extensive circulation of cinchona febrifuge was proposed as an economical and benevolent step. In October 1879, cinchona febrifuge was available for Rs. 16 per pound from the government stores. In comparison, the prevalent price of quinine in the Calcutta market was shown as Rs. 25 an ounce. Consequently, it was argued: 'If introduced instead of quinine a greater saving will be effected than if all the other drugs put together were purchased at half price...'.[134] The introduction of cinchona febrifuge into all the native hospitals of Bengal to an amount of 75 per cent in lieu of quinine, it was hoped, would effect a considerable saving.

The late 1870s witnessed a curious situation when a lesser substitute appeared to be favoured over the drug it tried to simulate. In the hierarchy of drugs, the status of cinchona febrifuge underwent substantial changes. It had begun competing with quinine in the drug market. Cinchona febrifuge seemed to displace drugs circulating as quinine from the government hospitals as the principal cure of malarial diseases. In December 1878 for example the medical officer of the 43rd Regiment Assam Light Infantry abandoned the use of quinine altogether in favour of cinchona febrifuge in both his military and civilian practice.[135]

Such acts of substitution were witnessed in military hospitals for Indian troops in the British imperial army in most presidencies. In the Bengal presidency, cinchona febrifuge displaced quinine to the extent of 75 per cent. Two-thirds of the stock of quinine was replaced by

---

[132] Beatson to the Officiating Secretary, the Government of India. Home, Medical, October 1879, 64–80 A (NAI).
[133] Ibid.   [134] Ibid.   [135] Ibid.

cinchona febrifuge in these hospitals in Bombay Presidency. By February 1879, Madras had not, however, agreed to such proposals.[136] In March 1879, W. Walker, Inspector General of the Civil Hospitals and Dispensaries, North-Western Provinces and Oudh, compared the therapeutic and economic values of the two drugs. On the basis of observations made in police and jail hospitals and dispensary practice, he suggested that cinchona febrifuge should be considered half as effective as quinine. He argued that so long the price of quinine remained more than double that of cinchona febrifuge, such acts of substitution made sense. On the basis of Walker's recommendations, the use of imported quinine and cinchona febrifuge was prescribed in the proportion of one-fourth and three fourths, respectively.[137]

Cinchona febrifuge was often blamed for causing harmful side effects, including intense nausea and gastric irritation. Howard attributed these reactions to the 'noxious properties' inherent in the 17 per cent of 'amorphous alkaloid' present in the drug. At a time when cinchona febrifuge had begun commanding considerable respectability, de Vrij wrote a report emphasising the 'desirability' of retaining such 'nauseating principles' in the drug. The elimination of the 'amorphous alkaloid', he suggested, could be an expensive process, which would 'frustrate the humane purpose of the government to procure a cheap febrifuge for the numerous population of India'. de Vrij went on to argue that the elimination of the 'nauseating principle' would require the mediation of 'different liquids'. Such 'offensive impurities' would contaminate the 'nature' of the alkaloids, he feared. The nauseous side effects associated with the cinchona febrifuge had to be tolerated then as necessary and even desirable.[138]

Successive Superintendents of the cinchona plantations in British Sikkim, the managers of the cinchona factory at Rungbee and their subordinates had since the late 1860s asserted themselves as experts on the alkaloid chemistry of the cinchonas. The extensive circulation of cinchona febrifuge in the late 1870s suggests that such claims acquired considerable credibility in different parts of British India. However, cinchona febrifuge had also aroused the interests and anxieties of officials, chemists and businessmen beyond the borders of mainland British India. J. E. Howard had grown intensely inquisitive about the functioning of the

---

[136] Government of Bengal, 'Register no. 1231, Diary no. 92 Medical', No. 937, 24 February 1879. Home, Medical, May 1879, 16–18A (NAI).

[137] W. Walker to the Secretary, Government of the North-Western Provinces and Oudh, No. 49, 3 March 1879 Lucknow. Home, Medical, May 1879, 19–21 A (NAI).

[138] 'Enclosure no 6'. Home, Medical, 1882, November, 67B.

cinchona plantations and factory in British Sikkim around 1878.[139] In August 1880, Lieutenant-Colonel T. Cadell, the Chief Commissioner of the Andaman and Nicobar Islands, ordered the issue of three grains of cinchona febrifuge daily to 1000 labouring convicts in the Northern districts of the island. In the southern districts, similar doses were to be made available to 500 labouring convicts. He argued that such distribution of febrifuge would reduce rather than enhance expenditure because those who received 'the cinchona febrifuge will not receive the much more expensive milk ration'.[140] Far away in Trinidad in May 1881, the Surgeon General was contemplating a substitution of quinine manufactured in England by cheaper cinchona febrifuge, for use in the island.[141] Earlier in April, Mr Mitchell, the Emigration agent for Trinidad in Calcutta, had suggested the same. He proposed that a supply of cinchona febrifuge could be secured at cost price directly from the government factory in British Sikkim. The drug would then be recommended to the indentured immigrants in Trinidad.[142] Cinchona febrifuge, thus, tended to serve the cost-effective managerial needs of the colonial medical bureaucracies. It was as well showcased as an object of 'botanical curiosity', and was solicited as an exhibit at the National Museum, Washington, in August 1881.[143]

Writing in 1888, J. A. Gammie claimed that cinchona febrifuge had inspired the manufacture of similar drugs in England and Holland. Those drugs, he suggested, circulated under the name quinetum, but credit for the preparation belonged to India: 'It is a remedy for which the whole world is indebted to India.'[144] Such assertive claims were followed by elaborate statistical detail, conveying the enormous scale of profit enabled by the venture of manufacturing cinchona febrifuge at the factory in Rungbee. Gammie claimed that the supply of cinchona febrifuge from the factory at Mungpoo increased from 1940 pounds in 1875–1876 to 87, 704 pounds in the late 1880s. The price of the commodity was shown as uniform; at 16 rupees 8 annas per pound. In the same period the average price of quinine in London appeared as 8s. 4 and ½ d. per ounce. Gammie added, 'The sterling value (calculated at this rate) of 87,704 pounds of quinine would be £587,616, while this

[139] Howard Private papers: ACC/1037/693/1–3 (LMA).
[140] T. Cadell to Officiating Secretary, Government of India, Home, Revenue and Agricultural Department, No. G426–448, 12 August 1880 Port Blair. Home, Port Blair, October 1880, 30–32 A (NAI).
[141] The Surgeon General to the Colonial Secretary, 27 May 1881, Trinidad. File 929, June–July 1881, IOR/L/PJ/6/42 (BL).
[142] Home, Medical, January 1882, 36 B (NAI).
[143] Home, Medical, April 1882, 20–22 A (NAI).
[144] Gammie, 'Manufacture of Quinine in India', 141.

quantity of febrifuge has actually been delivered to the Indian consumer for the sum of Rs. 14,47,116. The actual saving to India has, therefore, been very great, and the capital account of the plantations (about 11 lakhs of rupees) has been covered several times'.[145] Earlier, the Report of the Government cinchona plantation in Bengal and of the Government Quinologist for 1880–1881, had suggested that 'total savings' resulting from the substitution of cinchona febrifuge for quinine amounted to 'more than 16 Lakhs of rupees'.[146] In February 1888, George King similarly claimed that the saving to the government by the substitution of quinine by the febrifuge amounted to 25 lakhs of rupees, 'which is more than twice the total capital cost of the Sikkim plantation'.[147]

By the early 1880s, the managers of the cinchona plantations and the factory in British Sikkim started asserting considerable authority in the world of pharmaceutical chemistry as producers of cinchona febrifuge. It was hardly, however, an easy process. Cinchona febrifuge came under attack from different quarters. The proposal to substitute cinchona febrifuge for quinine was firmly resisted in the Madras Presidency by G. Smith, the Surgeon General, Indian Medical Department for Madras. Reports received from subordinate officials in the Presidency failed to convince him of the relative merits of cinchona febrifuge vis-à-vis quinine.[148] In the late 1860s, efforts at manufacturing medical preparations from cinchona barks began at Ootacamund and British Sikkim almost simultaneously. At this time J. F. Broughton was the Government Quinologist to the Madras Presidency and Thomas Anderson followed by C. B. Clarke were Superintendents in-charge of cinchona cultivations in Bengal. Early efforts were characterised by collaborations between them. They exchanged insights and travelled into plantations managed by one another.[149] I have already mentioned that efforts at manufacturing drugs were discontinued at Ootacamund in 1875. This made the position of the Quinologist of Madras redundant, and Broughton resigned. The post was not filled until the mid-1880s. Meanwhile, the factory at Rungbee had begun manufacturing cinchona febrifuge amongst other substitutes of quinine. Cinchona barks grown in Madras were instead made to travel into England, where they were auctioned and made available to the highest bidder. This was how long-standing pharmaceutical interests represented by the Howards or the

---

[145] Ibid., 141–142.   [146] Home, Medical, 15–16 A, August 1881 (NAI).

[147] G. King to the Secretary, Government of Bengal. Finance, Miscellaneous, August 1888, File M Q/1, Prog. 1–13 (WBSA).

[148] Home, Medical, March 1879, 55–57 A (NAI).

[149] Clarke, to the Secretary, Government of Bengal. Home, Public, 24 December 1870, 128–132 A (NAI).

Whiffens could access them as cheap raw materials for manufacturing quinine. Earlier associations between the plantations in the Niligiris and British Sikkim gradually faded. Instead, the managers of the plantations in the Nilgiris found themselves entangled in another network of pharmaceutical business marked by long-distant circulation of cinchonas. Madras was incidentally the only Presidency that had rejected the substitution of cinchona febrifuge for quinine. This decision may not have been entirely informed by apprehensions about the many vices associated with cinchona febrifuge.

It is then hardly surprising that the fiercest and most consistent voice against cinchona febrifuge should be J. E. Howards. In February 1879, for instance, Howard refused to consider the price charged for cinchona febrifuge by the managers of the factory at Rungbee as reasonable. He maintained that the government could be supplied with the 'mixed crystallised alkaloids' at the 'same or still lower price by the European manufacturers'.[150] In June 1881, he bolstered his earlier judgment by the following observation: '1 pound of sulphate cinchonine would cure 89 cases, at an expense of Rs. 5, whilst 1 pound of febrifuge might cure 65 cases, at an expense of Rs. 16, while with sulphate cinchonidine 101 cases would be cured, at an expense of less than Rs. 17 ... So much for the supposed cheapness of the febrifuge ...'.[151] In an earlier report he had asserted that the amorphous alkaloids inherent in the cinchona febrifuge 'are capable of producing death under a fearful aggravation of symptoms'.[152]

Medical bureaucrats in British India appeared to believe that cinchona febrifuge was not suitable for European soldiers. A senior member of the Indian Medical Service, Dr Ker Innes, recommended against the employment of cinchona febrifuge in the European military hospitals and in British hospitals in substitution or supersession of quinine. Reports from the members of the British Medical Department reflected similar impressions. Cinchona febrifuge was seen as a 'crude and coarse' preparation that could only cure the Indians.[153]

Such impressions were usually contested by medical bureaucrats representing the Bengal Presidency. These officials were located at various levels in the hierarchy, and included, for instance, medical officers

[150] J. E. Howard to Under Secretary of State for India, 22 February 1879, Tottenham. Home, Medical, June 1879, 17–19 A (NAI).
[151] J. E. Howard to the Under Secretary of State for India, 21 June 1881, Tottenham. Home, Medical, November 1882, 67B (NAI).
[152] J. E. Howard to the Under Secretary of State for India, 'Enclosure no. 2'. Home, Medical, February 1879, 53–57 A (NAI).
[153] J. M. Cunningham, 'Memorandum', 14 May 1878. Home, Medical, September 1878, 126–128 A; Home, Medical, November 1880, 111–119 A (NAI).

appointed by the East India Company, Dr Pilcher, the Surgeon to the Howrah Hospital, J. M. Cunningham, senior member of the Indian Medical Service and J. Irving, Surgeon General for Bengal.[154] Irving suggested that 'all medicines affect Europeans and Natives alike, and that the medicines which will cure fever or dysentery, or any other disease, in a native, will have the same effect on a European, I know of no facts to the contrary...'.[155] In a memorandum on cinchona febrifuge, Cunningham wrote, 'Papers... relating to the trial of the drug in European military hospitals... are disappointing. With exception of Lucknow and Delhi... the reports are against the use of this substitute of quinine amongst European soldiers... I confess that I do not understand the results, as I have taken the febrifuge frequently myself, and have seen other Europeans take it, with excellent results, and not a single symptom of nausea which is so much complained of'.[156]

Officials based in the Bengal Presidency did not always express themselves as a homogenous group in defence of cinchona febrifuge. In June 1879, cinchona febrifuge faced attack from its manufacturers themselves, when Wood once again claimed to have manufactured a much more efficacious drug at the factory in Rungbee. It came to be recognised as triple sulphate. Wood and George King recommended it as a much more effective substitute for quinine than cinchona febrifuge. While trying to highlight the relative efficiency of the triple sulphate over cinchona febrifuge, they ended up exposing some of the limitations associated with the latter: 'In every instance, the triple sulphate has been found to be quite efficacious as the febrifuge... and free from the objections that attach to the latter preparation. Some even regarding it as fully equal to quinine... in large doses the triple sulphate creates less constitutional disturbance than the cinchona febrifuge...'.[157] King and Wood's claims were opposed by certain sections of the medical bureaucracy within the Bengal Presidency. In May 1879, the Surgeon General of Bengal, J. F. Beatson, disagreed with King and Wood, noting 'There may perhaps be claimed for the "triple" febrifuge... a slight superiority over the cinchona febrifuge; but at what an extra expenditure – the former costs Rs. 29–9–8, the latter Rs. 16 per pound, – while the price of the former might at any time be increased'. A committee earlier appointed to examine the

---

[154] C. Macaulay to The Officiating Secretary, Government of India, Home department, No. 631, 14 February 1879, Calcutta. Home, Medical, March 1879, 58–60 A (NAI).

[155] J. Irving, to The Undersecretary to the Government of Bengal, Judicial, Political and Appointment Departments, No. 111. B G, 24 January 1879, Calcutta. Ibid.

[156] Home, Medical, November 1880, 111–119 A (NAI).

[157] G. King and C. H. Wood, 'Memorandum'. Home, Medical, October 1879, 64–80 A (NAI).

recommendations from King and Wood turned them down.[158] Wood resigned as Chemical Examiner and Quinologist to the Government of Bengal in April 1879.[159]

Drugs circulating as cinchona febrifuge thus faced opposition from a variety of quarters. Nonetheless, by the late 1870s, managers of the cinchona plantations and the factory in British Sikkim had begun engaging in effective negotiations with contending actors. The manufacturers of the extensively circulating cinchona febrifuge appeared to have acquired a set of allies and a vocabulary for articulating further ambitions. It was often recommended by various officials based in Bengal, for instance, that the practice of exporting Nilgiri barks to London be discontinued. Instead, the feasibility of converting these barks into cinchona febrifuge at the factory in British Sikkim was considered. Between June 1879 and May 1882, this suggestion was made at least twice.[160] Nothing much immediately emerged out of such proposals. However, they were symbolic of the esteem which products like cinchona febrifuge had brought to the factory at Rungbee. Such esteem, in turn, empowered its managers into indulging in the act of making more ambitious claims.

James Alexander Gammie succeeded Wood as the manager of the plantation and executive in-charge at the factory at Rungbee. In May 1881, George King asserted that Gammie's experiments at 'discovering processes for manufacturing quinine at a comparatively small cost' had proven successful. King suggested that Gammie had 'succeeded in turning out a crystalline preparation... free from the amorphous alkaloid... a pleasanter medicine than cinchona febrifuge in its present form... a very pretty preparation, being nearly as white as quinine itself...'.[161] He went on to argue the case for the drug: 'appearance is undistinguishable from, and which on analysis proves to be quite as pure as, the best English quinine...'.[162] King's claims appeared credible to several government officials in British India. Colonel R. H. Beddome, Conservator of Forests, Madras, visited the Darjeeling cinchona

[158] Beatson, to Officiating Secretary, Government of India. Ibid.; C. Bernard, Officiating Secretary to the Government of India to the Secretary, Government of Bengal, No. 385, 2 July 1879, Simla. Ibid.

[159] H. A Cockerell to the Officiating Secretary, Government of India, No. 1402, 24 July 1879, Darjeeling. Ibid.

[160] Home, Medical, June 1879, 43 B; C. Macaulay to Officiating Secretary, Government of India, No. 134, 23 January 1882, Calcutta. Home, Medical, May 1882, 58–61A (NAI).

[161] G. King, Nineteenth Annual Report of the Government Cinchona Plantations in British Sikkim, 28 May 1881. Home, Medical, August 1881, 15–16 A (NAI).

[162] G. King to Secretary, Government of Bengal, Medical and Municipal department, No. 65 Q, 14 May 1881 Darjeeling. Home, Medical, June 1881, 47–49 A (NAI).

plantations in December 1881. He recognised Gammie's preparations as 'very pure quinine'.[163] In July 1881, Dr Macnamara, the Examiner of the Medical Stores in Calcutta, presented a comparison between 'Mr Gammie's quinine' and 'Mr Whiffen's quinine'. He argued that 'Gammie's quinine' was of 'excellent quality' and 'in purity surpassed Mr Whiffen's manufacture'.[164] The response received from the office of the Secretary of State for India was, however, more lukewarm. It was admitted that the sample of 'Gammie's quinine' sent to England was indeed of 'excellent quality', but warned that Gammie's process would inevitably fail to extract the whole of valuable alkaloids from the barks, and could not profitably be undertaken on a 'large commercial scale'.[165] Drugs manufactured on a commercial scale at Rungbee would not be recognised unanimously as quinine until the late 1880s. However, it was agreed by many that Gammie's efforts in the early 1880s had resulted in considerable experimental success. It appeared that the art of manufacturing cheap and pure quinine no longer remained an elusive mystery to the managers of the factory at Rungbee. The increasing prominence of this factory was reflected in the shifting botanical identities of plants growing in the adjacent cinchona plantations.

'A Botanical Puzzle'

Along with alterations in equations of authority in the overlapping worlds of medical relief and pharmaceutical business, the botanical perceptions about particular cinchona plantations changed. In the early 1880s, King proposed a major shift in the geography of cinchonas growing in the British Indian plantations. I have already indicated that the barks of succirubra cinchona trees, which were believed to thrive in British Sikkim in the Bengal Presidency, were considered poor in quinine content. In contrast, cinchona plants belonging to the officinalis and calisaya varieties which abound in the Nilgiris were considered rich in quinine. Such impressions survived at least till June 1883.[166] This neat division was

---

[163] R. H. Beddome to Secretary, Government Revenue Department, 12 December 1881, Bombay. Home, Medical, February 1882, 42 B (NAI).

[164] 'Enclosure no. 7: Copy of a report by Dr Macnamara, dated 29 July 1881,' Home, Medical, November 1882, 67B (NAI).

[165] Secretary of State for India to the Governor General of India in Council, 30 March 1882 India Office London. Ibid.

[166] F. C. Daukes, 'Cinchona', 30 June 1883. Home, Medical, January 1884, 9–11 A (NAI).

however disputed by King on his return from an official visit to Dutch Java in November 1879.[167]

The greater part of King's report focused on a 'variety of calisaya'[168] in cultivation in Dutch Java. The bark of that particular variety was considered richer in quinine than any other bark ever imported from South America. Some of the Dutch samples had apparently revealed on analysis an extraordinary 13.7 per cent of quinine. That particular variety, King informed, was called ledgeriana. Disagreeing with preceding understandings, King asserted that quinine-rich varieties of cinchonas could thrive in the plantations at British Sikkim, suggesting that plants of ledgeriana had already survived there for more than a decade. The managers of the plantation, he claimed, had been unaware of its identity. His experience in Java apparently proved that 'three of our best kinds of calisaya are precisely the same as some of the forms of ledgeriana cultivated by the Dutch . . . '. He was satisfied that the 'true ledger calisaya' grew in Sikkim, and advocated that its cultivation should be maximised.[169]

King did not mention whether he had carried any sample of ledgeriana from Java for comparison with plants in British Sikkim.[170] He seemed to rely more on the authority of the claim itself, and showed little interest in establishing his claims. He suggested that cinchona barks that yielded the Dutch such an alarmingly high percentage of quinine were raised from a parcel of seeds purchased in 1866 by the Dutch government from an English collector named Charles Ledger. The presence and survival of such ledgeriana plants in British Sikkim, however, did not seem out of place to King. He claimed that 'a pinch of those seeds' was purchased from Ledger in the 1860s by J. W. B. Money, a private planter in British India, who exchanged those seeds for succirubra with McIvor, the head of the government cinchona plantations at Madras Presidency. McIvor, in turn, conveyed them to a colleague based in Bengal. King claimed that those seeds 'were obtained at second hand from the Nilgiris'.[171]

King appeared to project the plantations he managed as pregnant with unlimited sources of quinine. This coincided with the claim that Gammie had acquired the technical skills of manufacturing experimental samples of pure quinine. King's observations barely seemed absurd to his contemporaries. There was no official report dismissing or even

---

[167] G. King to Secretary, Government of Bengal, Revenue department, No. 96 C, 22 November 1879 Royal Botanical Gardens, Howrah. Home, Medical, January 1880, 24–26A (NAI).

[168] Ibid.   [169] Ibid.

[170] C. Bernard, Officiating Secretary, Government of India to the Secretary, Government of Bengal, 8 January 1880, Fort William. Ibid.

[171] J. H. Holland, 'Ledger Bark and Red Bark', *Bulletin of Miscellaneous Information (Royal Gardens, Kew)*, 1 (1932), 1–17.

questioning his claims. This could have been evidence of the authority King had begun commanding as the Superintendent of the cinchona cultivation in Bengal since late 1870s, and as a mentor to the increasingly significant cinchona factory at Mungpoo.

This also coincided with a phase of intense impasse in the botanical classification of cinchonas grown in the British Indian plantations. Robert Cross had been an associate of C. R. Markham in the exploration of the 'cinchona forests' of South America in the late 1850s. In 1879, Cross returned to South America to collect cinchona plants under instructions from the office of the Secretary of State for India.[172] On his return, Cross claimed to have discovered considerable discrepancies involving the 'true identities' and names of different varieties of cinchonas grown in the government plantations. 'The plant hitherto termed cinchona succirubra is micrantha...the tree known on the estates as "McIvor's hybrid" and "pubescens" is the true cinchona succirubra...the plant designated "magnifolia" is the pata de gallinazo of the red bark regions of South America'.[173]

Cross was not alone in asserting such discrepancies. Colonel R. H. Beddome, Conservator of Forests, Madras Presidency had similar reservations.[174] In 1881, Beddome was deputed to visit, inspect and report on the cinchona plantations in Ceylon and British Sikkim. He reported about similar confusion in identifying and naming plants in Ceylon. 'I was much interested to find the "pata de gallinazo" described by Mr Cross, the species hitherto known here as "magnifolia"... The same species is in Ceylon generally known as "hybrid" though it has other names and is sometimes called "condaminea"...'.[175] Lack of clarity about the identity of each species, argued Beddome, was detrimental to commercial interests. Having encountered a plantation of 'hybrid calisaya' near Nuwara Eliya, Beddome observed: 'The trees...would completely puzzle any botanist...whether they are distinct species or all forms of one very protean species...analysis is all important in a plantation of this sort, if profit is to be looked to...as forms apparently similar in every way may in some individuals be very rich in quinine and in others have no trace of it'.[176]

This questioning of plants and their identities provoked responses beyond India. The authorities at Kew Gardens initially tried to distance

[172] Home, Medical, June 1880, 26 B (NAI).

[173] Surgeon General Bidie to the Secretary to Government, Revenue Department, Madras, No.199, 3 March 1882. Home, Medical, April 1882, 80 B (NAI).

[174] W. T. Thiselton Dyer to L. Mallet, 24 January 1882 Royal Gardens, Kew. Home, Medical, May 1882, 37 B (NAI).

[175] Home, Medical, November 1881, 41 B (NAI).   [176] Ibid.

themselves, but later determined to resolve the confusion. The commercial value of cinchona trade appeared too great to allow such confusion.[177] This initiated a series of correspondence involving senior officials at Kew including Joseph Hooker, Thiselton Dyer, and Benj H. Paul of the Analytical laboratory in London, Hartington, the Secretary of State for India, Dr Trimen, the Director of the Botanic Gardens at Ceylon, Dr Bidie and the Superintendent, Central Government Central Museum at Madras.[178]

In this context King made two claims: first, the cinchona plants in the plantations in British Sikkim belonged as much to the calisaya varieties as they did to the succirubra species; second, the calisaya trees in British Sikkim actually belonged to the superior ledgeriana variety. It was a situation when the accepted identities of different varieties of cinchonas were subjected to intense scrutiny and revision. This explains why King's claims were not immediately denounced as absurd.

King's claims had their effects. The landscape of British Sikkim suddenly seemed compatible with the proliferation of quinine-yielding cinchonas. In 1881, he noted how the existing succirubra trees in British Sikkim were being gradually uprooted to make room for calisaya and ledgeriana.[179] Colonel Beddome, touring the plantations in British Sikkim in late 1881, noted that 200 acres had been assigned to plant 'young ledgeriana'. He found 150 calisaya and ledgeriana trees in British Sikkim as against 4,320,000 succirubra trees.[180] In the course of the 1880s, evidence suggests a gradual decrease in the number of succirubra trees in these plantations. This converged with a sharp rise in the number of quinine-rich yellow bark trees (i.e., ledgeriana, calisaya, verde, morada).[181] By 1885, quinine-rich yellow bark trees in these plantations numbered more than 1,200,000.[182] Writing in 1888, Gammie observed: 'Calisaya and its variety ledgeriana really thrives in Sikkim . . . succirubra has been supplanted by calisaya to the extent of about a million trees'.[183] Early 1880s onwards, the landscape of British Sikkim thus seemed particularly malleable to cultivate quinine-rich cinchona plants (see Figure 4.4).

[177] W. T. Thiselton Dyer to L. Mallet, 13 June 1882 Royal Gardens, Kew. Home, Medical, November 1882, 67 B.

[178] Ibid.

[179] From in-charge of the Cinchona cultivation in Bengal, No. 37, 28 May 1881, Home, Medical, August 1881, 15–16 A (NAI).

[180] Beddome to the Secretary to the Government. Home, Medical, February 1882, 42 B (NAI).

[181] 'Resolution', 30 May 1884 Darjeeling. Home, Medical, June 1884, 81–84 A (NAI).

[182] 'Resolution', 19 June 1885 Darjeeling Home, Medical, July 1885, 40–43 A (NAI).

[183] Gammie, 'Manufacture of Quinine in India', 142.

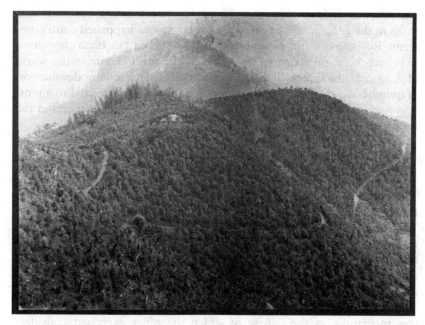

Figure 4.4 Photograph of a 'Ridge covered with Cinchona Ledgeriana in Munsong, British Sikkim'. Unnamed photographer. Credit: Wellcome Library, London.

Such impressions were reflected in a variety of official correspondence. In July 1882, for instance, a collection of plants and seeds belonging to the 'china cuprea' variety of cinchona, collected from South America and considered 'good quinine yielders' was sent to British Sikkim with the understanding that it would 'grow well' there.[184] In September 1883, a sample packet containing cinchona calisaya seeds was sent from South America through Messrs Christy of London to British Sikkim. The seedlings were eventually planted out, and 'thrived well'. Even when they were 'too young' to be classified with 'absolute certainty', Gammie preferred to identify them as ledgeriana.[185]

Since the early 1860s, quinine-yielding varieties of cinchonas were considered the exclusive privilege of a very few plantations and particular landscapes. In the 1880s, however, such trees appeared much

[184] E. N. Baker to Secretary, Government of India, Revenue and Agricultural Department, 7 June 1882 Darjeeling. Home, Medical, July 1882, 15–16 B (NAI).
[185] Acting Superintendent, Cinchona plantations, Darjeeling to the Officiating Under Secretary, Government of Bengal, Financial Department, 17 September 1883, Mungpoo. Home, Medical, April 1884, 46–47 B (NAI).

less rare than before. Newer assertions of pharmaceutical authority and shifts in the geographies of quinine-rich cinchonas happened simultaneously. Revisions in the botanical knowledge about cinchonas appeared to reflect the unprecedented prominence of British Sikkim in the world of drug manufacturers. This converged with a decade-long devaluation of quinine as a medical commodity which, in turn, was related to a temporary decay in the prestige commanded by the erstwhile experts in the manufacture of pure quinine.

An 'Experiment' in London

The year 1880 saw crucial changes in the office of the Secretary of State for India, as the Marquis of Hartington replaced Viscount Cranbrook. This office had been so long preoccupied with liaising efforts relating to the manufacture of pure quinine in British India. Correspondence between the managers of cinchona plantations and factories in British India and the European and Javanese experts on quinine were either received through this office or carried in its name. The most significant role performed by this office between the late 1860s and 1880 was mediation, in the course of which the office exercised considerable agency. Under Hartington, however, the office began intervening more directly, becoming more assertive in relation to contending actors. The tone was set by disagreement with some of the measures proposed by King. King's report on his trip to Java had concluded by proposing new sites where cinchona plantations might be contemplated, for instance, in the Andaman Islands, Khasia hills and Burma.[186] This was followed by extensive initiatives relating to King's proposed trip to the Andamans for supervising the selection of prospective sites.[187] The Secretary of State, however, considered King's proposals not 'necessary or desirable'.[188]

In September 1880, the Secretary of State proposed an 'experiment'. The auction of cinchona barks (exported from the government plantations in the Madras Presidency to the highest bidder) in London was to be discontinued. Instead, quinine and 'other alkaloids' were to be extracted from the Madras barks in London by 'established quinine

---

[186] King to Secretary, Government of Bengal. Home, Medical, January 1880, 24–26A (NAI).

[187] Home, Medical, February 1880, 53–54 B (NAI).

[188] Secretary of State for India to Governor General of India in Council, No. 85 (Revenue), 14 October 1880 India Office. Home, Medical, December 1880, 51 A (NAI).

manufacturers', on government account, precisely for the British Indian market. The experiment was supposed to be consonant with the declared governmental goal of distributing pure quinine in British India at the cheapest possible price. The Howards and the Whiffens were asked to tender and submit detailed responses. The Howards agreed to receive all the Nilgiri bark sent to London and in return to supply the government with as much quinine and alkaloids as they might require. They suggested the following conditions: 'Government would be their own analysts, and would receive a price proportional to such analysis;... and Government would also be gainers by the saving in brokerage and intermediate profits...'.[189] After 1880, auction of Nilgiri barks in London was discontinued, but the Howards retained convenient access to the Nilgiri barks. The alliance with the office of the Secretary of State for India was presumably profitable: in April 1883, having extracted 803 pounds of febrifuge from a consignment of 200 bags of red cinchona bark, Messrs Howard and Sons earned £441.[190]

In March 1882, the office of the Secretary of State reacted adversely to suggestions that the manufacture of quinine in Sikkim could be initiated on a large scale in accordance with the method proposed by Gammie. Recommendations that a large factory be set up in British Sikkim to utilise the Nilgiri barks in addition to the barks from Darjeeling were rejected on the grounds that the process was not new and had little to offer.[191] The Secretary of State instead suggested that barks from the Darjeeling plantations could be 'more profitably worked in England for the extraction of sulphate of quinine than in India'. He asked for 600 bales of different kinds of barks from Darjeeling in London to verify his assumptions. His suggestions in turn were firmly resisted by senior bureaucrats in Bengal,[192] including King, J. M. Cunningham and the Lieutenant Governor. In the early 1880s, it seemed that the managers of the cinchona factory in British Sikkim and the Office of the Secretary of State for India were competing for access to cinchona barks produced in British India.

[189] Secretary of State for India to Governor in Council, Fort St George, Madras, No. 39 (Revenue), 16 September 1880, London. Home, Medical, November 1880, 103–108 A (NAI).
[190] Secretary of State for India to Governor General of India in Council, No. 32 (Revenue), 8 May 1884 India Office. Home, Medical, June 1884, 50–54 A (NAI).
[191] Secretary of State for India to Governor General of India in Council, 30 March 1882, India Office London. Home, Medical, November 1882, 67 B dated 30 March India Office London, 1882. See especially 'No. 1 Enclosure. Report on the manufacture of Sulphate of Quinine and other Cinchona alkaloids on Government account'.
[192] Government of Bengal, 'Cinchona', No. 370, 15 February 1883. Home, Medical, April 1883, 38–40 A (NAI).

As I have indicated, the control of the Secretary of State over the barks grown in the Nilgiris was much more complete.[193] In the early 1880s, private business interests based in the Madras Presidency were keen on procuring cinchonas grown in the government plantations in Madras. By April 1882, Messrs Croysdale and Co., Messrs Parry and Co., Messrs Dymes and Co., and Messrs F Muraglia and Co. had made several applications to the Acting Commissioner of the Nilgiris to allow the auction sale of the Madras barks at Messrs Oaks and Co.'s salesrooms in Madras itself. Such sales were quite profitable, but were rarely organised. N. A. Roupell, Acting Commissioner of the Nilgiris explained the situation: 'It is the wish of the government that a local demand should be developed without interfering with the experiments now in progress in England for the manufacture of quinine and other alkaloids from the government plantation bark. It will be necessary, therefore, that the sales would be limited...'.[194]

While engaging the 'established manufacturers' in extracting quinine and other forms of febrifuge in London on its behalf, the office of the Secretary of State faced certain difficulties. Most of these related to transport insurance and irregularities involving freight charged on shipment.[195] However, the most irreparable oversight in relation to the Secretary of State's experiment surfaced in the official registers after June 1883. It was the fear of overproduction and wastage. It was admitted on behalf of the office of the Secretary of State for India that the 'result of the manufacture in London during the last three years has been to accumulate a stock both of quinine and other alkaloids, and of febrifuge, for which there is no immediate demand in India'.[196] The stock, it was feared, would outlast the anticipated demand in British India for many years. This could initiate a phase of unprecedented devaluation of quinine in British India.

However, it might be naïve to consider 'demand of quinine and febrifuge in British India' as a disinterested and objective description. Knowledge of such demand or the lack of it was contingent upon projections and mediations from officials based in British India. The agency of the managers of the cinchona factory and plantations in British Sikkim, senior officials in the medical depot and medical bureaucracy

---

[193] For an understanding of the varied terms and modalities of correspondences between the Madras Government and the Office of the Secretary of State for India see, Home, Medical, February 1882, 65B (NAI).

[194] Home, Medical, May 1882, 36 B (NAI).

[195] Home, Medical, February 1882, 53 B; Home, Medical, October 1881, 86 B (NAI).

[196] Secretary of State for India to the Governor General of India in Council, No. 68 (Revenue), 18 October 1883, India Office London. Home, Medical, January 1884, 9–11 A (NAI).

in Bengal, and their colleagues and subordinates towards circulating such perceptions can hardly be exaggerated.[197] In a memorandum titled 'Cinchona' submitted by the British Indian medical bureaucrat F. C. Danvers in June 1883, the accumulated excess stocks of quinine and cinchona febrifuge were reported as 3595 pounds and 7576 pounds, respectively.[198] As a trademark of the government, these had already been coloured with carmine before circulation in British India. These products were, therefore, considered 'unsaleable' in Europe.[199]

The manufacture of quinine and febrifuge on government account in London from Nilgiri barks continued and inevitably augmented the accumulated stock. Worse still, the office of Secretary of State for India was anticipating fresh shipments of barks from the Nilgiris. This alleged inability to maintain parity between anticipated demand in British India and manufacture in London was admitted as a source of collective embarrassment which the Howards, the Whiffens and the office of the Secretary of State for India shared. To reduce the accumulated stock of surplus cinchona barks from Madras, the Howards were requested to accept payment for manufacturing charges entirely in bark instead of money.[200] The remaining stock of barks consigned to the office of the Secretary of State from Madras, it was proposed, could be made available by 'the former system of sale by auction' in London. The Secretary of State for India was thus compelled to discontinue the experiment of engaging 'established manufacturers' to extract quinine and other alkaloids in London on government account from barks grown in the Nilgiris.[201] In March 1884, the Secretary of State thought it prudent to advise against any further shipment of cinchona barks from the Nilgiris to London.[202]

In the wake of this embarrassment, the Secretary of State for India was confronted with the challenge of distributing the accumulated stock of quinine and febrifuge in British India. It was a concern that plagued the office of the Secretary of State for India until November 1887. To get rid of the accumulated stock in London, the Secretary of State

---

[197] For instance, see A. J. Payne to the Secretary, Government of Bengal, Municipal Department, No. 2362, 9 April 1884, Calcutta. Home, Medical, June 1884, 36–43 A (NAI).

[198] F. C. Danvers, 'Cinchona', June 1883. Ibid.

[199] Secretary of State for India to the Governor General of India in Council. Home, Medical, January 1884, 9–11 A (NAI).

[200] Danvers, 'Cinchona', June 1883. Home, Medical, June 1884, 36–43 A (NAI).

[201] E. N. Baker, to the Secretary, Government of India, Home department, 15 May 1884 Darjeeling, Ibid.

[202] Secretary of State for India to the Governor in Council of Fort St. George, 27 March 1884, India Office. Home, Medical, June 1884, 30–31 B (NAI).

decided to make the 'English-made febrifuge' available in 'special localities especially affected with malaria at a nominal price'. It was believed
that it could reach out to the 'very poor classes who are unable to buy
the Sikkim febrifuge'. The Secretary of State's proposals were driven
by an aspiration to replace the Sikkim febrifuge by the 'English-made
febrifuge' as the most benevolent face of medical governance in British
India. It was feared by the Secretary of State that the 'English-made
febrifuge' might not readily be purchased in British India even when
offered at a nominal price. Alternatively, the stock of 'English-made
febrifuge' could be considered for 'gratuitous distribution'.[203] It was
decided to distribute the 'English-made febrifuge' to 'out of the way
places where the Indian febrifuge does not now reach'.[204]

The desperation with which the Secretary of State for India set out
to dispose of the accumulated stock of quinine and febrifuge into dispensaries in British India was striking. It is hardly surprising that the
managers of the factory and plantations in British Sikkim should use
this opportunity to assert their relative superiority as manufacturers. In
February 1885, King described the febrifuge manufactured in London
as a lesser drug. He feared that the circulation of an inferior drug under
the same name might tarnish the image of the febrifuge he was associated
with. He proposed a couple of measures to enable the convenient delineation of these drugs as two different commodities. He suggested that
either the London drug be purified in the Bengal factory or be coloured
before issue to distinguish it from the Sikkim version. These comments
suggest how British Indian bureaucrats had subjected the 'English-made
febrifuge' as well as its manufacturers to vigorous condescension in the
mid-1880s.[205]

In June 1884, following recommendations from the Secretary of State
for India, it was decided to distribute the stock of quinine and febrifuge
accumulated in London amongst the Bengal, Bombay and Madras Presidencies. A quarter of the stock was to be sent to the government of
Madras. Another quarter went to the government of Bombay. The
remaining half was to be sent to Calcutta for distribution in the Bengal Presidency. Subsequently, it was predicted on behalf of the government of India that the proposed transfer of accumulated stock of
quinine would suffice for the requirements of the Medical Department

---

[203] E. N. Baker to the Secretary, Government of India, Home department, 15 May 1884,
Darjeeling. Home, Medical, June 1884, 36–43 A (NAI).

[204] E. N. Baker to the Surgeon General Bengal, No. 262 T-M, 19 April 1884, Darjeeling.
Ibid.

[205] G. King to the Secretary, Government of Bengal, Financial department, No. 23 Q, 19
February 1885, Howrah. Home, Medical, May 1886, 83–86 B (NAI).

in British India for many years to come, and would make any further indents unnecessary in the foreseeable future.[206] In the mid-1880s then the image of quinine underwent crucial changes in the pharmaceutical market of British India. It ceased to be seen as a rare and expensive drug. By the latter half of the decade, quinine revealed itself as a commodity in overabundant supply. It was going through a phase of considerable depreciation in value. These were reflected in the price charged for the commodity.

An Expensive Substitute

Official reports from Bengal claimed that the price of cinchona febrifuge manufactured in British Sikkim remained relatively stable through the course of the 1880s, in contrast to the drastic reduction in the price of quinine imported from England.[207] The difference between the price of quinine and cinchona febrifuge appeared considerably less than before. Quinine now figured as a much more affordable commodity, and cinchona febrifuge began to be considered an expensive substitute for a relatively cheap commodity. 'At present quinine can be bought freely in Calcutta for Rs. 2–1 per ounce. There is therefore comparatively little inducement to the public to buy febrifuge at about half that price. It was quite a different matter quite a few years ago when the bazaar rate of quinine was seven or eight times higher than at present...'.[208]

In November 1888, A. P. MacDonnell, the Secretary to the Government of India, expressed concern about the 'present high price of cinchona febrifuge' manufactured in British Sikkim. He pointed out that King had promised to sell quinine at the rate of Rs.1 per ounce or Rs. 16 per pound. By contrast, the Sikkim febrifuge was being sold at Rs. 16–8 per pound, a price which, he suggested, was introduced when the price of quinine was high enough to alienate the poorer classes. He argued that decline in the price of quinine should be followed by a corresponding reduction in the price of cinchona febrifuge.[209]

In response to such criticisms, King recommended the reduction of the price of cinchona febrifuge from Rs. 16–8 per pound to Rs. 14 per pound.[210] Quinine supplied to the Bombay depot in early 1889 was

---

[206] The Government of India to Secretary of State for India, No. 31, 13 June 1884, Simla. Home, Medical, June 1884, 36–43 A (NAI).

[207] Home, Medical, September 1886, 57–59A (NAI).   [208] Ibid.

[209] Home, Medical, November 1888, 43–44A (NAI).

[210] G. King to the Secretary, Government of Bengal, Financial Department, No. 2 Q, 3 January 1889, Seebpore. Home, Medical, March 1889, 117–118 A (NAI).

invoiced at Rs. 16–7–9. In view of such a 'phenomenally low' price for quinine, the substitution of cinchona febrifuge for quinine made little sense. The Surgeon General of Bombay suggested that the proportion of such acts of substitution should be diminished from 75 per cent to 50 per cent.[211]

An annual report of the government cinchona plantation and cinchona factory in Bengal, published earlier in June 1887, took note of the 'extraordinary cheapness of quinine'. This cheapness was explained in terms of a 'series of years of depression' in the cinchona planting business.[212] The 'real cause' was thought to be 'abnormal export' of cinchona from Ceylon. The planters in Ceylon were apparently uprooting cinchona trees to make room for tea. Such trees were feared to have become 'almost universally unhealthy'. The export of cinchona plants from Ceylon in the preceding three years, it was suggested, averaged a staggering fifteen million pounds annually.[213] The relative decline in the price of quinine vis-à-vis cinchona febrifuge also began to be felt beyond the shores of British India. Mr Butler, the Keeper of the Medical Stores in Jamaica, for instance, mentioned in 1887 that the cost of buying one ounce of cinchona febrifuge from British Sikkim was higher than importing equal amount of quinine from London. The Medical department of Jamaica reportedly paid Rs. 2–10 1/2 per ounce for Sikkim febrifuge as opposed to Rs. 2- 9 3/8 per ounce for quinine.[214] In the distant United States, the decline in the price of quinine in the ten years following 1879 was reported as 'magical'. In five years it had fallen from $3.40 per ounce to $1.23 and in ten years to 35 cents.[215]

From 'Discovery' to 'Invention'

It was in this context of an extensive slump in the price of quinine that Gammie claimed to have discovered a process for manufacturing cheap and yet 'very best and pure' quinine at the factory in Mungpoo.[216]

---

[211] G. King to Secretary, Government of Bengal, Financial Department, No. 106 Q, 22 July 1889, Seebpore. Home, Medical, October 1889, 19–21 A (NAI).

[212] G. King to Secretary, Government of Bengal, Financial department, No. 25, 9 June 1887, Seebpore. Home, Medical, December 1887, 63–65 A (NAI).

[213] C. Macaulay, 'Resolution', 22 November 1887, Calcutta. Ibid.

[214] W. Fawcett to the Secretary of State for the Colonies, No. 1837, 6 June 1887, Jamaica. Home, Medical, October 1887, 64–70 A (NAI).

[215] I. M. Tarbell, *The Tariff in Our Times* (New York: The Macmillan Company, 1911), 93, 280 quoted in F. W. Taussig, 'Public Finance, Taxation and Tariff', *The American Economic Review*, 2, 1 (March 1912), 132–134.

[216] J. A. Gammie to Secretary Government of Bengal, Financial Department, No. 43c, 2 July 1888, Mungpoo. Home, Medical, January 1889, 38–41 A (NAI).

Erstwhile contenders of such claims did not voice much dissent. The alliance between the 'established manufacturers' and the office of the Secretary of State for India had just ended in crucial miscalculations and shared embarrassment. In the latter half of the 1880s, the Howards and the Whiffens appeared to distance themselves from questions concerning quinine manufacture in British India in pursuit of other preoccupations. Thomas Whiffen acquired the business of George Atkinson and Co. in 1887 and diverted more attention towards the manufacture of antimony compounds, clove oil, mercury sublimate, almond oil, vermilion, iodine, iodides, iodoform, bromides and camphor.[217] The Howards similarly found themselves entangled into other concerns. John Eliot Howard died at the age of 75 in 1883. David Howard, a nephew of J. E. Howard, and William Dillworth Howard, J. E. Howard's son, took over. J. E. Howard's death was preceded by considerable imprecision and confusion within the family, relating to clauses in the articles involving partnership. Hierarchical distinctions involving 'partner', 'senior partner' and 'sleeping partner' were subjected to probe and revision.[218] By April 1886, the Howards were considering suggestions for investing in synthetic preparations of quinine.[219]

Parallel claims for manufacturing pure quinine were, however, received from private interests based in the Madras Presidency. Government efforts at manufacturing quinine had been abandoned at Ootacamund in the mid-1870s. The post of the Quinologist to the Government of Madras remained unoccupied for more than a decade. By the mid-1880s, supplies of Nilgiri barks exceeded the demand and were declared unwanted in the London market. Firms like Messrs Arbuthnot and Co. were keen on accessing and investing in those barks for the manufacture of quinine at a private factory in the Madras Presidency. A group of 'English capitalists' hired a scientific chemist, Dr E. L. Cleaver. Experimental manufacture began under his supervision at Calicut by September 1885.[220] In response, the office of the Secretary of State for India and the senior officials in the Madras Presidency were discouraging. The Secretary of State appointed D. Hooper as the Government Quinologist of Madras. Under his supervision, attempts at manufacturing quinine at a government factory in Madras were resumed. Such efforts

[217] Rupert S. Law, *The End of a Chapter: The Story of Whiffen and Sons Limited, Fine Chemical Manufacturers* (London: Fisons, 1973), 7 (WL).
[218] Howard Private Papers. ACC/1037/706/2 (LMA).
[219] Howard Private Papers. ACC/1037/707/1,3 (LMA).
[220] Note no. 1016 (Revenue), 11 September 1885. Home, Medical, November 1885, 52–54 A (NAI).

promised to consume the bulk of the cinchona barks cropped in the Nilgiris. Hooper claimed to have prepared a drug 'fluid cinchona febrifuge' and in July 1886, the Deputy Surgeon General with the Madras Government, G. Bidie, offered generous comments on the preparation. He described the product as 'efficient, safe, stable and cheap'.[221] Samples of quinine manufactured by Dr Cleaver on behalf of Messrs Arbuthnot and Co. were subjected to analysis by Dr Cornish, the Surgeon General of Madras and Hooper. Cornish found it 'so far . . . not very satisfactory'.[222] Hooper predicted that the commercial value would be 'greatly impaired' in the 'present dogmatic state of the market'.[223] Private interests in the manufacture of quinine based in the Madras Presidency failed to resist the claims of Gammie.

Such undermining of private initiatives towards extracting quinine in the Madras Presidency was hardly new. Proposals for setting up a private quinine manufactory had been mooted by one Colonel Henderson, a resident of Devala in the Nilgiri district in July 1882.[224] Similar proposals were repeated in a detailed letter addressed by Messrs H. Stranborough, Hinde and others to the Under Secretary of State for India in January 1884.[225] These failed to receive sympathetic consideration from the Office of the Secretary of State for India. The Office denied private proprietors of a proposed local factory on the Nilgiris the right to import alcohol free of duty, or to supply them with fuel at cost price or concessions in acquiring land.[226]

Thus the attitude of officials associated with British Indian governments towards private interests had been various and ambiguous. At one level, pharmaceutical families like Howards or Whiffens were recognised as 'established manufacturers' of quinine. Until the mid-1880s, the Office of the Secretary of State for India looked up to them for deriving legitimacy and initiating respectable alliances. This is not to overlook the different ways officials based in British India set limits to the authority asserted by these families.

---

[221] G. Bidie to the Secretary, Government of Madras, (Revenue), No. 0–276, 16 July 1886, Ootacamund. Home, Medical, May 1887, 44–51 A (NAI).

[222] M. A. Lawson to Secretary, Government of Madras (Revenue), No. 28, 9 July 1885, Ootacamund. Home, Medical, November 1885, 52–54 A (NAI).

[223] M. A. Lawson to the Secretary, Government Revenue Department, No. 7, 1 May 1885, Ootacamund. Home, Medical, March 1886, 8–9 B (NAI).

[224] F. Henderson to the Private Secretary to the Governor of Madras, 10 June 1882, Devela. Home, Medical, November 1882, 9B (NAI).

[225] Note dated 21 January 1884, 9 Mincing Lane, London. Home, Medical, May 1884, 8–11 A (NAI).

[226] Secretary of State for India to the Governor in Council, Madras, No. 29 (Revenue), 28 August 1884 London. Ibid.

Through the course of the 1860s, the usual attitude of the government towards private planters in British India, on the other hand, was one of patronage. This gave way to frequent bouts of competition, allegation and denial.[227] At the same time, the office of the Secretary of State for India, as I have just noted, was more dismissive and discouraging towards private initiatives for extracting quinine in factories based in British India. Thus, different constituents and layers within the British Indian governments had to engage with diverse sets of private interests. These engagements manifested in a variety of ways over time. Ironically, as I will point out in what follows, the managers of the factory at Mungpoo vindicated their 'discovery' by evoking the private manufacturing interests based in British India.

In July 1888, Gammie claimed credit for having discovered a 'cheap process' for the manufacture of 'pure sulphate of quinine'.[228] Both Gammie and King admitted that the market price of quinine had slumped into an unprecedented low in the latter half of the 1880s. In such a situation, the discovery of a cheap process might not have been considered an extraordinary achievement. Colman Macaulay, Secretary to the Government, observed that Gammie's process would never cost more than Rs. 25 per pound. However, he added, that quinine was then obtainable in the open market at similar or lower rates anyway.[229] King predicted that the product resulting from this 'new process' could be circulated at Rs. 1 per ounce. In comparison, 'Howard's quinine', he continued, was 'obtainable in the open market at the unprecedented low rate of one rupee and nine annas per ounce'.[230]

However, both Macaulay and King acknowledged that the decline in the market price of quinine had been caused by 'entirely exceptional circumstances' – the 'abnormal exports' of cinchona barks from plantations in British Ceylon and Dutch Java. As a result, they argued, the barks from South America had been almost driven out of the market. This converged with the excessive production of quinine in London on government account. Macaulay and King predicted that such a situation would not continue for very long. The market would revert back to

---

[227] For instance, see G. King to Secretary, Government of Bengal, Financial Department, 30 May 1881, Howrah. Home, Medical, June 1881, 47–49 A (NAI); Secretary of State for India to the Governor General of India in Council, No. 68 (revenue), 18 October 1883, London. Municipal, Medical, File 1, Prog.1–16, April 1884 (WBSA). See especially the allegations made by J. W. B. Money on 28 June 1875.

[228] Gammie, to Secretary, Government of Bengal, Financial Department. Home, Medical, January 1889, 38–41 A (NAI).

[229] Gammie, 'Manufacture of Quinine in India', 142.

[230] G. King to the Secretary, Government of Bengal, Financial Department. Finance, Miscellaneous, August 1888, File M Q/1, Pros 1–13 (WBSA).

the 'ordinary course'. The 'new process', it was argued, would enable the price to remain low despite the unpredictability of the market. The novelty in the discovery, it was claimed, lay in its ability to impose a 'permanent reduction' in the price of quinine.[231]

Such apparent novelty inspired the government of Bengal to file an application requesting a patent for the process. It was communicated to the Bengal Government by T. T. Allen, Superintendent and Remembrancer of Legal Affairs, that such a petition could only be filed by an 'individual' in accordance with the Section 15 of Act XV, 1859. Such 'exclusive privilege' could only be granted to the 'inventor'.[232] Such legal compulsions necessitated the refashioning of the 'discovery' as an 'invention'.[233] Gammie was chosen to file the application on behalf of the Bengal government citing himself as the 'inventor'. G. C. Paul, the Advocate General, advised the Bengal Government that once the patent had been granted it could be purchased from Gammie. The government could thereafter become the patentee by assignment and be entitled to all the rights and benefits accruing from the patent.[234]

Despite the application for patent, neither Gammie nor King appeared absolutely certain about the technical originality of the process. Neither the title of the 'invention' nor its description in the application mentioned the word quinine: 'A process for the extraction of the alkaloids from cinchona bark by means of alkalis and oil . . .'.[235] King seemed confident that the process resembled the 'European oil processes' already in use. His detailed narrative of the history of the discovery acknowledged debt to the German quinine makers. He admitted that on his trip of Europe in 1884, he set out to 'discover' the process used in Germany.[236] The *Calcutta Gazette* observed that the process was 'an adaptation of a Dutch plan of manufacture'.[237] Wood himself admitted elsewhere that during his stay in Holland, King 'had acquired some valuable

---

[231] Gammie, 'Manufacture of Quinine in India', 142.

[232] T. T. Allen to Under Secretary, Government of Bengal, Finance department, No. 1489, 7 March 1888, Calcutta. Finance, Miscellaneous, File M Q/1, Pros 1–13 August 1888 (WBSA).

[233] Government of Bengal, 'Diary no. 251', No. 1386, 27 March 1888. Home, Patents, June 1888, 166–169 A (NAI).

[234] T. T. Allen to Under-Secretary, Government of Bengal, Finance, No. 395, 22 June 1888, Calcutta. Finance, Miscellaneous, August 1888, File M Q/1, Pros 1–13 (WBSA).

[235] R. L. Upton to the Under-Secretary to the Government of India, No. 2487, 24 March 1888, Calcutta. Home, Patents, June 1888, 166–169 A (NAI).

[236] King to the Secretary, Government of Bengal, Financial Department. Finance, Miscellaneous, August 1888, File M Q/1, Pros 1–13 (WBSA).

[237] J. Gammie to the Secretary, Government of Bengal, Financial Department. No. 9, 1 June 1888, Mungpoo. Ibid.

information regarding the paraffine oil process as used in the continental oil factories'.[238]

What Gammie and King considered original, unique and novel in their discovery was the declared intention. By indulging in the rhetoric of benevolence the managers of the factory at Mungpoo emphasised a place for themselves in the world of quinine manufacturers. The Bengal government rhetorically denied any desire to derive profit from the discovery.[239] King suggested that quinine makers in England and Germany had so far concealed the process of making quinine as a 'trade secret'. Despite considerable increase in the consumption of quinine in the latter half of the 1880s, the manufacture of quinine was still restricted allegedly to an exclusive club of manufacturers. Only two firms in England and a few others in Germany claimed to manufacture it. This, King argued, was responsible for the high price usually commanded by quinine in the market. He justified the patent application as a means to protect private efforts in British India from the 'quinine-makers in Europe'.

King appeared to fear that the 'Mungpoo process' could be closely similar to methods pursued by European firms. Once the details of the 'Mungpoo process' reached Europe, King predicted, 'quinine-makers' could try to prevent its use by patenting an exactly similar process in British India. This could be a danger to the 'private cinchona growers' who might effectually be prohibited from using this process. This could leave the project of circulating cheap and pure quinine in British India incomplete. 'Government should patent the Mungpoo process and announce that it does so with the intention of allowing it to be freely used by any one in India'.[240] A month later, in March 1888, Colman Macaulay, the Secretary to the Government of Bengal rephrased King's words: '. . . The application has been submitted on behalf of the Government of Bengal, with the view of only preventing any one concerned in the manufacture of quinine from obtaining a monopoly in India. Mr Gammie's application is merely filed as a bar to any other claim to patent the process in question . . .'.[241]

The claim of 'inventing a new process' at the Mungpoo factory was thus founded on the promise of 'permanent reduction' in the price of quinine. The apparent insistence on a humanitarian agenda made

---

[238] C. H. Wood, 'Memorandum on the fusel oil process of manufacturing quinine'. Rev-Agriculture, Agriculture, November 1891, 29 B (NAI).

[239] Gammie, 'Manufacture of Quinine in India', 142–143.

[240] King to Secretary, Government of Bengal, Financial Department. Finance, Miscellaneous, August 1888, File M Q/1, Pros 1–13 (WBSA).

[241] Government of Bengal, 'Diary no. 251'. Home, Patents, June 1888, 166–169 A (NAI).

the managers of the factory accountable to a range of scrutiny. Price emerged as a crucial index around which the credibility of manufacturers could be measured. 'What has been the average price of quinine for the year?'[242] Was Mungpoo indeed supplying quinine at the cheapest possible price? Such questions began to be asked from different quarters: the British parliament,[243] contending private manufacturers,[244] and officials based in the Madras Presidency.[245] The question of price predictably figured while assessing the initiatives of the Madras Government towards manufacturing quinine. In response to such attempts in October 1890, one Dr Rice wrote: 'I don't understand why the manufacture of these alkaloids by Government should be so costly, it should be enquired whether the selling price of them is not kept up so as to cover losses in other branches of the department...'.[246]

The early 1890s witnessed the return of the Howards to prominence in British India. Henry Wellcome set up a few quinine depots in British India in the late 1890s. Manufacturers based in Dutch Java also started exploring the market in British India. They brought with them competitive conceptions of quinine and its fair price, and recurrently alleged that government quinine continued to remain more expensive than the market price. Focusing on the two decades following 1889, the next chapter will examine, amongst other questions, how the managers of the factory at Mungpoo negotiated these allegations.

Conclusion

The recognition that commercially produced drugs manufactured at the cinchona factory in British Sikkim in the late 1880s was quinine was thus an intensely political process. The discovery/invention attributed to Gammie was not an exclusively scientific event which reflected unprecedented pharmaceutical craft. It did not indicate a glorious ending to a straightforward teleological journey: from relative ignorance to more improved technology. Nor was it achieved within the walls of an insulated colonial factory. The discovery/invention of the process for manufacturing cheap and pure quinine in British Sikkim was instead founded on legal manoeuvrings, imperial rhetoric, strategic revisions in the

---

[242] Rev-Agriculture, Agriculture, December 1893, 14 C (WBSA).   [243] Ibid.

[244] Deputy-Secretary, Government of India to the Surgeon General, Government of India, No.166/7, 10 February 1888, Fort William. Finance, Miscellaneous, M 1R/27, December 1890, 3–6 B (WBSA).

[245] A note from the Madras Government No. 706 A., dated 4 September 1890. Rev-Agriculture, Agriculture, November 1891, 29 B.

[246] Ibid.

botanical identification of cinchonas, the increasing (political and commercial) preeminence of Mungpoo in the world of drug manufacturers, and the transitory retreat of contending actors (particularly the Howards, the Whiffens, the office of the Secretary of State for India, private manufacturing interests in Madras) at a time when the decade-long devaluation of quinine had reached its apogee.

Focusing particularly on the first half of the twentieth century, historians have justifiably argued that allegations about impurity, corruption and adulteration of quinine were made to explain the inefficacy of the drug in contemporary medical practice in British India.[247] I have hinted that this tendency also existed in the two decades following the first establishment of quinine factories in British India in the late 1860s. However, what is especially noteworthy is that imperial officials in colonial departments, factories, laboratories and plantations across South Asia and beyond carried out the more fundamental debate about what could be considered pure quinine itself even as the drug continued to be recommended to patients as an efficacious remedy.

The mere convergence of prevalent techniques and necessary material ingredients could not inevitably guarantee a product the status of quinine in the second half of the nineteenth century. Whether manufactured in Ootacamund, Mungpoo or London such products could receive various labels, such as, 'Brown viscid quinium' or 'yellowish grey powder amorphous quinine', or white pure quinine. The various labelling of these products were contingent upon the shifting configurations of authority in the overlapping worlds of pharmaceutical business, colonial governance and scientific knowledge. Hierarchies between the expert manufacturer and the factory-in-tutelage were hardly absolute, stable and inflexible. Instead, these hierarchies indicated specific relations, which could be altered and reconfigured, between contending actors.

Thus, perceptions about who could or couldn't act as legitimate custodians of pure quinine varied along with these shifting relations of authority and subordination. In the preceding pages I have explored the myriad assertions, contestations and the emergence of newer nodes of authority to explain the shifting status of the factory at Mungpoo. Although initially ridiculed by the Howards to be producers of amateurish drugs like 'brown viscid quinium', this factory was recognised eventually in the early 1880s as manufacturers of 'a pretty preparation' which closely resembled the 'best English quinine'. Neither was the subordination of

---

[247] See especially P. Barton, 'Powders, Potions and Tablets: The "Quinine fraud" in British India, 1890–1939' in J. H. Mills and P. Barton (eds.), *Drugs and Empire: Essays in Modern Imperialism and Intoxication, c. 1500–1930* (Basingstoke: Palgrave Macmillan 2007), 144–161.

the factory at Mungpoo to dismissive judgments from various European and Dutch experts of pure quinine permanent nor was the authority asserted by the Howards or Whiffen or de Vrij absolute. British Indian officials set limits to the reputation of the Howards in significant ways. Most glaringly in 1885, one might recall, George King discredited the London febrifuge manufactured by the Howards to be an inferior drug, which required further purification in the factory at Mungpoo.

Such fluctuating configurations of authority and subordination were both engendered by and reflected in the vibrant careers of drugs which were described as substitutes of pure quinine. Without addressing the history of these substitutes it is difficult to make sense of the historical commodification of pure quinine in British India. Pure quinine is an example of a commodity which was constructed in significant ways in reference to what were considered its substitutes. Producers of 'substitutes' like cinchonidine, cinchonine, quinetum, cinchona febrifuge, quinidine and mixed triple sulphate were crucial in delimiting, defining and contesting the prestige of pure quinine and its reigning experts. In the process these producers ended up asserting their own contending claims to authority over pure quinine.

For much of the period, pure quinine continued to figure widely in official correspondence as a rare, relatively inaccessible, distant drug. The imperial medical marketplace consisted of a plethora of widely circulating signifiers of pure quinine. It was suggested that pure quinine's physical characteristics, taste and therapeutic efficacies could be measured by mapping the more tangible substitutes like quinine brute, rough quinine, Darjeeling quinine and amorphous quinine. The insurmountable superiority of pure quinine, officials maintained, could be gauged comparatively from the perceived inadequacies of the substitutes: 'Cinchonidine is one-third the value of quinine'.[248] Mixed triple sulphate 'is less intensely bitter than quinine; (it is a) white crystalline substance closely resembling quinine in appearance'.[249] Cinchona febrifuge 'tastes nearly that of quinine... (is) less powerful than pure quinine... half as effective as quinine'.[250]

In the end, pure quinine, as a commodity-in-the-making in British India, was occasioned by Empire. This is why it tells us a lot about

---

[248] Clarke to Secretary, Government of Bengal. Home, Public, 12 March 1870, 157 A (NAI).

[249] Beatson to the Officiating Secretary, Government of India. Home, Medical, 64–80 A, 1879 October (NAI).

[250] Cockburn to Howell, Home, Medical, August 1875, 49–58 A (NAI); Walker to the Secretary, Government of the North-Western Provinces and Oudh. Home, Medical, May 1879, 19–21 A (NAI).

Empire. The imperial assemblage that constructed pure quinine was constituted of a network of humans and nonhumans. The project of manufacturing it held together not only the contending aspirations of European pharmaceutical families, office of the Secretary of State for India, chemical examiners, peripatetic geographer-botanists, cinchona planters, mangers of colonial factories, but also properties attributed to cinchona barks, alkaloids, colouring matter, alkalis, alcohol, oil, paraffine, labelled bottles, sealing wax and carmine. The history of manufacturing and maintaining pure quinine reminds us that such chains of human/nonhuman enmeshes could be amongst the indispensible constituents of Empire.

Pure quinine not only reinforced Empire as a profit-making enterprise couched by the rhetoric of benevolence, but also revealed it as a 'commodity spectacle': Administrators, planters and factory managers located in places as distant as Andaman, Ceylon, India, Java, Jamaica, Sumatra, Samaran and Trinidad were bound up by their preoccupations to produce and protect the purity of cheap quinine.[251] Apart from exposing an extensively interconnected imperial space, the history of manufacturing pure quinine reconfirms existing historiographical insights about the fault-lines and 'tensions of empire'.[252] The history of quinine manufacture contests the impression that Empire was characterised by unidirectional and uncomplicated flows of authority from London to the rest of the world.[253] The question of pure quinine cemented alliances as well as deepened conflicts between the office of the Secretary of State, pharmaceutical business houses, and managers of colonial plantations and factories. Pure quinine thus immensely fractures the homogenous and monolithic image of Empire.

Pure quinine attracted the attention of a range of imperial workaholics across extensively dispersed geographical locations for more than three decades. Having acquired somewhat of a larger-than-life status, it nonetheless found itself embroiled in broader dehumanising processes. The production and distribution of pure quinine or its substitutes stoked various narratives of racial discrimination. Cinchona febrifuge, for example, was considered too 'crude and coarse' to suit for the delicate

---

[251] For commodity-spectacle, see A. McClintock, *Imperial Leather: Race, Gender and Sexuality in the Colonial Context* (New York and London: Routledge, 1995), 56.

[252] A. L. Stoler and F. Cooper, 'Introduction: Between Metropole and Colony: Rethinking a Research Agenda', in A. L. Stoler and F. Cooper (eds.), *Tensions of Empire: Colonial Cultures in a Bourgeois World* (Berkeley/Los Angeles/London: University of California Press, 1997), 1–46.

[253] In the history of science this model has been epitomised by G. Basalla in 'The Spread of Western Science', *Science*, 156 (May 1967), 611–622.

constitutions of European soldiers serving in British India.[254] In contrast, following a recommendation in 1880, Indian labouring convicts in the Andaman and Nicobar islands were not only forced to consume the same drug every day, but as an effective cost-cutting measure, on each such occasion they were denied their daily milk ration.[255]

The perceived material configurations of pure quinine closely indicate how scientific racism and what Anne McClintock in another context calls 'commodity racism' converged and sustained one another.[256] Pure quinine was projected consistently in official sources as a 'white substance'[257] which crystallised as 'beautiful, long needles', was bitter in taste and had a sweet smell. This metaphorical correlation of whiteness with purity is particularly striking considering impure quinine was frequently associated with yellow and brown. For example, 'amorphous quinine', which was produced by Broughton at Ootacamund was discarded by Howard as a 'yellow stuff, sticky like resin... on the whole a very impure preparation'.[258] Similarly quinium, which was manufactured at Rungbee by Anderson in the late 1860s, was declared impure by officials on the basis of its 'brown viscid' appearance.[259] In the process, pure quinine and its impure substitutes were anthropomorphised as they were shown to personify racial hierarchies of colour.[260] It is further revealing to recall that yellowness, blackness and brownness figured around this time in various imperial reports as colours most closely associated with malaria.[261]

Colonial bureaucrats warned that the purity of white quinine could be contaminated when exposed to Indian weather and the natives. As

---

[254] Cunningham, 'Memorandum'. Home, Medical, September 1878, 126–128 A; Home, Medical, November 1880, 111–119 A (NAI).

[255] Cadell to Officiating Secretary, Government of India, Home, Revenue and Agricultural Department. Home, Port Blair, October 1880, 30–32 A (NAI).

[256] For commodity racism, see McClintock, *Imperial Leather*, 31–33.

[257] Cockerell to the Secretary to the Government of India, Home, Revenue, and Agricultural departments. Home, Medical, October 1879, 64–80 A (NAI).

[258] J. E. Howard to the Under Secretary of State for India, 21 June 1881, Tottenham. Home, Medical, November 1882, 67 B (NAI).

[259] Anderson to the Secretary, Government of Bengal. Home, Public. 12 March 1870, 157 A (NAI).

[260] For the links between scientific racism and whiteness see W. Anderson, *The Cultivation of Whiteness: Science, Health and Racial Destiny in Australia* (Durham: Duke University Press, 2006). For a recent commentary on the nineteenth-century racialisation of yellow see, M. Keevak, *Becoming Yellow: A Short History of Racial Thinking* (New Jersey: Princeton University Press, 2011), 70–122.

[261] J. Macculloch, *Malaria: An Essay on the Production and Propagation of this Poison* (London: Longman, Rees, Orme, Brown and Green, 1827), 429–430; G. Dodds, 'Tropical Malaria and its Sequels', *Edinburgh Medical Journal*, 23 (1887–1888), 1094; E. A. Parkes, 'Report on Hygiene for 1867', *Army Medical Department Report for the year 1866*, Volume viii, 1868, 316–317 (WL).

Broughton observed in 1871, 'The purest and whitest alkaloids I have been able to prepare become coloured brown when exposed to the Indian sunshine...'.[262] It was feared that quinine became potentially impure whenever accessed by the native doctors, indigenous hospital assistants, fake patients or other handlers in the vernacular marketplace. The need to deploy a range of protective mechanisms including sealed bottles, carmine, patrol boats, police stations and glass cases with extra strong patent locks thus loomed large in the bureaucratic imagination.

This chapter has thus alerted us to details which histories dedicated exclusively to analysing either materiality or social construction of scientific facts often miss. Scientific knowledge about pure quinine, the material configurations of pure quinine and imperial politics were not only intimately entangled, but also co-constituted.

---

[262] J. Broughton, 'Chemical and Physiological Experiments on Living Cinchonaey', *Philosophical Transactions of the Royal Society of London*, 161 (1871), 8.

5   Of 'Losses Gladly Borne'
Feeding Quinine, Warring Mosquitoes

> ...Possibilities in the direction of any permanent improvement in price (of quinine)...one being...constantly increasing the consumption of quinine, combined with the opening up of the world's dark places, which is so steadily going on year by year, month by month, almost day by day, may in the end lead to consumption overtaking supply...[1]

> Malarial parasites...are as natural amongst primitive races as flea infestation is to a dog.[2]

The various social lives of government quinine in British India were not confined within the walls of insulated colonial factories and laboratories. Quinine was reconstituted through the predicaments and processes of circulation. The decades following 1890 were marked by a unique phase in the history of colonial governance in British India. They witnessed unprecedented governmental rigour in enforcing consumption of the imperial drug quinine across the subcontinent, whilst the corresponding diagnostic category of malaria itself was redefined beyond recognition: from an elusive cause of many diseases to the name of a specific mosquito-borne fever disease. Ironically, therefore, the colonial state retained and enforced the drug quinine as a quintessential remedy at the precise moment when the corresponding problem of malaria was radically reinvented and ascribed with newer meanings. This converged with official lamentation about an enduring slump in the wider imperial economy of quinine, apparently the result of an excessive supply of cinchona barks from Dutch Java into the European markets, overproduction of quinine and a consequent shrinking of demands. British India emerged, by the 1910s, as the world's largest quinine consuming market.

Many scholarly works have explained such reconfigurations of knowledge about malaria by focusing on the agency of individual scientists

---

[1] 'Cutting from the "Civil and Military Gazette"', 3 November 1910. 'Notes', Rev-Agriculture, Agriculture, February 1911, 37–39 A (NAI).

[2] *Proceedings of the Third Meeting of the General Malaria Committee at Madras November 1912* (Simla: Government Central Branch Press, 1913), 13.

and their networks of collaborators.[3] Knowledge of malaria and quinine (extracted from the bark of cinchona plants) has usually been studied as parts of separate and mutually exclusive histories.[4] Early twentieth-century colonial officials involved in killing mosquitoes and those engaged in distributing quinine have appeared in prevailing studies as antagonistic and oppositional groups.[5]

In the 1900s, quinine, mosquitoes and malaria emerged as intrinsic components of shared, symbiotic and interdependent histories.[6] The social and physical attributes associated with quinine were refashioned once it was made to interact in the 1890s and 1900s with a range of situations and sites, including colonial factories, prisons, plantations, military barracks, high schools, mofussils, government offices, post offices, imperial conferences, bazaars, legal codes, forms of punishments and primary school curricula. Meanwhile, mosquitoes had emerged as a subject of enduring attention in the disparate fields of entomological science, sanitary governance, plantation economy and vernacular literature. The reconfiguration of malaria into a mosquito-borne fever disease at the turn of the century can be attributed to the metamorphoses of mosquitoes into a subject of overwhelming public spectacle. Unprecedented enthusiasm relating to the newer meanings conferred

---

[3] See for instance, J. Guillemin, 'Choosing Scientific Patrimony: Sir Ronald Ross, Alphonse Laveran and the Mosquito Vector Hypothesis for Malaria', *Journal of the History of Medicine*, 57 (2002), 385–409.

[4] For a recent sophisticated work on cinchona and its economy of substitutes in an eighteenth- and early nineteenth-century British imperial context, see P. Chakrabarti, 'Empire and Alternatives: Swietenia Febrifuga and the Cinchona Substitutes', *Medical History*, 54, 1 (2010), 75–94. See also, P. Burton, 'Powders, Potions and Tablets: The "Quinine Fraud" in British India, 1890–1939' in J. H. Mills and P. Barton (eds.), *Drugs and Empire: Essays in Modern Imperialism and Intoxication, c. 1500–1930* (Basingstoke: Palgrave Macmillan 2007), 144–161; L. H. Brockway, *Science and Colonial Expansion: The Role of the British Royal Botanic Gardens* (New Haven: Yale University Press, 2002), 104–125; R. Drayton, *Nature's Government: Science, Imperial Britain, and the 'Improvement' of the World* (New Haven: Yale University Press, 2000), 207–210, 230–231; K. Phillip, *Civilizing Natures: Race, Resources and Modernity in South Asia* (Hyderabad: Orient Longman, 2004) 238–272; A. Mukherjee, 'The Peruvian Bark Revisited: A Critique of British Cinchona Policy in Colonial India', *Bengal Past and Present*, 117 (1998), 81–102.

[5] See for instance, H. Evans, 'European Malaria Policy in the 1920s and 1930s: The Epidemiology of Minutiae', *Isis*, 80, 1 (March 1989), 40–59.

[6] A recent essay has hinted that quinine distribution and mosquito eradication in early twentieth-century British India often happened simultaneously. N. Bhattacharya, 'The Logic of Location: Malaria Research in Colonial India, Darjeeling and Duars, 1900–30', *Medical History*, 55, 2 (April 2011), 183–202. The works of James Webb and Frank Snowden address together both the themes of malaria and its cure. J. L. A., Webb Jr, *Humanity's Burden: A Global History of Malaria*, (Cambridge: Cambridge University Press, 2008); F. M. Snowden, *The Conquest of Malaria: Italy, 1900–1962* (New Haven: Yale University Press, 2006). Extending their insights I comment on how the medicalisation of mosquitoes and the unprecedented circulation of quinine in the 1900s informed and shaped one another.

upon mosquitoes and malaria augmented rather than displaced the significance of quinine as an object of enforced consumption in various parts of British India.

Such historical imbrications of mosquitoes, quinine and malaria were produced and sustained by the enduring overlaps between the worlds of pharmaceutical commerce, scientific knowledge, colonial governance and vernacular cultures. In these many-layered worlds held together by Empire malaria, mosquitoes and quinine were reshaped as vibrant, commodious and entangled entities, deserving of attention, intervention and investment. At the same time, while being produced by the discourses and enactments of imperial politics, mosquitoes, quinine and malaria emerged as indispensable subjects and constituents of Empire. This chapter continues to engage histories of empire with science studies to suggest the ways in which histories of insects, commodities, disease and empire interacted and shaped one another. It goes beyond celebrating mosquitoes and quinine as historical actors, and more critically examines the processes and perceptions through which these were endowed with enduring medical attributes in the imperial archive and beyond. Thus, it raises methodological questions about how the historical inscriptions of nonhumans (like mosquitoes or quinine) can be narrated while retaining a critique of the links between empire and the production of scientific knowledge.

'Cheapest Possible Quinine'

By the early 1890s, government factories based in Mungpoo and Nedivattam claimed that they were capable of supplying pure quinine at the cheapest possible price. The validity of these claims was queried by a number of contenders. Indeed, the prices levied by these factories on quinine were subjected to vigorous scrutiny in the following decades. The managers of these factories, in turn, continued to reiterate programmatic statements, which had been associated with the introduction of cinchona into British India since the 1860s. These factories manufactured quinine, it was suggested, not for profit but as charitable ways to offer medical relief. Such efforts presumably reflected the benevolent and humanitarian face of the colonial state in British India. The government resolved to distribute quinine at much less than the ruling market rates – at or even below the cost of production. The possibility that commercial 'losses' could be incurred was acknowledged. Such 'losses', it was promised, 'shall be gladly borne by the government'.[7]

---

[7] H. Wheeler, Secretary, Government of Bengal, Municipal (Medical) Department to Secretary, Government of India, Home department, No. 74. Home, Medical, June 1909, 105–107 A (NAI).

Despite this, contemporary government correspondences reveal sustained efforts towards averting such losses. Officials had to deal with allegations about the *higher* price of quinine supplied from the factories at Mungpoo and Nedivattam. The price of government quinine allegedly exceeded the rates charged by private sellers in European markets from the early 1890s.[8] Writing in 1892, the civil surgeon of Akyab in Burma, for example, lamented that the price of government quinine was higher than that charged by European dealers.[9]

It is doubtful whether the rates charged by the government factories in British India were ever considered an index of fair, normative price of quinine. The managers of the factory at Mungpoo claimed to have invented a process for manufacturing the cheapest possible quinine in 1889. By 1890, official files began to reflect efforts at curbing the rising price of government quinine, by placing greater trust on the prices charged by influential private operators in Europe. It was decreed in 1890, for instance, that government quinine should be 'offered' at the 'market rate quoted for Howard's quinine by the latest mail from London, converted into Indian currency at the annual rate of exchange for the adjustment of financial transactions between the Imperial and Indian governments'.[10]

In course of the following two decades, the price of government quinine remained consistently higher than the rates charged by private European firms. In July 1909, Rai Saheb B. L. Kabra, who worked as the Chief Medical Officer for the Poonch State, released a comparative table of prices of sulphates of quinine levied by various firms. These included besides the government factory in Calcutta, Burroughs Wellcome and Co. and Dakin Brothers Limited of London, Ferries and Co. of Bristol, and agents for a German manufacturer in Bombay. The table suggests that alternative sources of quinine continued to supply the drug at cheaper rates.[11]

In the official papers the higher price of government quinine was justified in terms of its 'assured purity'. In June 1892, David Prain, then acting superintendent of the royal botanic gardens in Calcutta provided an elaborate defence of the 'slight difference' in the price of quinine. He referred to the British pharmacopoeia to suggest how the commercially

---

[8] Rev-agriculture, Agriculture, September 1892, 8–9A (NAI).
[9] Civil Surgeon, Akyab to the Secretary and Engineer, Akyab Municipality, No. 399, 19 January 1892. Rev-Agriculture, Agriculture, April 1892. 12 A (NAI).
[10] Deputy Secretary, Government of India to the Surgeon General, Government of India, 10 February 1888, Fort William. Financial Department, Miscellaneous branch, December 1890, M 1R/27, Prog. 3–6 B (WBSA).
[11] B. L. Kabra to W. R. Edwards, Superintending Surgeon, Poonch State, Gulmarg. No. 206, 20 July 1909. Home, Medical, October 1909, 131–135 A (NAI).

agreeable form of the drug was required to contain at least 95 per cent of the alkaloid, quinine. He claimed that the percentage of 'pure alkaloid' was higher in the government quinine than in the 'best commercial samples'. 'The extra pie', he argued, 'procured the purest quinine available'.[12]

In August 1897, George King warned of extensive practices of adulteration in the medical market. King suggested that the drug offered by the 'banneah and druggist' in the stores possibly contained little or no quinine. Under the prevailing circumstances, he thought, the bazaar quotations for Howard's or Herring's quinine had to be considered with caution. He alleged that shopkeepers in the Calcutta bazaar frequently adulterated or even replaced quinine with inferior preparations of the cinchona barks such as muriate of cinchonine or sulphate of cinchonidine. These 'inferior preparations', he claimed, were indistinguishable both in appearance and taste from quinine except by chemical analysis. Empty quinine bottles with Howards' or Herring's labels on them, he feared, could bring a price in to the bazaar far beyond their intrinsic value. By contrast, King considered government quinine which was distributed by carefully designated officials as 'absolutely pure'.[13]

A range of medical bureaucrats considered the higher price of government quinine not only unavoidable, but also desirable, since it conformed to certain political commitments of the British government. The sale of government quinine below the market rate was shown to have been detrimental to the ideologies of free trade and to the profit-maximising interests of private enterprise. It was feared it might lead to unpleasant competitions with private firms. Excessively cheap government quinine could have driven 'the private firms out of the field' by undercutting them. 'Unjustifiable interference' with private enterprise, it was argued, was 'opposed to the policies of the government of India'. The higher price of government quinine was thus projected as one way of ensuring the prospects of privately initiated quinine trade in British India.[14]

The bureaucrats preferred uniformity in the pricing of the drug to lowering the cost of government quinine. Concessional rates, it was apprehended, were liable to be abused by middlemen interested in speculating

---

[12] D. Prain, Acting Superintendent, Botanic Garden, Calcutta to the Officiating Under Secretary, Government of Bengal, Financial Department. No.316S.G, May–June 1892, Seebpore. Rev-agriculture, Agriculture. September 1892. 8–9A (NAI).

[13] G. King to the Secretary, Government of Bengal, Municipal department, No. 9 S.Q/P.P, 21 August 1807, Seebpore. Municipal, Medical, March 1898, Progs. 66–69, File Q/1 (WBSA).

[14] Rev-agriculture, Economic-products, February 1901, 3–6 A (NAI); Kabra to Edwards, Home, Medical, October 1909, 131–135 A (NAI).

in quinine. It was suggested that 'native druggists' or 'traders with enterprise and capital' could exploit differences in price. Such groups could
buy up cheaper government quinine at concessional rates and retail them
at profit. Enforcing uniformity in the price of quinine was thus highlighted as one way of purging corrupt speculative ventures out of the
market.[15]

However, the most persistent set of justifications about the higher
price of government quinine referred to the cinchona plantations in
British India. The state-owned plantations in British India were shown
to have been in decline since the mid-1890s. In the ten years ending in
1894–1895, the total number of plants in the government plantations
allegedly fell from 17 1/4 million to 9 3/4 million.[16] Tea planters in the
Darjeeling Terai who were earlier drawn towards cinchona cultivation
were now contemplating investments in cocoa plants.[17] Even the government plantation and factory at Mungpoo began devoting some space
to the experimental cultivation of cocoa and manufacture of cocaine.[18]
As a result, the most subsidised and concessional source of raw materials for the state-run quinine factories seemed gradually to wane and the
factories were compelled to fall back on alternative sources in the open,
local and competitive market within British India.

This effectively meant that government quinine factories in Madras
and Bengal emerged as rival buyers in a cinchona market dominated by
private planters.[19] This situation was invoked recurrently well into the
second decade of the twentieth century to explain the ever-increasing
price of government quinine. It was suggested that demand in British
India for quinine had outstripped the 'producing powers' of the government cinchona plantations. As a result, the government factories had
to purchase expensive bark from private growers. This in turn, it was
argued, caused an abrupt increase in the cost of production.[20]

By 1908, the price difference between quinine manufactured in government factories in British India and its counterparts in Europe was
sharp. In 1908, government quinine in British India reportedly sold at

[15] Ibid.; R. E. V. Arbuthnot 'Note dated 21–01–190'. Rev-agriculture, Economic-
    products, March 1902, 1–2 A (NAI).
[16] Rev-agriculture, Economic-products, April 1896, 10–12 C. 9 (NAI).
[17] J. Gammie to Secretary, Government of Bengal, Financial department, 20 May 1892,
    Mungpoo-Kurseong. Rev-agriculture, Agriculture, July 1892, 12 A (NAI).
[18] C. E. Buckland to the Government of India, Revenue and Agriculture department, 14
    October 1890, Darjeeling. Financial, Miscellaneous, November 1890, File M 1C/3;
    5–6 B (WBSA).
[19] Rev-agriculture, Economic-products, May 1898, 1–7 A (NAI).
[20] G. King to the Secretary, Government of Bengal, Financial department, 9 February
    1898, Shibpur. Financial, Miscellaneous, August 1898, M 1Q/1, 1–9 (WBSA).

Rs. 15–10 per pound, while Burroughs Wellcome and Co. had agreed to supply the drug wholesale at Rs. 9–8 per pound.[21] In 1909, quinine supplied from official sources in British India was shown to vary between Rs. 12 per pound and Rs. 13–10 per pound. By contrast, Europe-based private distributing firms including Messrs Burgoyne Burbidges and Co., Messrs Smith Stanistreet and Co., Messrs Peake Allen and Co. sold quinine in British India at around Rs. 10 per pound.[22]

In view of this, officials in charge of various government institutions in British India began contemplating the direct purchase of quinine from the open market. The government of East Bengal and Assam, for instance, started negotiations with Messrs Parke Davis and Co., an American firm, for an annual supply in April 1910.[23] Messrs Turner, Morrison and Co. had been sugar merchants based in Calcutta with considerable stakes in Dutch Java. In January 1907, it was proposed that they could, if required, act as a liaison between the Bengal government and manufacturers of quinine based in Dutch Java.[24] In September 1909, the Superintendent of the District Jail at Aligarh purchased 2000 pounds at Rs. 8 per pound from Messrs Burroughs Wellcome and Co.[25] Such officials found it strange that profit-seeking business firms could supply quinine cheaper than factories harbouring charitable pretensions.[26] These years witnessed 'careful consideration' of proposals concerning the discontinuation altogether of government cinchona factories and plantations in British India.[27]

A range of colonial bureaucrats, including managers of the reportedly dwindling government cinchona plantations in British India, resisted such proposals. They described the availability of cheaper varieties of quinine in the open markets of Europe and Java as a transitory phase in the history of the commodity. The gradual deterioration of the government cinchona plantations in British India, it was suggested, coincided with a phase of overproduction of cinchona barks in the island of Java, which had glutted the European market. In 1906 alone Java exported more than 16 million pounds of barks; and between 1898 and 1904,

---

[21] J. C. Fergusson, 'Note Dated 5-2-1906'. Rev-agriculture, Agriculture, September 1908, 44–71 A (NAI).

[22] Rev-agriculture, Agriculture, February 1909, 36–39 A (NAI).

[23] Rev-agriculture. Agriculture, December 1910, 15 B (NAI).

[24] F. Noel Paton 'Note dated 03-01-1907'. Revenue and Agriculture, Agriculture, September 1908, 44–71 A (NAI).

[25] A. G. Cardew to Secretary, Government of India, 26 May 1910, Ootacamund. Rev-agriculture, Agriculture, September 1910, 40–43 A (NAI).

[26] Rev-agriculture, Agriculture, February 1909, 36–39 A (NAI).

[27] H. Stuart to Secretary, Government of Punjab, Home department, 23 May 1909, Simla. Rev-agriculture, Agriculture, June 1909, 10 A (NAI).

shipments from Java averaged 12 million pounds annually. Such enormous outturn was described as unprecedented and which considerably exceeded the demand for the barks. This, it was argued, initiated a cascading effect which caused the price of quinine in the European markets to fall drastically.

Yet, British Indian bureaucrats like A. T. Gage, the superintendent of the cinchona cultivation in Bengal, asserted that a return of high price of quinine in the open European market was imminent. An agreement between dominant Javanese planters deliberately restricting the supply of cinchona barks, it was feared, could reinvigorate the price of quinine in the wider imperial world. Besides, shifts in the priorities of the Javanese planters could displace cinchona by sugarcane or rubber as the predominant object of investment. It was thus predicted that government quinine manufactured in British India would not retain its higher price indefinitely.

Bureaucrats like Gage considered it imprudent to discontinue government plantations and factories under such circumstances. Instead, they recommended that the government should purchase superior breeds of Javanese cinchona barks at cheaper rates from Holland. However, this was to be considered a 'temporary expedient and not a permanent policy'.[28] It was further instructed that the government plantations in British India should not only be retained, but also extended. Potential sites for new state-owned cinchona plantations in North Bengal, the North East and the Andamans were contemplated.[29] The retention and extension of government cinchona plantations in British India were conceived as measures to guarantee adequate supply of cinchona at reasonable rates once imports from Java shrank. Meanwhile, the additional expenditure involved in purchasing from the factory and retaining the government plantations, it was suggested, 'must be regarded as the premium for an insurance against the creation of a monopoly'.[30]

'Within the Reach of the Poorest'

By 1905, the significance of British India as a cinchona-growing and quinine-manufacturing territory was on the decline. Statistics released at the beginning of the twentieth century situated it amongst many colonial

---

[28] Fergusson, 'A Note dated 5–2–1906'. Rev-agriculture, Agriculture, September 1908, 44–71 A (NAI).

[29] A. T. Gage, 'A Note dated, 25–11–1910'. Rev–agriculture, Agriculture, January 1911, 15–16 A (NAI).

[30] Stuart to Secretary, Government of Punjab, Home department. Rev-agriculture, Agriculture, June 1909, 10 A (NAI).

locations including Ceylon, Africa and South America where governments had initiated cinchona plantations. By then, however, the subservience of British India to the superiority of Dutch Java in the world of cinchona planters was complete.[31] Java was reported to produce more than 90 per cent of the world's cinchona plants in the first decade of the century,[32] whilst factories in British India did not figure in a list of fifteen leading quinine factories in the world released in 1905.[33]

Nonetheless, British India remained significant in the world of quinine trade. The basis of that significance, however, had shifted considerably. British India figured in many accounts as one of the largest markets for quinine in the world in the first decade of the twentieth century.[34] In 1912, British India was reported to account for about one-sixth of the world's annual quinine consumption, and was one of the world's most dominant importers of quinine. Despite the government's persistence with Indian cinchona plantations and quinine factories, in effect, only 12 per cent of the enormous consumption was supplied by the dwindling factories in India.[35]

The years 1890–1910 witnessed declining prices, shrinking demand and overproduction of quinine in most of the world. Private firms and colonial governments searched for new markets for the drug. In this context, extensive distribution and effective governance of quinine appeared as much more relevant than planting cinchonas and manufacturing quinine. Colonial governments in British India initiated elaborate and enduring ways of distributing quinine in these decades, which yielded the desired results. In sharp contrast to the situation elsewhere, the demand and price of quinine in British India was higher than ever before. As a result, British India remained significant in global quinine trade. 'Constantly increasing the consumption of quinine' appeared as one of the most plausible ways of effecting a 'permanent improvement in the price' of the commodity.[36]

Bureaucratic correspondences in British India in these decades reveal an irony. The governments within British India were at one level tied with the wider efforts of 'improving' the price of quinine. At the same time, the officials felt compelled to lament the higher price of government

[31] W. R. Dustan to J. Wilson, Secretary, Government of India, 25 July 1907. Rev-agriculture, Agriculture September 1908, 44–71 A (NAI).

[32] The Editor of *The Chemist and Druggist* to F. Noel-Paton, Ibid.

[33] Dustan to Wilson, Rev-agriculture, Agriculture, September 1908, 44–71 A.

[34] C. A. Innes, 'Report dated 22–09–1907', 24, Ibid.

[35] 'Note on Cinchona policy'. Rev-agriculture, Agriculture, March 1912, 22 B (NAI).

[36] 'The Price of Quinine', Cutting from the 'Civil and Military Gazette' dated the 3 November 1910, 'Notes'. Rev-agriculture, Agriculture, February 1911, 37–39 A (NAI).

quinine in British India. This contradiction emerged from the government's compulsion to speak in the language of charity whilst acting in the interests of profit.

This section and the next explore how quinine was reconstituted through the government's efforts at distributing, popularising and ensuring its consumption in British India. The production of quinine was thus not confined within the walls of factories and laboratories. But rather, quinine was transformed through the processes and predicaments of circulation.

The energies and investments of the colonial state were geared towards sustained attempts at distributing the drug in 1890s and 1900s. Various categories were invoked to describe the vigour, extent and depth of the efforts to circulate quinine beyond the factories, hospitals, urban enclaves and official institutions. Quinine emboldened the government to reach out to the 'remote districts,'[37] 'the poorest,'[38] 'poorer classes,'[39] 'the interiors,'[40] 'small road side stations,'[41] 'the general public,'[42] 'the Santhal Parganas,'[43] 'remote' locations within British India, which apparently lay 'beyond the reaches of the market'.[44]

The project of reaching out to the 'genuine consumers',[45] however, was not an invention of the 1890s. In the late 1860s and the early 1870s, successive Sanitary Commissioners of the Bengal Presidency prescribed various ways of selling imported quinine in the 'mofussil' at a reasonable price.[46] These efforts were sporadic and fleeting. Sustained official efforts were resumed and reinforced only in the 1890s. Prior to this, imported quinine and its indigenous substitutes circulated in the 'interiors' along the networks of a proliferating vernacular medical market. As I will explore in the epilogue, cures and potions for malarial diseases constituted a thriving vernacular market, for instance, in Bengal. The colonial state's efforts in the 1890s did not represent the first or the only attempts towards distributing quinine. The routes conceived by the colonial state for the convenient circulation of quinine had been traversed

---

[37] 'Enclosure No. 1' Home, Medical, July 1893, 55–58 A (NAI).
[38] 'Appendix', Rev-agriculture, Economic-products, September 1896, 1 A (NAI).
[39] Home, Medical, July 1892, 38–40 A (NAI).   [40] Ibid.
[41] KW No. 224, 27 January 1893. Municipal department, Medical branch, March 1893, 2M/3, 5–6 (WBSA).
[42] Home, Medical, June 1895, 18–21 A (NAI).
[43] Rev-agriculture, CVA, December 1903, 15 B (NAI).
[44] 'Enclosure No. 1', 30 October 1894, Rangoon. Home, Medical, October 1897, 285–297 A (NAI).
[45] Ibid.
[46] Home, Public, April 1872, 508 A; H. H. Risley, Officiating Secretary to the Secretary, Government of India, 12 April 1892, Calcutta. Home, Medical, July 1892, 38–40 A.

already by various actors in the vernacular markets. However, after 1890 the colonial governments designed strategies of distributing quinine with unprecedented vigour.

The reinforcement of state initiatives in the early 1890s began with an acknowledgment of past failures. The sales of imported quinine, it was alleged, had been so far confined within the district and subdivisional headquarters. 'Special arrangements' were now proposed to bring quinine 'within easy reach of the rural population . . . to popularise the use of quinine amongst the poorer classes in the provinces'.[47] As noted earlier, the colonial state pledged to distribute government quinine in the 'interiors', which figured as locations without any druggists' shops or easy means of transport.[48] But the distribution of quinine, government officials feared, was not necessarily followed by acts of consumption. To flesh out such apprehensions, the prospective consumers in the interiors were variously stereotyped in the official files. Attempts to enforce the consumption of quinine in the 1890s thus emerged as yet another occasion for the imperial projection of the inhabitants of the interiors as 'backward and conservative in their habits and ideas', 'averse from innovations' and characterised by 'primitive ignorance'.[49] The governments, therefore, exercised considerable care in selecting agents for distributing quinine: Who were best placed to act as vendors and to convince the intended consumers about the merits of consuming quinine? Answers to this question revealed the colonial governments' various understandings about how questions of political legitimacy and acceptability might have been perceived by the intended consumers.

European officials and physicians were assumed to have authority over colonised Indian consumers. Such officials, it was suggested, were considered exotic characters and most frequently associated with institutional power. Insistence from such officials could carry the weight of a regulation.[50] However, it was eventually decided that it would be prudent to engage the lowest rung of officials from within the different communities. The purchase and consumption of quinine, it was suggested, should not appear as an outcome of rigorous punitive imposition but of voluntary appreciation. The arrival of quinine then mustn't be projected as an exceptional event in the life of communities inhabiting the

---

[47] Risley to the Secretary, Government of India, Home, Medical, July 1892, 38–40 A (NAI).
[48] 'Resolution', Enclosure no. 2. Home, Medical, July 1893, 55–58 A (NAI).
[49] Secretary, Government of Burma to Secretary, Government of India, 14 August 1897, Rangoon. Home, Medical, October 1897, 285–297 A (NAI).
[50] Ibid.; See also, A. J. Payne to the Secretary, Government of Bengal, Medical and Municipal department, 17 August 1881, Calcutta. Home, Medical, January 1882, 41–43 A (NAI).

'interiors', but accommodated instead within the prevailing rhythms of the everyday as an effortless and routine process. This explains why officials recommended that quinine required to be 'sold at places where people were likely to frequent in ordinary course of business'.[51]

In the early 1890s, the elaborate distribution of government quinine began in Bengal and through the 'pice packet system'. According to codes of monetary circulation in contemporary British India, one pice referred to three pies and 'to the smallest coin in daily use amongst the public'. Quinine manufactured in the government factory at Mungpoo was to be made up into very small packets. Each packet, according to government instruction, was to contain 5 grains, worth 1 pice each. 'Packing factories' or central depots were set up at the Hazaribagh Reformatory School and the jail depot at Calcutta. Juvenile delinquents at the school and convict labourers at the depot were entrusted with receiving quinine from the factory, preparing the envelopes and filling them with quinine.[52]

The government of Bengal initially decided to sell quinine through all 'public offices in the interior of the districts', such as police outposts, dispensaries and offices of the managers of wards' estates. However, the intricate network of post offices was eventually considered the most 'convenient and effective agency' for the enforcement of the consumption of quinine amongst the inhabitants in the interiors. The consent of the Post Master General of Bengal was sought. It was recommended that the packing factories at Hazaribagh and Calcutta would supply every post office in Bengal with a permanent stock of a sufficient number of packets. When a postmaster found that his stock was running short he was directed to requisition the packing factory for a fresh supply. The central depots were expected to comply with the requisition order by sending the required number of packets which the postmaster paid for on receipt. The postmaster was expected to finance the procurement of new supplies from the sale of previously received quinine. A nominal remuneration was proposed to induce the postmaster to encourage sales, initially fixed at one *anna* for every sale amounting to one rupee.[53]

By the late 1890s, this intricate and elaborate 'system' had been extended to almost every province within British India, including Assam, Burma, Madras, Central Provinces, Sind and Baluchistan, Punjab, United Provinces, Bombay, North Western Provinces and Oudh. The government factory at Madras was responsible for the supply of quinine

---

[51] Home, Medical, July 1892, 38–40 A (NAI).

[52] Ibid.; See also, E. Hutton to All Postal Officials, Bengal Circle, 12 November 1892, Calcutta. Home, Medical, July 1893, 59–63A (NAI).

[53] Ibid.

to Burma, the United Provinces, Central Provinces and Bombay. Quinine was supplied to the remaining provinces from the factory at Mungpoo.[54] More packing factories were soon set up at jails in Aligarh,[55] Mandalay and Rangoon.[56] In official correspondence, the post office figured as a site which the 'poorer classes in the interiors' were likely to frequent 'in ordinary course of business'. The village post office was described as 'a popular place of meeting, where people assemble to hear the news and discuss matters of common interest.' The postmasters and the postal peons, it was hoped, would be able to conduct sales of quinine without interfering with their 'ordinary duties'.[57] The village postmen were instructed to carry a few quinine powders with them when making their rounds. This was conceived as a convenient way of bringing quinine to the 'doors' of the malarial patients.[58] The government considered it more prudent to employ postmasters and the postmen over the subordinate revenue officials and the lower rank policemen as vending agencies in the villages. Postmen were considered better distributed across the rural interiors of the districts in British India than officials associated with the revenue or police departments. The 'universal' presence of the subordinate postal officials in the villages, it was argued, aroused much less suspicion amongst the people than the occasional and significant visits of the police or revenue officials. The 'poor in the country', officials suggested, lived in 'constant fear' of the police and the revenue officials. The government was keen to resist the impression that increased sales of quinine were enforced by the imposition of authority or coercion by the colonial state: 'Postmasters are free from this objection; postmasters are universal, they exercise no authority, they are poor men as a rule, and the inducement held out in the shape of commission will be an incentive to pushing the sales'.[59] The recruitment of lower vernacular officials in the postal department, government officials thought, would make the distribution of quinine effortless, routine, regular and more acceptable to the people. These intentions are echoed in a contemporary signboard (see Figure 5.1) issued by the postal department across eastern India,

---

[54] 'Notes'. Home, Medical, October 1903, 109–112 A (NAI).

[55] Secretary, Government of the North-Western Provinces and Oudh to Postmaster General, North-Western Provinces, 23 October 1895. Home, Medical, December 1895, 105–108 A (NAI).

[56] Chief Commissioner of Burma in the General Department, 'Proceedings', 30 October 1894, Rangoon. Home, Medical, March 1895, 16–18 A (NAI).

[57] Home, Medical, July 1892, 38–40 A (NAI).

[58] W. Standen, to Secretary to the Government, Revenue Department, 31 August 1897, Ootacamund. Rev-agriculture, Economic-products, November 1897, 8 B (NAI).

[59] W. F. Defabeck to the Secretary to Government, Revenue department, 9 September 1892, Madras. Home, Medical, November 1893, 78–79 B (NAI).

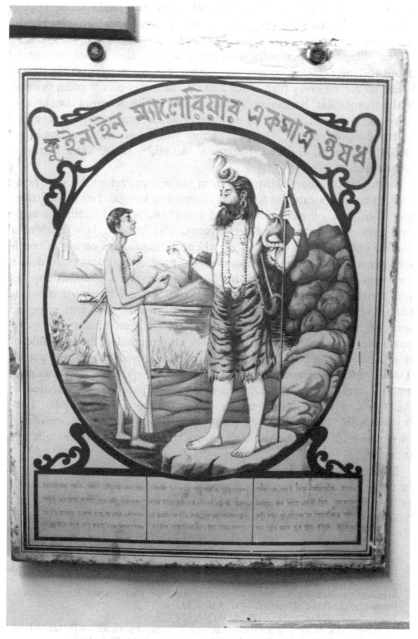

Figure 5.1 Signboard on malaria containing the caption 'Quinine the only cure for malaria'. Credit: Philatelic Museum, General Post Office, Kolkata.

presently in the custody of the Philatelic Museum at the General Post Office in Calcutta, which portrays quinine as a panacea gifted by Hindu deity Lord Shiva to the villagers of Bengal.

The village postmen were also instructed to disseminate awareness about the 'pice-packet system' by pasting relevant notices on the notice board adjoining every post office and circulating copies,[60] often printed in the 'vernacular' languages.[61] Instructions to the potential consumers, price and dose were inscribed on a paper which was used to wrap every pice packet of quinine. The information was eventually translated into Bengali, Marathi, Gujarati, Kanarese, Sindhi,[62] Tamil[63] and Burmese languages.[64]

Strategies of quinine distribution in various provinces did not, however, blindly replicate the 'system', initiated in Bengal. Nor were strategies of enforcing the consumption of quinine subsumed within the intricate networks of the postal department. The 'pice-packets' enabled a flexible system, which could enlist, whenever required, a variety of familiar figures in accordance with the varying provincial situations in different parts of India and beyond. In Burma, for instance, a range of agents was considered in November 1892, including the Myooks or subordinate magistrates in charge of towns, forest officers, sergeants of police stations, thugyis or headmen of circles or villages, bazaar gaungs or headmen, and vaccinators. It was also recommended that the sale of quinine could be popularised by the police constables on beat patrol. These vendors were to be supplied with one parcel each containing 102 packets of quinine. The worth of every parcel was estimated at Rs. 1–9–6. However, the vendors were likely to receive it at Rs. 1–8–0 per parcel. The balance of 1 *anna* and 6 pies was to be considered as remuneration for the vendor's efforts.[65] Later this profit margin was increased.

Dissemination of knowledge about the drug through the medium of released convicts was also proposed, besides extensive distribution of handbills. Non-official vendors of quinine, like stallholders and 'respectable shop keepers' were considered for almost every bazaar in

---

[60] E. Hutton to All Postal Officials, Bengal Circle, Home, Medical, July 1893, 59–63A (NAI).

[61] Standen to Secretary to the Government, Revenue Department. Rev-agriculture, Economic-products. November 1897, 8 B (NAI).

[62] Home, Medical, September 1904, 49 B (NAI).

[63] W. F. deFabeck, to the Secretary, Government, Revenue department, 9 February 1892, Nungumbakum. Rev-agriculture, Agriculture, July 1892, 25–28 A (NAI).

[64] Chief Commissioner of Burma in the General Department, 'Proceedings', Home, Medical, March 1895, 16–18 A (NAI).

[65] 'Enclosure No. 2', Home, Medical, July 1893, 55–58 A (NAI).

the province.[66] Within Bengal itself, the postal network apart, quinine was sold through the railway stationmasters at 'small roadside stations', vaccination establishments and the dispensaries located in the 'mufassals'. Private employers, including zamindars, indigo and tea planters were also permitted to procure quinine from the Superintendent of Jail Manufactures and sell the drug.[67]

The government devised means of distributing quinine in locations not connected by the post. In the 'interiors' of Sind and certain native states, quinine was distributed through the political officers or political agents, circle inspectors, patel of villages and salt licensees.[68] In June 1905, the chief commissioner of Assam recommended the enlisting of village schoolmasters, village headmen and village chaukidars as salesmen of quinine in the rural areas of the province.[69]

Quinine in the 'interiors' figured as an agent of Empire. Its arrival was both mobilised and predicated upon a series of transformations, at least momentarily: prisons became packing factories, juvenile delinquents became convict labourers, released prisoners turned into reformed volunteers, post offices became dispensaries, peons became vaccinators and an entire network of *mofussil* appeared co-opted into the state's regime of distribution as 'vending agents'. Quinine emboldened the government with an object (and an objective) with which to reach out to the interiors. Government correspondence, in turn, described quinine and the interiors as alien to and yet intimately adaptive with one another.

Such arrangements for governing a 'thing-in-motion', conjured up fetishist intimacies between quinine and the people inhabiting the interiors.[70] Quinine was projected as compatible with the prevailing bonds of a shared language, locality, community and the rhythms of daily life. Apart from resulting in a communalisation of quinine, exigencies of circulation reconfigured some of its physical attributes. However, as the following section shows, as a commodity-in-motion, quinine was not only reconstituted, but also, in turn, exposed fractures and tensions in between provincial governments, besides revealing various imperial prejudices.

[66] Secretary, Government of Burma to the Secretary, Government of India, 14 August 1897, Rangoon 'Enclosure 4.' Home, Medical, October 1897, 285–297 A (NAI).
[67] J. A. Bourdillon, Secretary, Government of Bengal to the Secretary, Government of India, 5 September 1893, Darjeeling. Home, Medical, October 1893, 29–31 A (NAI).
[68] Home, Medical. September 1904, 49 B (NAI).
[69] L. J. Kershaw to the Secretary, Government of India, 22 June 1905. Home, Medical, August 1905, 67–68 A (NAI).
[70] For things-in-motion, see A. Appadurai, 'Introduction: Commodities and the Politics of Value', in A. Appadurai (ed.), *The Social Life of Things: Commodities in Cultural Perspective* (Cambridge: Cambridge University Press, 1986), 5. For commodity fetishism, see A. McClintock, *Imperial Leather: Race, Gender and Sexuality in the Colonial Context* (New York and London: Routledge, 1995), 207–225.

Policing Purity

In establishing new distribution networks, the government was keen to police against the possibility of corruption of the purity of quinine. These anxieties went back to the early 1880s, when the state had begun distributing anti-malarial drugs in the form of cinchona febrifuge. These acts of policing often resulted in punishment. In January 1882, for example, Dr Bensley, the civil surgeon of Nuddea in the Bengal Presidency, was suspended for misappropriation of cinchona febrifuge in the interest of private trade. He gave the drug a Bengali name – 'jvarer mahaushadhi' or 'the sovereign remedy for fever' – altered the label on the seal and adopted his own mode of accounting. These measures, Bensley argued, were deliberate innovations to attract a rural Bengali clientele belonging to 'all classes'. He mentioned that as part of his innovative strategies of distribution he had trained and sent out 33 kavirajas to various parts of the district with the mixture: 'My object in carrying out this plan was simply to place the remedy within the reach of those who had no medical aid, and would probably have perished'.[71]

Nonetheless, the higher authorities went ahead with the punishment. They did, however, acknowledge the merits of some of the measures initiated by Bensley. In view of the remarkable popularity of the drug dispensed by Bensley, they observed, 'the people seem to prefer a made-up draught to the Cinchona febrifuge'. Innovations by officials located in the interiors often made the distribution of state-manufactured drugs more convenient. This opened up the intriguing administrative challenge of distinguishing between acceptable forms of innovation and corruption. Such tensions survived and were augmented in the following decades with the state-initiated efforts of distributing quinine into the interiors.[72]

Retailers and speculators also were often suspected of buying subsidised government quinine in bulk in the garb of 'genuine consumers'. It was feared that they could then package it as more expensive forms of European quinine and re-sell it at greater profit. Official files referred to 'low paid compounders',[73] 'druggists', 'petty native chemists in towns' as the potential suspects.[74] Preventing the identity and 'purity' of

[71] Payne to the Secretary, Government of Bengal, Medical and Municipal department. Home, Medical, January 1882, 41–43 A (NAI).

[72] Ibid.

[73] C. A. Galton, Secretary, Government of Fort St George to Secretary, Government of India, 28 April 1893, Ootacamund, Home, Medical, November 1893, 78–79 B (NAI).

[74] M. Hammick to the Secretary, Government of India, 18 July 1902, Ootacamund. Rev-agriculture, Economic-products, July 1902, 3 A (NAI).

government quinine from being tampered with emerged as issues of consistent concern.

Labelling the physical appearance of government quinine with an inerasable and distinctive marker figured as a credible way of ensuring purity. To that effect, most of the quinine manufactured by the government in Madras was coloured pink between 1893 and 1904. Pink colour thus emerged as a label for government quinine manufactured in Madras while serving as an assurance of purity.[75] The 'caste natives', it was claimed, considered 'pinkness' as a sign of legitimate, credible, established, recognised, trustworthy, protected version of pure quinine.[76] Private manufacturers of quinine based in Europe, including the Howards, sought permissions repeatedly from the Indian government to export 'pink coloured quinine' into India. These requests, however, were turned down.[77]

Pink quinine revealed interprovincial tensions between Madras and Bengal. In March 1904, David Prain, then Director of the Botanical Survey of India and erstwhile Superintendent of the Botanic gardens in Calcutta, questioned the prudence of such acts of colouring. He failed to appreciate any 'excessive virtue' in pink quinine. He lamented the conversion of pink quinine into an 'official fetish', and instead described 'white' as the 'natural colour of pure quinine'. Any additional colouring of the drug, he feared, would constitute a more expensive and long process.[78] Officials representing the two provinces differed on the question of 'natural colour of pure quinine'. In a polemical retort, a bureaucrat based in Madras refused to consider 'whiteness' as the 'natural colour' of quinine. He argued that like pink quinine, 'whiteness' was manufactured through long, tedious and expensive processes.[79] The Director General of post offices, in turn, showed that the colour of the quinine supplied by private European manufacturers and sold by druggists across British India was white. Contrary to the claims of officials representing Madras, he thought that the public more generally associated the best forms of the drug with whiteness.[80]

By the late 1900s, antagonism between officials reached new depths over the difference in price charged for government quinines

[75] Secretary of State for India, 'Telegram dated 23 August 1904', Notes, Rev-agriculture, Economic-products, September 1904, 7 A (NAI).
[76] H. O. Quin to the Secretary, Government of India, 9 November 1906. Home, Medical, December 1906, 54 A (NAI).
[77] Director General of Stores, 'Memorandum', 6 June 1907. Rev-agriculture, Agriculture, September 1907, 14 B (NAI).
[78] 'Notes', 18 March 1904. Home, Medical, April 1904, 46–47 A (NAI).
[79] J. N. Atkinson to the Secretary, Government of India, 1 February 1904. Ibid.
[80] 'Notes', 7 August 1903. Home, Medical, October 1903, 109–112 A (NAI).

manufactured in the two provinces. In January 1909, the price for quinine supplied by the Bengal government was fixed in accordance with the average wholesale price of Howard's quinine prevalent in the preceding year. This amounted to Rs. 10 per pound. Meanwhile, the Madras government broke away from the prevalent convention of determining the price of government quinine. Instead, it proposed to adopt a 'different system' which was to be regulated by the cost of production. Accordingly, a price of Rs. 8 per pound was set for government quinine manufactured in Madras. This was considered much lower than the existing market rates. This could, it was alleged by Bengal, disturb the uniformity in the price of the commodity, drive private enterprise out of the British Indian market, and undermine the credibility of the government factory in Bengal. For a while, officials in Bengal protested in vain for the price of Madras quinine to be raised. Thereafter they turned combative.

Pink quinine could be sold at the cheaper price, it was alleged on behalf of the Bengal government, as it was relatively impure: 'The Madras article contained only 75 per cent of the sulphate of quinine, the rest being water crystallisation; the percentages for Bengal quinine being 98 and 2, and for Howard's quinine 92 and 8, respectively'.[81] Successive chemical analyses conducted in Europe and India under the initiatives of the Bengal government suggested that pink quinine was impure.[82] It was alleged to contain a cinchonidine content of 7.84 per cent. This appeared to exceed the permissible limit allowed by the British pharmacopeia, that is, 3 per cent. Thus, pink colouration, it was suggested, could not be considered a guarantee of purity.[83] The impression of 'pinkness' as an indicator of purity was, according to A. T. Gage, Superintendent of the cinchona factory in Bengal, 'misleading, a delusion, a snare'.[84] Pinkness, according to these officials, provided a distinctive label for the quinine manufactured on behalf of the Madras government, but could not serve as proof of the purity of the commodity.[85]

While British officials in India were debating the physical appearance of pure quinine, greater clarity emerged on the colour of less pure and ineffective forms of quinine. Once exposed to 'adverse conditions' in the 'plains of India', it was argued in January 1912, quinine – 'no matter of what brand' – could be converted into 'an inert form known as quiniretin'. Enduring exposure to heat and light, it was suggested, could

[81] 'Notes', 21 October 1909. Rev-agriculture, Agriculture, December 1909, 17–18 A (NAI).

[82] H. D. Holme, 'Note dated 03–08–10'. Home, Medical, January 1911, 43 B (NAI).

[83] E. D. Maclagan to the Secretary, Government of Madras, 17 September 1910, Simla. Rev-agriculture, Agriculture, September 1910, 24–26 A (NAI).

[84] C. P. Lukis, 'Note dated 7.7.1910', Ibid.   [85] 'Note dated 17 September', Ibid.

initiate a series of 'molecular transformations' in the drug: 'Quiniretin is the name given to an undefined *brown* product of the action of sunlight on an aqueous solution of quinine alkaloid'.[86]

Colouring quinine was certainly not the only safeguard adopted by the governments in British India towards protecting its purity from potential abuse, when the drug was being circulated beyond the secure confines of chemical laboratories and factories. A range of other steps was considered to protect the commodity from being retailed or abused. It was recommended, for instance, that no consumer should be sold more than a certain number of packets of government quinine.[87] Each packet contained very small quantities of quinine varying from 5 grains to 7 grains. 'The small profit and great labour involved in opening an infinite number of small packages' was considered by itself a significant disincentive against fraud. To guard against tampering with quinine packets or the substitution of quinine by inferior articles, routine inspections of post offices were conducted.[88] A variety of government stamps were attached upon 'firmly closed covers' and packets to secure the purity of the product. They usually included a seal of the 'royal arms'[89] or a seal bearing the mark of the packing factory, for example, 'Yerrowda Prison'.[90] It was often suggested that a certificate endorsing the purity of the drug be enclosed in the packets, along with relevant instructions for the prospective consumers.[91] After sale, strict vigilance was recommended to prevent the recycling of empty labelled packets for fraudulent purposes.[92]

These careful safeguards notwithstanding, desperate acts of fraud – ranging from attempts to forge government labels and packets to selling adulterated forms of the drug – continued to figure in official correspondence. One such case was reported in May–June 1905. Mahim Chandra Dutta and his son Shashi Kumar were joint proprietors of a grocery business, and owned a shop at Sapar Hat in the jurisdiction of Matbaria thana in the Pirojur subdivision of the Backergunge district in Bengal. On the days of the weekly bazaar, they sold groceries at the Tushkhali Hat. A branch post office located in Tushkhali sold government quinine in pice packets of 5 grains each to the public. In June 1904, the

[86] A. T. Gage, 'Note dated 27-02-1912', Rev-agriculture, Agriculture, May 1912, 21 B (NAI).

[87] Hammick to Secretary, Government of India. Rev-agriculture, Economic-products, July 1902, 3 A (NAI).

[88] Bourdillon to Secretary, Government of India. Home, Medical, October 1893, 29–31 A (NAI).

[89] H. M. Kisch, 'A Note dated 7.8.1903'. Home, Medical, October 1903, 109–112 A (NAI).

[90] A. U. Fanshawe, 'A Note dated 10 June 1896'. Home, Medical, July 1896. 144–145 A (NAI).

[91] J. P. Hewett to the Chief Commissioner, Assam, 15 July 1896, Simla. Ibid.

[92] 'Enclosure no. 2', Home, Medical, November 1893, 78–79 B (NAI).

postmaster of that branch reported to the manager of the jail depot in Calcutta accusing Sashikumar of engaging in fraudulent acts. For more than a year, Sashikumar had been apparently selling a 'white powder' in packets exactly similar in size and shape as the government ones. Such packets bore the same inscriptions with an addition of 'S. K. Dutta' typed in very small fonts. On instruction from the Inspector General of Jails, the postmaster sent 32 packets of S. K. Dutta's quinine for analysis by the chemical examiner. This revealed that S. K. Dutta's 'powder' consisted chiefly of 'flour or other starchy matter with traces of quinine sulphate and arsenic'. Subsequently, Pyar Mohun Biswas, a police inspector, was deputed to raid Shasikumar Dutta's shop. Amongst many other items, he found some packets of government quinine, a tin containing white powder, rubber stamps and pads and ink for putting the impression on the envelopes. Shasikumar was tried and convicted on charges framed under sections 274, 275, 276 and 417–511 of the Indian penal code and under sections 6 and 7 of the Merchandise Marks Act 1889. The convictions were upheld, it was observed, because Sashikumar had falsely claimed that the packets contained pure quinine. He was sentenced to six months of rigorous imprisonment.[93]

The details of this case are suggestive. A network of post officials, chemical analysts, police inspectors and legal clauses were in place to detect, report, investigate, convict and punish acts of fraud in relation to quinine. Despite this, the image of quinine as a profitable commodity seems to have excited the imaginations of a range of actors in marketplaces across Bengal.

'War of Mosquitoes'

The social and physical characteristics associated with quinine were reconstituted, while the state arranged for the travel of the drug from government factories to the 'doors' of potential consumers. Ironically, meanwhile, the corresponding diagnostic category, malaria, itself underwent considerable mutations. The increasing recognition of a range of microorganisms by the early 1900s as the generic cause behind different forms of diseases brought insects into the centre of public health discourse.[94] Bugs of various shapes and sizes began being suspected

---

[93] Rev-agriculture, Agriculture, June 1905, 12 B (NAI).

[94] For an insightful intellectual history, see M. Worboys, *Spreading Germs: Disease Theories and Medical Practice in Britain, 1865–1900* (New York and Cambridge: Cambridge University Press, 2000). See also, M. Worboys, 'From Miasmas to Germs: Malaria 1850–1879', *Parassitologia*, 36 (1994), 61; P. Chakrabarti, *Bacteriology in British India: Laboratory Medicine and the Tropics* (Rochester: University of Rochester Press, 2012), 8.

as carriers of different types of invisible (without a microscope) disease-causing germs between human bodies, and this resulted in a series of nosological reconfigurations. In this process, the category malaria was retained, but redefined in various quarters as the name of a fever disease caused by parasites. Although the redefinition of malaria from a generic cause of many diseases to an insect-borne fever disease was far from complete in the first decade of the twentieth century, the category became more associated with parasites, insect vectors, fevers and blood samples than ever before. It was not achieved in a day, or by the brilliance of any particular individual, or through the initiative of any specific institution. It reflected the scientific investments and political priorities of an entire generation.[95]

The initiatives of Ronald Ross constituted a crucial moment in that history. Ross, in significant ways, was a product of the British Empire. His father was a Scottish officer in the British Indian army, and Ross was born in the year of the Sepoy Mutiny in Almora in northern India. As a trained physician, Ross served the colonial Indian Medical Service in different parts of the subcontinent for about two decades (1881 to 1899). Ross's microscope-based findings in the late 1890s (corroborated by his British collaborators and Italian detractors) contributed eventually to the identification of certain species of mosquitoes as the vectors for transmitting malarial parasites between human bodies. However, the process through which Ross's findings acquired wider currency and credibility was long and chequered, and was not confined to the laboratory. The widespread recognition acquired by the theory that mosquitoes were the insect vectors for malaria, this section argues, need to be situated within the broader history of enduring prejudices held towards insects more generally, and mosquitoes in particular, in colonial India and beyond. Contentious laboratory speculations were validated and reinscribed retrospectively through elaborate efforts of application by sanitary officials in the 'fields of practice'; anticipated by anxieties amongst managers of colonial plantations; and sustained considerably by articulations in the realm of vernacular literary production.[96] Certain concerns of

[95] Worboys, 'From Miasmas to Germs', 61–68; Guillemin, 'Choosing Scientific Patrimony'. On the early history of parasitology and its interactions with the medical knowledge of diseases, see for example, J. Farley, 'Parasites and the Germ Theory of Disease', in C. E. Rosenberg and J. Golden (eds.), *Framing Disease: Studies in Cultural History* (New Jersey: Rutgers University Press, 1992), 33–49; S. Li, 'Natural History of Parasitic Disease: Patrick Manson's Philosophical Method', *Isis*, 93 (2002), 206–228. For a magisterial survey W. D. Foster, *A History of Parasitology* (Edinburgh and London: E&S Livingstone Ltd., 1965).

[96] The expression 'fields of practice' had been attributed to a 'leading Italian authority on malaria', Professor Celli. See correspondence from the Secretary of State for India,

colonial medical entomology were shared by the worlds of imperial sanitary governance, and commercial plantations, and colonial vernacular literature.[97]

A range of visitors to Ross's laboratory in Calcutta in the late 1890s, from J. W. Daniels to Leonard Rogers, were deeply impressed with him but left unmoved by the hypothesis. Studying the suburbs of Calcutta, Rogers found the presence of anopheles mosquitoes in 'inverse proportion to the amount of fever'.[98] Despite such informed scepticisms, by the early 1900s Ross had mobilised unforeseen funds from the British state and the industry to employ his findings in restricting malaria. A series of campaigns or what he termed 'mosquito brigades' and 'malaria expeditions' were launched, proclaiming the goal of suffocating and exterminating mosquitoes. Initiated in 'cantonments, towns, plantations' across Sierra Leone, Lagos and Cape Coast Castle in the West Coast of Africa, such efforts were extended subsequently to Ismailia, Hong Kong, Staten Island, Havana and Mian Mir in British India amongst many other locations.[99] Ross's expeditions, amongst other features, consisted in revisiting locations established firmly as malarial in the prevalent medical geographies and finding evidence in favour of the theory he was so keen on establishing.[100] Through such expeditions, Ross prophesised, 'the winged insects will vanish as if by magic'.[101]

Insects attracted variously the attention of British officials in India from late eighteenth century: as objects of collection, cataloguing,

---

No. 153 (Revenue), 30 September 1904. 'Notes', Home, Medical, June 1905, 200–204 A (NAI).

[97] While commenting on these historical specificities which shaped medical knowledge about mosquitoes around the 1900s, this chapter adopts an approach that is different from those evident in the important works of environmental historians like J. R. McNeill, *Mosquito Empires: Ecology and War in the Greater Caribbean* (Cambridge: Cambridge University Press, 2010) and Webb, *Humanity's Burden*, 32–49, and historical demographers like M. Dobson, '"Marsh Fever": The Geography of Malaria in England', *Journal of Historical Geography*, 6, 4 (1980), 357–380.

[98] 'J. W. Daniels report to the Secretary of the Malaria Investigation Committee of the Royal Society, London,' 23 January 1899, Calcutta. Home, Medical, May 1899, 156–159 A (NAI); L. Rogers, 'The relationship of the water supply, water-logging, and the distribution of Anopheles Mosquitoes to the prevalence of Malaria north of Calcutta', *Journal of the Asiatic Society of Bengal*, 69 (2), No. iv. (1900), 474–476.

[99] Home, Medical, December 1901, 69–72 A (NAI); R. Ross, *Mosquito Brigades and How to Organise Them?* (London: Longmans, Green, 1902).

[100] Ross, *Mosquito Brigades*, 69; For greater detail, see N. H. Swellengrebel, 'How the Malaria Service in Indonesia came into being, 1898–1948', *The Journal of Hygiene*, 48, 2 (June 1950), 148–150; J. Western and S. Frenkel, 'Pretext or Prophylaxis? Racial Segregation and Malarial Mosquitoes in a British Tropical Colony: Sierra Leone', *Annals of the Association of American Geographers*, 78, 2 (June 1988), 214–17.

[101] Ronald Ross to the Under Secretary of State for India, 2 October 1901. Home, Medical, December 1901, 69–72 A (NAI).

and exchanging,[102] as items of commerce,[103] as means of punishing suspected criminals,[104] and rarely yet strikingly as sources of food.[105] However, in proposing such hawkish measures, Ross echoed and appealed to some of the contemporary biases prevalent in the British Empire about insects. As the historian Richard Jones has recently shown, protection from insects, particularly mosquitoes, mobilised a range of commodities from the end of the nineteenth century.[106] A series of advertisements (see Figures 5.2, 5.3, 5.4 and 5.5) reveal that imperial encounters with mosquitoes necessitated particular forms of houses, cones, nets, iron bedsteads, soaps and creams.[107]

From the 1860s, insects were projected as notorious destroyers of commercially relevant vegetation: preying on 'woods and forests', inflicting agriculture with plant diseases, and most consistently, as detrimental to the tea, cinchona, coffee, sugarcane and cotton plantations.[108] Collecting and cataloguing insects on behalf of the Asiatic Society, Bombay Natural History Society and Europe-based imperial museums continued. However, from the 1890s onwards, plantation money was used to fund travel to research insect pests, affecting industrially relevant vegetation. In September 1894, E. C. Cotes, the Deputy Superintendent of the Indian Museum, was deputed to tour almost every province in British India. Over a period of three years, Cotes was expected to study and report on the various insects that were alleged to destroy agricultural crops and commercially valuable plants. It is revealing to note that the Indian Tea Association elaborately sponsored his extensive entomological tours.[109] The department of Economic Entomology was instituted

---

[102] T. Horsfield and F. Moore, *A Catalogue of the Lepidopterous Insects in the Museum of the Hon. East India Company* (London: W. H. Allen, 1857).

[103] T. W. Helfer, 'On the Indigenous Silkworms of India', *Journal of the Asiatic Society of Bengal*, 6, 1 (January 1837), 38–47.

[104] N. Chevers, *A Manual of Medical Jurisprudence for India* (Calcutta: Thacker, Spink and Co, 1870), 260, 350, 386, 564–567.

[105] V. M. Holt, *Why Not Eat Insects?* (London: Field and Tuer, 1885), 36–48.

[106] R. Jones, *Mosquito* (London: Reaktion Books, 2012).

[107] 'Advertisement for Southalls' Mosquito Cones', *Times of India* (4 January 1894) and 'Advertisement for Barff Boro-Glyceride', *Times of India* (2 December 1909) See M. Srivastava (ed.), *Branding New: Advertising Through the Times of India* (Faridabad: Thomson (India), 1989), 158 and 191.

[108] R. Thompson, *Report on Insects Destructive to Woods and Forests* (Allahabad: Government Press, 1868); Rev-agriculture, Agriculture, August 1894, 18–34 A (NAI); E. T. Atkinson, 'On Pests Belonging to the Homopterous family of Coccidae, which Attack Tea, Cinchona and Coffee Trees', *Journal of Asiatic Society*, 55 (1886), 121–123; Rev-agriculture, Agriculture, April 1892, 29 B; Rev-agriculture, Economic-products, October 1904, 10 A (NAI).

[109] J. Buckingham to the Acting Secretary, Indian Tea Association, 13 October 1894, Amgoorie. Rev-agriculture, Agriculture, January 1895, 1–8 A (NAI).

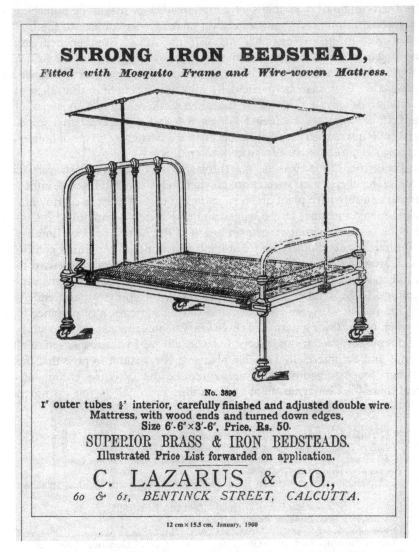

Figure 5.2 Advertisement of 'Strong iron bedstead fitted with mosquito frame'. January 1900. R. Ray Choudhuri, *Early Calcutta Advertisements, 1875–1925: A Selection from the Statesman* (Bombay: Nachiketa Publications, 1992), 400. Credit: The Statesman, Kolkata.

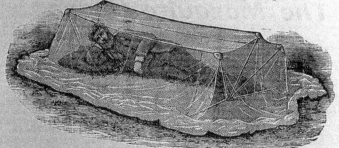
Figure 5.3 Advertisement of 'The Folding Hood of Mosquito Net by
White and Wright'. Reproduced in R. Ross, *Malarial Fever, Its Cause,
Prevention and Treatment* (London: Longman, Green and Co, 1902).
Credit: Wellcome Library, London.

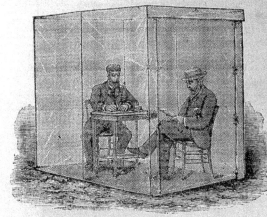
Figure 5.4 Advertisement of The Mosquito House by White and Wright. Reproduced in R. Ross, *Malarial Fever, Its Cause, Prevention and Treatment* (London: Longman, Green and Co, 1902). Credit: Wellcome Library, London.

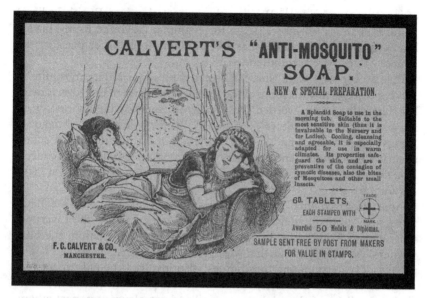

Figure 5.5 Advertisement of 'Calvert's "Anti-Mosquito Soap" showing one woman covered in mosquitoes while another is free from them', c. 1890. Credit: Wellcome Library, London.

in 1902. E. P. Stebbing, the erstwhile Deputy Conservator of Forests, was appointed the first Economic Entomologist to the government of India.[110] Earlier in February 1901, Stebbing was ordered by the Inspector General of Forests to 'conduct investigations regarding insects injurious to forests'.[111] In the same year, at the insistence of the United Planters' Association of South India, George Watt, the Reporter on Economic Products, was deputed for six months to investigate the relation between 'plant diseases' and 'insect pests'.[112] On similar insistence from the planters' community, the Mysore durbar appointed a mycologist and an entomologist to supervise the protection of sandal trees.[113]

To encourage institutionalised killing of insect pests, the Deputy Superintendent of the Indian Museum, Cotes was deputed to the USA to study insecticides and other appliances geared towards the 'destruction' of insects.[114] The Central Provinces prohibited by law the slaughter

[110] 'Notes', Rev-agriculture, Agriculture, November 1902, 2–5 A (NAI).
[111] Rev-agriculture, Forests, February 1901, 8–10 A (NAI).
[112] Secretary, United Planters' Association of South India to the Secretary, Government of India, 31 August 1900, Madras Rev-agriculture, Economic-products, February 1901, 1–2 A (NAI).
[113] Rev-agriculture, Agriculture, October 1905, 11B (NAI).
[114] Rev-agriculture, Agriculture, November 1894, 8–12 A (NAI).

of insectivorous birds.[115] Besides, the importation into British India of
'natural enemies' of insect pests, for example, ladybirds from Hawaii,
hyacinths like Azolla and fishes like Millions from other parts of the
United States were recommended.[116]

Ross's proposals were thus not isolated pleas for killing mosquitoes.
Having converged with some of the broader priorities of the government,
his suggestions were worded with recurrent military metaphors: 'wag-
ing war against mosquitoes', 'crusades', 'flags', 'volunteers', 'brigades',
'gangs', 'expeditions' and so on.[117] Metaphors which described action
against mosquitoes and military intervention continued to overlap through the interwar period and into the Korean War (see
Figure 5.6).

Apart from colonial governments, as hinted already, Ross's expeditions were funded extensively by industrial concerns like the Liverpool
Chamber of Commerce, the Steamship Owners' Association, the Ship
Owners' Association and the West African Trade Association.[118] The
project of 'exterminating mosquitoes' also involved the enlistment of a
range of commodities: nets, Keating's insect powder, quicklime, char-
coal and gallons of phenyl, kerosene, oil and petroleum, amongst others.
Killing mosquitoes further required support from 'insectivorous' plants,
fishes and birds. Mosquitoes mobilised a hierarchy of regular and part-
time labourers: 'commissioned' district-level officials serving the municipal and public works departments, Indian troops serving in Hong Kong,
the police, assistant surgeons, hospital assistants, peons, 'daily recruited
local labour', and a range of 'native agents' including village headmen,
workmen, 'gangs of coolies', 'sweepers', convict labour, tinsmith and
so on.[119]

Such extensive recruitments metamorphosed mosquitoes into subjects of unprecedented attention, observation and interest, beyond the

---

[115] Home, Public, July 1890, 95–97 A (NAI).

[116] For details about the use of the aquatic plant Azolla for the killing of mosquitoes, see
Home, Medical, June 1909, 242–245 A; for colonial requisition for a consignment
of a fish called Millions see Home, Sanitary, 150–152 A, July 1909; see also Rev-
agriculture, Agriculture, September 1897, 3–5 A (NAI).

[117] Ross, Mosquito Brigades, vi, 88; For political implications of the deployments of mil-
itary metaphors vis-à-vis insects, see E. P. Russell III, '"Speaking of Annihilation",
Mobilizing for War against Human and Insect Enemies, 1914–1945', The Journal of
American History, 82, 4 (March 1996), 1505–1529.

[118] Anonymous, 'The Malaria Expedition to West Africa', Science, New Series, 11, 262 (5
January 1900), 36–37; For details about 'The Committee of the Liverpool School of
Tropical Medicine' see Home, Medical, July 1909, 56–57A (NAI).

[119] Home, Medical, June 1909, 242–245 A; Home, Sanitary, July 1909, 150–152 A; Ross
to Under-Secretary of State for India, Home, Medical, December 1901, 69–72 A;
'Noted dated 17 March 1903', Bombay Castle. Home, Medical, April 1903, 2–3 A
(NAI); Ross, Mosquito Brigades, 65, 74.

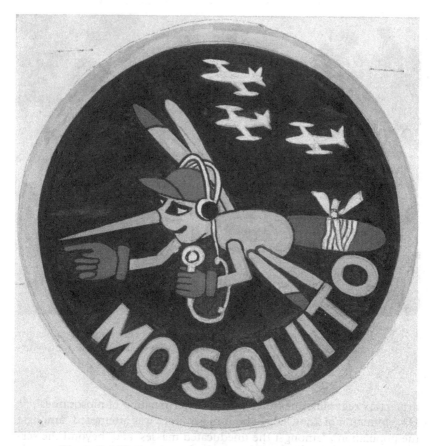

Figure 5.6 'Copy of the original artwork used to create the Mosquito patch during the Korean War', c. 1950–1955. Credit: National Museum of the US Air Force photo.

usual confines of entomological laboratories and naturalists (see Figure 5.7). In January 1902, the government of Bombay offered four prizes for a year's observations on the distribution and habits of mosquitoes in certain towns in the Presidency. The prizes ranged from Rs. 100 to Rs. 400. The competition was not restricted to the government servants. The Bombay Natural History Society was requested to adjudicate the prizes.[120] Circulars were distributed amongst certified sanitary

[120] 'Noted dated 17 March 1903', Bombay Castle. Home, Medical, April 1903, 2–3 A (NAI).

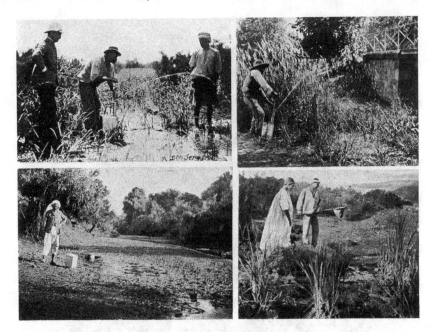

Figure 5.7 Photograph of sanitary measures being undertaken against mosquitoes. From R. Ross, *Prevention of Malaria* (London: John Murray, 1910). Credit: Wellcome Library London.

inspectors regarding measures for the 'extermination of mosquitoes'.[121] Dissemination of knowledge about mosquitoes was attempted 'amongst the population', 'amongst the uneducated masses' and 'beyond the services'. Teachers in the public schools were instructed to 'impart their scholars the rudiments of the malaria doctrine'.[122]

Neither Ross's discovery nor the expeditions initiated by him in the early 1900s revealed radically new arenas in the prevailing geographies of malaria. On the contrary, such expeditions were precisely organised in locations that had been labelled as notoriously malarial in the medical geographies of empires from the mid-nineteenth century. Ross's expeditions also constituted of revisiting such locations to find evidence in favour of the theory he was so keen on establishing.[123] In certain ways, the organisation of 'mosquito brigades' and the firmer entrenchment

[121] 'Circular no. 2109A-S' Home, Medical, September 1901, 139 A (NAI).
[122] Ross, *Mosquito Brigades*, 72–73.
[123] Ross, *Mosquito Brigades*, 69. For greater detail see, Swellengrebel, 'How the Malaria Service in Indonesia Came into Being, 1898–1948', 148–150.

of Ross's theory involving the insect vector of malaria were symbiotic processes. The mosquito brigades occasioned a spectacular network of correspondences, reports, recruitments, travels, subscriptions, fund collections, methods and personnel between various sites in British India, British Western and Central Africa, Hong Kong, Havana, New York, Dutch Java and German Africa.[124] The launch of expeditions to 'exterminate' mosquitoes in these locations reaffirmed their notoriety as malarial landscapes. But these expeditions equally emerged as occasions to establish the validity of laboratory speculations. Such speculations derived greater currency through confirmations acquired in the 'fields of practice'.

Thus the extensive mobilisation of disparate actors played a part in providing retrospective legitimacy to Ross's 'malaria doctrine'. In his book on the 'mosquito brigades' he referred to the 'investigations' he had led in the fields of Sierra Leone, Robert Koch's efforts in certain German tropical possessions, and the 'American campaigns described by L. O. Howard'. These, Ross acknowledged, provided as much recognition to his theory as the accomplishments attained within the enclosed spaces of the laboratory.[125] By 1904, earlier detractors and sceptics like Leonard Rogers had revised their opinions.[126]

In apparent contrast to such grim images, the deeply layered world of literary production, for instance in Bengali, featured mosquitoes as ubiquitous objects of fun, satire and irritation. Mosquitoes featured in the works of a range of authors: from a novel written by civil servant cum writer of fantasies Trailokyanath Mukhopadhyay in the 1890s to some of Rabindranath Tagore's poems in 1940–1941. Painful, irritating yet funny encounters between human skin and mosquitoes' stings remained an enduring theme in a range of fables, fantasies and poetry.[127]

Certain recurrent tropes, however, appeared amicably to speak to, draw upon and reinforce the more prosaic worlds of bureaucratic correspondence. In the 1880s, objects associated with mosquitoes began figuring in texts like *Moshari Rahasya (Mystery of the Mosquito Curtain)*

---

[124] W. MacGregor, 'The Fight Against Malaria: An Industrial Necessity for our African Colonies', *Journal of the Royal African Society*, 2, 6 (January 1903), 152–160; Ross, *Mosquito Brigades*, 64, 69, 70.

[125] Ross, *Mosquito Brigades*, 61–63.

[126] L. Rogers, 'Special Report on Fever in Dinajpur District', *Journal of the Asiatic Society of Bengal*, Supplementary volume (1904), 51.

[127] See for instance, T. Mukhopadhyay, *Kankabati* (Calcutta: Kebalram Chattapadhyay, 1892); R. Thakur, 'Likhi Kichu Saddho Ki' (How shall I write?), *Rabindra Rachanabali* (written in 1941) Volume 12, (Kolkata: Vishwabharati, 1995), 55; R. Thakur, 'Moshak Mangal Gitika', (Ode to Mosquitoes), *Rabindra Rachanabali* (written in 1940), Volume 12, (Kolkata: Vishwabharati), 55–56.

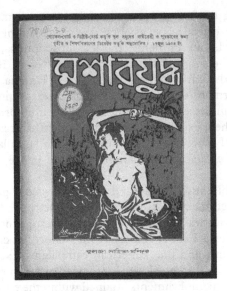

Figure 5.8 © British Library Board. Cover page of a Bengali book by Ksitishchandra Bhattacharya entitled *Moshar Juddho* (*War of Mosquitoes*), 1922. British Library, Shelfmark: Ben.B.6300.

as a metaphor for domestic scandals, immorality and decadent social practices.[128] Decades later, 'Mosha' figured as the name of an elusive serial killer in a detective fiction called *Moshar hul*, i.e., *The Sting of Mosquito*.[129]

Moreover, Ross's insistence on a war on mosquitoes was parodied variously, for instance, in educational pamphlets like *Moshar Juddho* (*War of Mosquitoes*) published in 1922 (see Figure 5.8).[130] The possible transformation of mosquitoes into deadly and invincible enemies to humans was alluded to in the first of the legendary Ghana-da stories written by Premendra Mitra. Published in 1945, it was titled 'Mosha', that is, 'Mosquito'.[131] Insufferable mosquito bites featured in Annada Sankar Ray's unforgettable poem 'Kaduni' ('In tears') as the nemesis of

---

128 S. Saphari, *Moshari Rahasya* (*Mystery of the Mosquito Curtain*) (Calcutta: Chandi Charan Basu, 1887); see also, J. Mukhopadhyay, *Korakey kit ba Somaj Chitra* (*Worm in a Flower Bud*) (Calcutta: Bamacharan Dutta. 1877).
129 D. Ray, *Moshar Hul* (*The Sting of Mosquitoes*) (Meherpur: Manasi Press, 1922).
130 K. Bhattacharya, *Moshar Juddha* (*War of Mosquitoes*) (Calcutta: Kulja Sahitya Mandir, 1922).
131 P. Mitra, 'Mosha', in S. Dasgupta (ed.), *Ghanada Samagra 1* (Kolkata: Ananda Publishers, 1945/2000), 21–30.

Japanese soldiers in northeastern India during World War II.[132] Earlier, as Figure 5.9 suggests, an illustrated anthology of Bengali short stories published in 1911 depicted the stomach of mosquitoes as a stage where bitter human animosities could be enacted.

Such literary images caricatured, mimicked and sustained suggestions about a potentially harmful, nonhuman world of quotidian insects. As a recurrent trope and a subject of enduring concern, mosquitoes thus held together the disparate worlds of entomological laboratories, literary production, sanitary governance and plantation economy.

Countable and the Accountable

The emergence of mosquitoes to prominence in the vocabulary of public health administration altered considerably the meaning of the word malaria. Indeed, 'malarial fever' in the 1900s, it was argued in certain quarters, differed radically from what was understood as malaria for much of the nineteenth century. Writing in December 1901, John H. McCollom, a professor in contagious diseases at Harvard, for instance, considered the retention of the term malarial to refer to the disease described by Ross and his collaborators as a 'misnomer'. Instead, he proposed the name 'gnat (mosquito) fever'.[133] For others like Patrick Manson, the establishment of mosquitoes as the vector for transmitting malarial parasites between human bodies represented a moment for rectifying prevailing diagnostic 'ignorance' and acknowledging what malaria really meant. Writing in April 1907, Manson recalled how in the nineteenth century an enormous variety of diseases, ranging from black water fever to sleeping sickness, were mistakenly clubbed under 'a very big name – malaria'. Since the early 1900s, he argued, 'the great block of African disease, called malaria', had gradually 'disintegrated into a number of independent, essentially different diseases.'[134] The delineation of these various 'new diseases cut out of the malarial block' found reflection in the mortality figures of the colonial governments.[135] Leonard Rogers referred to the mortality figures in British India as 'incorrectly returned' and 'grotesquely inaccurate', ridiculing the practice of combining deaths

---

[132] A. S. Ray, 'Kaduni' ('In tears'), in Buddhadeva Bose (ed.), *Adhunik Bangla Kabita* (*Modern Bengali Poems*) (Calcutta: M. C. Sarkar and Sons Private Limited, 1940/73), 148–150.

[133] J. H. McCollom, 'The Role of Insects in the Propagation of Disease', *The American Journal of Nursing*, 2, 3 (December 1901), 183.

[134] P. Manson, 'The Malaria Parasite', *Journal of the Royal African Society*, 6, 23 (April 1907), 226–228.

[135] Ibid.

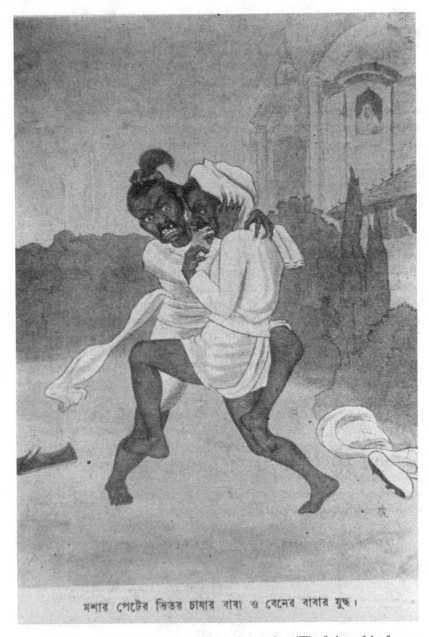

মশার পেটের ভিতর চাষার বাবা ও বেনের বাবার যুদ্ধ।

Figure 5.9 Illustration containing the caption, 'The father of the farmer engages in war with the father of the bania within the stomach of a mosquito'. Illustrator: Upendrakishore Chatterjee, in Ramananda Chatterjee (ed.), *Hindustani Upakatha* (Calcutta: Prabasi Karjalaya, 1912). Credit: Hites Ranjan Sanyal Collections, Centre for Studies in Social Sciences, Calcutta. Shelfmark: EJ 94.

from dysentery, diarrhoea, bowel complaints, 'born feeble', dropsy, child birth, old age, malignant tumours, small pox, cholera, epilepsy, measles, liver abscess, asthma, snake bite, syphilis, drowning, rheumatic fever, meningitis and rheumatic fever under 'the very elastic heading fever'. Most of these causes of death, he suggested, could be considered as autonomous diseases which deserved to be reported separately.[136] In October 1909, J. T. W. Leslie, the Sanitary Commissioner with the government of India, made a similar point: 'Many people believe that all these fever deaths are due to malaria, but a very cursory examination will show that this assumption is erroneous'.[137]

In the 1900s therefore, malarial fever often appeared as a 'new disease' emerging out of nosological reconfigurations. Ross's version of the 'story of malaria' began in 1880. That was the year when Alphonso Laveran 'discovered the parasites of this disease'. This, according to Ross, was followed by 'independent conjectures' until 'facts of leading importance were obtained solely' by his research between 1895 and 1899.[138] However, these 'boastful statements' converged with various other attempts of constructing longer histories of malarial fevers in different contexts. At this time, malarial fevers were described as intrinsic features of the classical antiquity of various nations. It was claimed in Bengali medical journals, for instance, that the ancient Ayurvedic texts made several references to malarial fevers and parasites.[139] Published in 1907, W. H. S. Jones' *Malaria, A Neglected Factor in the History of Greece and Rome* was the first amongst many books which proposed malarial fevers to be a recurrent feature of 'ancient Greco-Roman past'.[140] In these narratives, it was argued that Ross drew upon received wisdom and his projection of his discovery as an abrupt, unforeseen breakthrough was seriously dispelled.[141]

However, the transformation of the diagnostic category malaria remained incomplete in the early 1900s in significant ways.[142] I have argued that the organisation of 'mosquito brigades' reinforced the

[136] Rogers, 'Special Report', 23, 28, 31, 32.
[137] J. T. W. Leslie, 'Malaria in India', *Proceedings of the Imperial Malaria Conference held at Simla in October 1909* (Simla: Government Central Branch, 1910), 3 Home, Sanitary, May 1910, 189–231 A (NAI).
[138] Ross, *Mosquito Brigades*, 61.
[139] P. Bhattacharya, 'Ayurvedey Malaria', *Bhisak Darpan*, 21, 12 (December 1911), 443–467.
[140] W. H. S. Jones, *Malaria, a Neglected Factor in the History of Greece and Rome* (Cambridge: Macmillan & Bowes, 1907).
[141] McCollom, 'The Role of Insects', 181.
[142] Many senior officials associated with the 'mosquito brigades' were not entirely convinced with Ross' approaches in the early 1900s. See, W. F. Bynum, 'An Experiment That Failed: Malaria Control at Mian Mir', *Parassitologia*, 36 (1994), 107–120.

prevailing political geographies of malaria. Besides, in clinical deployments malaria retained much of the elasticity ascribed to it in the nineteenth century. The detection of parasites in the blood through microscopic tests, for instance, did not become the only diagnostic practice in identifying malarial patients.[143] The retention of the term malaria (with its roots in the Italian word *mal-aria*, meaning bad air) itself, as a contemporary Bengali writer observed, indicated how memories of pre-parasitological conceptions persisted into the twentieth century.[144] The failure to detect parasites in the blood samples, it was argued as late as 1915, could not guarantee the absence of malarial infection in a body.[145] Malaria continued being invoked to explain a variety of maladies including chronic dysentery, diarrhoea, pulmonary tuberculosis, chronic gastritis,[146] syphilis, phthisis,[147] pneumonia, gastric and anaemia.[148] Such expressions, it was suggested, could manifest in the body two, ten or even fifteen years after it had encountered malaria.[149]

Similarly, malaria sustained its prior associations with urban insanitation, poverty, labouring classes, agricultural stagnation and racial degeneration.[150] By the mid-1900s, however, more than ever before fevers, blood samples, mosquitoes and gradually parasites had begun to be compatibly accommodated within such prevailing definitions.[151]

---

[143] Detection of parasites were often not conducted even when the 'mosquito brigades' were in operation. See correspondence from the Secretary of State for India, No. 153 (Revenue) dated 30 September, 1904. 'Notes'. Home, Medical, June 1905, 200–204 A (NAI).

[144] N. Majumdar, 'Malaria Rahasya', *Hahnemann*, 9, 11 (c. 1910), 584–585. On the persistence of neo-Hippocratic ideas in other contexts, see M. A. Osborne and R. A. Fogarty, 'Medical Climatology in France: The Persistence of Neo-Hippocratic Ideas in the First Half of the Twentieth Century', *Bulletin of the History of Medicine*, 86, 4 (Winter 2012), 547–548. For emphasis on the theme of 'continuities rather than change' with relation to an earlier period see Worboys, 'From Miasmas to Germs', 68.

[145] Anonymous, 'The Diagnosis of Latent Malaria', *Lancet*, 186, 4805 (2 October 1915), 768.

[146] Anonymous, 'Latent Malaria', *Lancet*, 170, 4376 (13 July 1907), 100.

[147] P. Manson, 'The Diagnosis of Malaria from the Standpoint of the Practitioner in England', *Lancet*, 159, 4107 (17 May 1902), 1378.

[148] Anonymous, 'The Diagnosis of Latent Malaria', 768.   [149] Ibid.

[150] S. R. Christophers, 'On Malaria in the Punjab', *Proceedings of the Imperial Malaria Conference held at Simla in October 1909* (Simla: Government Central Branch, 1910), 29–39 and J. T. W. Leslie to Secretary to the Government of India, No. 1148, 11 June 1909, Simla. Home, Sanitary, May 1910, 189–231 A; A. W. Chaplin to L. J. Kershaw, 29 November 1909. Home, Sanitary, April 1910, 47–67 A (NAI).

[151] E. Buck, 'Report on the Control and Utilisation of Rivers and Drainage for the Fertilisation of Land and the Mitigation of Malaria', Rev-agriculture, Agriculture, July 1907, 38–48 A; 'Circular no. 2109A- S', Home, Medical, September 1901, 139 A; Leslie, 'Malaria in India', Home, Sanitary, May 1910, 189–231 A (NAI); *Proceedings of the Third Meeting of the General Malaria Committee at Madras November 1912*, 13.

Mosquitoes now emerged as the defining feature, which shaped the malarial identity of most of these conditions. Mosquitoes, malaria and these conditions appeared congenial with one another and inseparable. Earlier aetiological judgments were reiterated and retrospectively justified by an invocation of the figure of mosquitoes. For example, their abilities to 'encourage the growth of mosquitoes' reconfirmed the status of stagnant 'trivial puddles' as sites generative of malaria.[152] In the 1900s, schemes of agricultural improvements were emphasised yet again as the 'sovereign remedy' of malaria. Such continuing faith was now restored on the basis of a novel explanation. It was hoped they could 'obliterate all the conditions under which the mosquito can survive'.[153] Mosquitoes were thus centrally and emphatically inscribed into the existing medical ecologies of malaria. Similarly, colonial bureaucrats often explained the proclivity of certain poorer groups of people to malarial diseases by asserting the attributes they apparently shared with mosquitoes. Senior officials in British India, Captain S. R. Christophers and Dr C. A. Bentley, for instance, argued that anopheles mosquitoes proliferated and the urban industrial labourers dwelt under 'analogous conditions'.[154] 'Urban mohullas swarming with the lowest classes living in a very overcrowded and squalid condition', bad housing, impure water supply figured as shared habitats of mosquitoes, malaria and urban industrial labourers.[155]

Likewise, the category parasite was incorporated into the continuing racialised prejudice of stereotyping 'primitives' and 'aboriginals' as immune from the effects of malaria. It was suggested that malarial parasites and 'primitives' were happily and conveniently wedded with one another. Explaining the immunity of the so-called primitives from malaria, a statement attributed to Bentley described 'primitives' as 'parasite laden races'. Malaria parasites, it continued, were 'as natural amongst primitive races as flea infestation is to a dog'.[156] In the same decade, reports from colonial Philippines argued that Filipino soldiers and children were the 'source of fatal infection to white men' in malarial

---

[152] 'Circular no. 2109 A-S'. Home, Medical, September 1901, 139 A (NAI).

[153] Buck, 'Report on the Control and Utilisation of Rivers', Rev-agriculture, Agriculture, July 1907, 38–48 A (NAI).

[154] Leslie, 'Malaria in India', Home, Sanitary, May 1910, 189–231 A (NAI).

[155] Christophers, 'On Malaria in the Punjab', Home, Sanitary, May 1910, 189–231 A; A. W. Chaplin to L. J. Kershaw, 29 November 1909. Home, Sanitary, April 1910, 47–67 A (NAI).

[156] *Proceedings of the Third Meeting of the General Malaria Committee at Madras November 1912*, 13.

localities although they were themselves racially immune from the effects of malaria parasites.[157]

Such insinuations that parasites and certain colonised people were intimately associated should be seen in the context of an enduring European tradition in which the expression parasites was regarded as a derogatory symbol. 'Parasites' was often used as a label to demean marginalised as well as ostensibly unethical groups of people. The anthropologist Hugh Raffles has drawn on the work of Alex Bein to show that the word parasite was used not just to express modern anti-Semitic contempt for Jews. In Greek comedy as well as in early modern European vernacular literature the expression parasite was also used to indicate 'destitute persons' and 'persons who fawn on the rich', respectively.[158] Victorian literary accounts compared parasitic existence with human indolence;[159] while theological texts published from London in the 1830s argued that parasites were a demonstration of the fact that man 'has fallen from his original state of integrity and favour with God'.[160] Therefore, like mosquitoes, parasites already constituted a vibrant social category when they were incorporated within the shifting aetiologies of malaria.

At the same time, the increasing recurrence of mosquitoes and parasites in literature about malaria transformed it into a more visible, tangible and precise phenomenon than ever before. Reports on malarial fevers began listing different varieties of anopheles mosquitoes which were held to cause different degrees of malarial fevers. Different 'kinds of malarial fever', that is, malignant tertian, benign tertian, quartan, it was suggested, could be associated with precise varieties of anopheles mosquitoes (i.e., *A. Fuliginosus, A. Rossii, A. Listoni*, etc).[161] Further, as early as 1903, fever patients at the penal colony of the Andamans had to get their blood samples microscopically tested for malarial parasites on a daily basis.[162]

---

[157] W. Anderson, *Colonial Pathologies: American Tropical Medicine, Race and Hygiene in the Philippines* (Durham: Duke University Press, 2006), 208–209.

[158] H. Raffles, 'Jews, Lice and History', *Public Culture*, 19, 3 (Fall, 2007), 527.

[159] A. Zwierlein, 'Unmapped Countries: Biology, Literature and Culture in the Nineteenth Century' in A. Zwierlein (ed.), *Unmapped Countries: Biological Visions in Nineteenth-Century Literature and Culture* (London: Anthem Press, 2005), 11. For more on the imagination of parasites in Victorian culture, see J. Samyn, 'Cruel Consciousness: Louis Figuier, John Ruskin and the Value of Insects', *Nineteenth-Century Literature*, 71, 1 (2016), 89–114.

[160] Quoted in J. Farley, 'The Spontaneous Generation Controversy (1700–1860): The Origin of Parasitic Worms', *Journal of the History of Biology*, 5, 1 (Spring, 1972), 103.

[161] Rogers, 'Special Report', 41, 48–49.

[162] T. E. Tuson to the Secretary to the Government of India, 13 October 1903. Home, Medical, April 1904, 42 A (NAI).

Mosquitoes and parasites made malaria quantifiable. Malaria could now be expressed as a number to be counted, controlled and compared. For example, from the early 1900s the 'spleen rates' which were supposed to reflect the intensity of incidence of malaria in any particular locality began to carry the weight of mathematical accuracy and precision. The precise 'percentage of infected children' could now be confirmed from the occurrence of parasites in samples of blood (apart from measuring the size of spleens). Such figures enabled the comparison of 'endemicity' in the villages in Dutch East Indies, Lagos, Sierra Leone in West Africa or the Duars in British India in a commensurate register.[163] Further, diagnosis on the basis of detecting parasites in blood samples resulted in the quantification of losses incurred from malaria. Writing in 1904, Ross reported that 'a total of about 250,000 days were lost to the public service as a result of this malady amongst the European troops (in India) alone . . . 676 men or over 1 per cent of the strength were constantly sick from malarial fever'.[164]

Efficiencies of various anti-malarial actions could now as well be expressed in terms of numbers. 'Diminishing the number of mosquitoes' figured as a consistent feature of anti-malarial measures initiated in West Africa and British India.[165] Reports about anti-mosquito projects, for instance, often contained such statements: 'In Sierra Leone six men can clear fifty houses and remove ten cart-loads of broken bottles and empty tins daily'.[166] Performances of the colonial governments in tackling cases of malaria could now more effectively be judged.

Although frequent references to mosquitoes and parasites delimited the category in various ways, malaria nonetheless acquired unprecedented visibility in the official registers. Mosquitoes, parasites, blood samples and fevers: these newer tangible, precise and even numerable indicators appear to have suited the managerial instincts of the colonial governments. These empowered them with more definite targets against which to act as accountable agents.[167] In the first decade of the century,

---

[163] J. W. Stephens and S. R. Christophers, 'An Investigation Into the Factors Which Determine Malarial Endemicity', *Report to the Malarial Committee of the Royal Society*, Seventh Series (1902), 23–24.

[164] R. Ross, 'The Prevention of Malaria in India', 'Notes', Home, Medical, June 1905, 200–204 A (NAI).

[165] 'The Malaria Expedition to West Africa', 36; See also Ross to Under Secretary of State for India, Home, Medical, December 1901, 69–72 A (NAI).

[166] Ibid.

[167] See for instance, Stephens and Christophers, 'An Investigation into the Factors Which Determine Malarial Endemicity', 23–24. See also A. Appadurai, 'Number in the Colonial Imagination', in C. Breckenridge and P. Van der Veer, (eds.), *Orientalism and the Postcolonial Predicament: Perspectives from South Asia* (Philadelphia: University of Pennsylvania Press, 1993), 314–339.

malaria was reasserted across South Asia, especially in Bombay, Punjab and the United Provinces, as a major public health concern.[168] This decade also witnessed overwhelming energy across the Empire in convening high-profile conferences, committees and funds towards studying and managing malaria.[169]

The list of academic and administrative committees set up in the early 1900s for the enhancement of knowledge on malaria includes the Society for the Study of Malaria set up in Italy, the Malaria and the Tsetse Fly Committee of the Royal Society, the Drainage Committee of Bengal, the Anti-Malaria League of Greece and the Malaria Advisory Committee of the Government of India. Books on malaria written by colonial officials witnessed unforeseen circulation. Captain S. P. James wrote a pamphlet titled 'Causation and prevention of malaria' in 1903. Within a year, two editions of 5000 copies each were sold out. James received an honorarium of Rs. 750 from the government of India in recognition of the success of his book.[170]

Anti-malarial projects provided occasions to test the fundraising abilities of various members of royal families. The King of Greece and Princess Christian of Great Britain, for instance, personally raised subscriptions in support of the Anti-Malarial League of Greece.[171] In July 1903, the British Colonial Office proposed the setting up of a 'general fund' for 'promoting researches into the origin and propagation of malarious diseases'. This was conceived as a consolidated fund for the British Empire. Contributions were solicited from various parts of the Empire. The Lords Commissioners of the Treasury were instructed to contribute £500 per year for five years from the Imperial Funds on behalf of the Exchequer-aided colonies and protectorates. Similarly, a sum of £1500 a year for five years was to be made available on behalf of the Crown colonies. In addition, both the governments of Gambia and Sierra Leone promised to each contribute a sum of £100 per year to the fund for five years, while the governments of Gold Coast and Southern Nigeria each

---

[168] M. Harrison, *Disease and the Dilemmas of Development: A Malaria Strategy for Bombay Presidency, 1902–42* (Calcutta: Estate and Trust Officer, University of Calcutta, 2011), 4,6,7, 9.

[169] B. Franklin to Secretary, Government of India, 15 December 1903. Home, Medical, March 1904, 38–39 A; L. O. Howard, 'Recent Important Anti-Malaria Work', *Science*, New Series, 24, 623 (December 7, 1906), 746; Home, Medical, October 1904, 53–54 A (NAI).

[170] Franklin to Secretary to the Government of India, Home, Medical, March 1904, 38–39 A (NAI).

[171] Howard, 'Recent Important Anti-Malaria Work', 746.

promised a sum of £200 and the governments of British India and Lagos promised amounts of £500 and £150, respectively.[172]

Amid such a workaholic ambience, the figure of quinine was not banished as an irrelevant relic from an obsolete past; it was not rejected as unsuitable to address the 'new disease' emerging from redefinitions of malaria. On the contrary, quinine distribution and killing mosquitoes, often literally, happened hand in hand.[173] In fact, the government prioritised quinine distribution over other concerns. There were attempts, for instance, to divert funds from the Indian People's Famine Trust to aid the distribution of quinine in the villages of Ajmer-Merwara province in British India.[174]

Indeed, along with shifts in insights about malaria, the status of quinine appeared almost equally malleable. Having been variously projected as an anti-periodic febrifuge, a prophylactic tonic, an antiseptic or a germicide in different moments in the nineteenth century,[175] quinine was ascribed, by the mid-1900s, the newer trait of being 'inimical to the *plasmodium malaria* parasites in the blood of man'.[176] Writing in 1902, Patrick Manson hinted at the relevance of quinine in the diagnosis of malarial infections in contemporary clinical practice.[177]

The recognition of mosquitoes and parasites as subjects worthy of enduring attention thus stoked unprecedented enthusiasm for antimalarial schemes. But it was alleged by certain sections of the 'Indian public' and 'native editors' that beneath these altruistic efforts the government was involved in a 'secret conspiracy' to push the sales of quinine. It was further alleged that the government was selling quinine at Rs. 6 per pound more than the market rates to replenish an otherwise bankrupt exchequer.[178] Indeed, officials were certain that recommendations extracted through zealous initiatives like the 1909 Imperial Malaria Conference at Simla would augment the demand for quinine and ensure

---

[172] Home, Medical, October 1904, 53–54 A (NAI).

[173] Ross, *Mosquito Brigades*, 72–73; 'Circular no. 2109A-S' Home, Medical, September 1901, 139 A (NAI); MacGregor, 'The Fight Against Malaria', 157; R. Ross, *The Best Antimalarial Organization for the Tropics* (Leipzig: Johann Ambrosius Barth, 1909) [Shelfmark: WC750 1909R82b. WL].

[174] Rev-agriculture, Famine, February 1903, 6–7 A (NAI).

[175] Surgeon O. G. Wood, 'Remark on the subject of the Microorganisms on the Disease', *Indian Medical Gazette*, 17 (1 March 1882), 60–62.

[176] 'Circular no. 2109A-S' Home, Medical, September 1901, 139 A (NAI).

[177] Manson, 'The Diagnosis of Malaria', 1378.

[178] Comment attributed to Mr Lawrence from *Proceedings of the Imperial Malaria Conference held at Simla in October 1909* (Simla: Government Central Branch, 1910), 87, Home, Sanitary, May 1910, 189–231 A (NAI).

its greater consumption in British India.[179] Such hopes reflected the government's concern with addressing a continuing slump in quinine trade.

> ...Possibilities in the direction of any permanent improvement in price...one being...constantly increasing the consumption of quinine, combined with the opening up of the world's dark places, which is so steadily going on year by year, month by month, almost day by day, may in the end lead to consumption overtaking supply...[180]

Thus, such commitment to push the sales of quinine in British India did not necessarily indicate disinterested altruism on the part of the state. Two decades earlier, as I have noted in the previous chapter, prisoners in the Andaman and Nicobar Islands who were subjected to the trial of anti-malarial drugs including quinine and cinchona febrifuge were denied their share of the more expensive daily milk ration. Therefore, while encouraging the purchase and consumption of quinine, state departments proposed various adjustments to make sure that they were not the ones suffering financially for it.[181]

'Experimental Demonstration Camps'

Quinine widely emerged as an object of enforced consumption in British India in the late 1900s. Wider governmental alacrity in addressing questions concerning malaria was reflected in a series of *strategies* in ensuring greater consumption of quinine. These, in turn, manifested in firmly punitive, carefully accommodative and exhaustively pedagogical efforts to access and regulate incompletely colonised bodies. While detailing such various faces of imperial biopower this final section suggests how, in the process, quinine itself underwent further reconstitutions. These efforts should not however be explained as immediate expressions of overwhelming economic logics, while admitting their unmistakable relevance. Although regimes of biopower and political economy conversed they were not reducible to one another. Taken together they considerably constituted what functioned as empire in British India in the 1900s.

Quinine began to figure as a necessary element in the inmates' timetable through which stricter discipline could be mobilised. In the

---

[179] C. A. Innes, Letter dated 17–02–10 and A. T. Gage, Letter dated 2–3–10, 'Notes II', Home, Sanitary, May 1910, 189–231 A (NAI).

[180] Cutting from the 'Civil and Military Gazette', 3 November 1910, 'Notes'. Rev-agriculture, Agriculture, February 1911, 37–39 A (NAI).

[181] T. Cadell to Officiating Secretary, Government of India, Home, Revenue and Agricultural Department, No. G426–448, 12 August 1880, Port Blair. Home, Port Blair, October 1880, 30–32 A (NAI).

official itineraries of quinine, high schools, military barracks and especially prisons featured amongst inescapable sites. Official correspondence cherished them as enclosed and 'analogical' spaces, where 'regularly ordered' bodies under 'skilled control' could be conveniently accessed.[182]

Quinine thus revealed a hierarchy of disciplinary institutions in British India. High schools like the Delhi Normal School, for example, compelled staff and the pupils to consume biweekly doses of seven grains of quinine.[183] However, meticulously monitored and intensely regimented 'quinine parades' organised daily in some prisons amongst the inmates, officials, cooks, sweepers and hospital attendants were projected as inspirational for other institutions.

Quinine parades were daily conducted under the supervision of the jailor and the hospital assistant in every prison in Punjab. They oversaw the accuracy of dosage, prevented any act of tampering, made sure that wastage by spillage could be reduced to a minimum and that 'each prisoner actually swallowed the quinine'. The jailor was responsible for ensuring the presence of all prisoners in their respective yards, enclosures and cells prior to every quinine parade. He counted all prisoners who actually received the mixture. This number was supposed to correspond to that at 'count out' in the morning or lockup in the evening. Finally, the jailor had to certify, under his signature in the hospital assistant's journal, the number of prisoners who had been dosed. Quinine was then distributed amongst the officials, cooks, sweepers and hospital attendants.[184]

The question of quinine enabled officials to project prisons as ideal sites which guaranteed freedom from malaria. Death rate from malaria amongst prisoners was shown to be one-fifth of what it was amongst the 'general population'. Out of every one thousand victims of malaria, it was suggested, merely one could be considered a prisoner. In the abstruse logic of medical governance, jails were projected as a model which should be replicated everywhere to ensure the safest and most beneficial abodes for colonial subjects. A 'free man' appeared more vulnerable to malaria than a prisoner. 'Why is it that a disease which is so rarely fatal to a prisoner should be so often fatal to a free man?'– officials wondered. Confinement within the prison, it was argued, provided the inmates a position of 'greater advantage'. Lives in the prison were projected as 'regularly ordered', more regimented and ideal for the

---

[182] G. Deleuze, 'Postscript on the Societies of Control', *October*, 59 (Winter, 1992), 3.

[183] W. S. Hamilton to the Secretary to the Government of India, 18 March 1909. Home, Jails, January 1910, 11–15 A (NAI).

[184] G. F. W. Braide to All Superintendents of Jails in the Punjab, 31 July 1907. Ibid.

disciplined distribution of quinine.[185] Prisons were compared to the barracks, which housed the Indian soldiers in the British imperial army. In both these sites, bodies of men were subjected to 'skilled control'. However, the most stringent measures of distributing quinine, it was argued, were more plausible in the jails than in the regimental lines. This seemed to explain how the prisoners appeared more protected from malaria than the soldiers, despite their 'inferior physique' and 'lower social status'.[186]

Enforced consumption of quinine was pursued by officials beyond the prisoner's cell and the native soldier's bunk. The Special Anti-Malarial Measures Act for India of 1907, for instance, recommended mandatory consumption of quinine in 'highly malarious areas', and 'removal of houses inhabited by persistently infected individuals from the neighbourhood by bodies of disciplined men and government institutions'.[187] In addition, denial of 'casual leave' was proposed in Punjab for government servants who refused to consume quinine regularly.[188] In a report published in 1912, one Major MacGilchrist mentioned similar punishments claiming to have fined people who visited him in the hospital for malaria treatment.[189] Similarly, in another context in the early 1900s, the German foreign office proposed an agreement with colonial officers in Africa, making it mandatory for every officer to consume quinine once in every eight or nine days. The agreement also suggested that the salary of a German officer in Africa could be stopped 'during the period of an illness that might have been avoided by reasonable care'.[190] In other parts of the world later in the 1910s, particularly during the British intervention in Salonika during World War I, as Figure 5.10 indicates, consumption of quinine continued to feature as an everyday protocol to enforce military discipline. Further, quinine calendars were also in vogue to indicate the number of occasions in which soldiers and officials had missed their mandatory dose of quinine.[191]

Quinine, however, was not fed exclusively through punitive measures or in situations of confinement. The 'free and unindentured' labourers

[185] Leslie, 'Malaria in India', 4, 5, 9. Home, Sanitary, May 1910, 189–231 A (NAI).
[186] Ibid.
[187] W. G. King, 'The Difficulties Which Beset the Practical Application of Anti-Malarial Measures', *Proceedings of the Imperial Malaria Conference held at Simla in October 1909* (Simla: Government Central Branch, 1910), 52, 53, 54. Home, Sanitary, May 1910, 189–231 A (NAI).
[188] C. A. Gill, 'A Summary of Anti-Malaria Measures in the Punjab', 67, Ibid.
[189] *Proceedings of the Third Meeting of the General Malaria Committee at Madras November 1912*, 20.
[190] MacGregor, 'The Fight Against Malaria', 157.
[191] Photograph of 'Medical Card Recording the Administration of Quinine, 1914–1945' (Credit: Wellcome Library, London. L0011627EL).

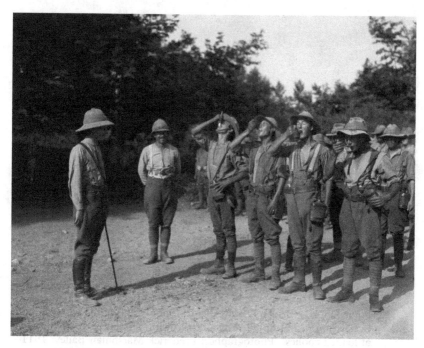

Figure 5.10 © Imperial War Museum (Q 32160). Photograph of 'British troops taking their daily dose of quinine', Salonika, July 1916.

in the Duars plantations, for instance, were persuaded not through codified contracts. In these plantations, the government was able to access the most 'ignorant, superstitious and backward of aboriginal tribes' as 'coolies'. Five-grain doses of quinine were 'served out' to them while conducting everyday acts of leaf-weighing or at muster by the managers' 'moral force of personal influence'. It was hoped, that once the 'headmen' began taking doses of quinine it would appear as a 'custom' for the rest, who with 'sufficient docility' would engage in acts of consumption.[192] Similarly, German medical officers in Togo and the Cameroons proposed the construction of 'quinine stations' on caravan routes which connected various African villages. In a remarkable demonstration of colonial desire for corporeal control, it was hoped that such stations would enable officers 'to put quinine on the tongue of each negro

[192] 'The Indian Tea Industry: The Labour Question, Malaria as a Factor', Cutting from *The Statesman*, 1 January 1909. 'Notes IV', Home, Sanitary, May 1910, 189–231 A (NAI).

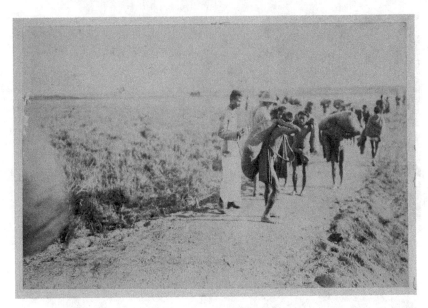

Figure 5.11 © British Library Board. Photograph of 'Sadiya. Captain Robertson and Hospital Assistant throwing quinine into the mouths of loaded coolies'. Photographer: Frederick Marshman Bailey; 1911–1912. [India Office Select Material, British Library]. Shelfmark: Photo 1083/34 (163).

passing by'.[193] Similar language has been used to describe enforced consumption of quinine in Northeast India. The caption of Figure 5.11 taken in 1911 or 1912 suggests a desperate scene in which a British official and a hospital assistant were 'throwing quinine into the mouths of loaded coolies'.

The state's intent to persuade its subjects into consuming quinine was evident in a range of accommodative gestures: during quinine parades, quinine was served by a 'high caste Hindu convict warder', who was assisted by a 'convict official of similar caste'; during ramzan in the Punjab prisons, quinine was distributed only after sunset; the standard dosage of quinine was often relaxed to prevent 'unpleasant consequences' amongst female prisoners.[194] Further, to make quinine more 'attractive' and 'palatable' to suit the 'taste' of prospective consumers, various innovations were prescribed. Messrs Burroughs Wellcome and

---

[193] MacGregor, 'The Fight Against Malaria', 157.
[194] G. F. W. Braide to All Superintendents in Punjab, 31 July 1907 and 4 July 1908. Home department, Jails Branch, January 1910, 11–15 A (NAI).

Co. began distributing 'sugar coated tabloids' in British India.[195] Two tablet-making machines capable of turning out 25,000 tablets a day were purchased for use in the Lahore Central Jail.[196] Thus the usually bitter and cumbersome quinine solutions were remade in more manageable forms of pills and compressed tablets, served as wine; made tastier by coating such tablets with sugar and sold under the cover of chocolate and sweetmeat. Particularly, to attract the children, solutions of quinine were sweetened with syrup and sugar, while powdered forms were often blended with condensed milk.[197] Thus, where British Indian subjects could not be regimented into consuming regular doses of quinine, the drug itself was repackaged to reach out to them. Figures 5.12 and 5.13 indicate how some of these innovations were advertised.

These elaborate initiatives coexisted with commentaries from officials who mentioned that certain marginalised groups within Indian society performed 'ghastly' religious rites to resist epidemics.[198] For example, in the 1910s, British Indian colonial ethnographer E. H. Hunt, through diary entries and photographs (see Figure 5.14), graphically asserted that the 'low caste inhabitants' of the village of Mettaguda near Secunderadad in Southern India resorted to practices like buffalo slaughter to prevent malarial epidemics.[199] Such ethnographic denunciation of the 'lowest outcastes... aboriginal peoples of India' almost coincided with the contemporary celebration of the enlightened benevolence of the colonial state.[200] Photographs (such as Figure 5.15) taken in the same decade from Northeastern India upheld quinine as a civilising object through which primitive tribes inhabiting the imperial frontiers could be reformed into a state of modernity.

Unsurprisingly, quinine became the focus of various pedagogical programmes. Already in 1909, the statistical officer to the government, S. P. James, for example, proposed an exhaustive pedagogical network, the 'experimental demonstration camps'. The 'primary objective' was to 'devise a scheme for increasing enormously the demand for quinine in the small villages' in British India. The camps were designed to

---

[195] 'The Indian Tea Industry: The Labour Question, Malaria as a Factor', Cutting from *The Statesman*, 1 January 1909. 'Notes IV', Home, Sanitary, May 1910, 189–231 A (NAI).

[196] Gill, 'A Summary of Anti-Malaria Measures in the Punjab', 66, Ibid.

[197] Ibid.; 'The Indian Tea Industry'; 'Extract from the Pioneer', 12 April 1909, 'Notes I', Home, Sanitary, May 1910, 189–231 A (NAI).

[198] E. H. Hunt, 'The Sacrifice: A Sketch Founded on Real Facts', 6–8, 1917. Unpublished manuscript. MSS Eur. F222/11 (BL).

[199] E. H. Hunt, 'E. H. Hunt and the Buffalo Sacrifice', 1917. Unpublished manuscript. MSS Eur. F222/11 (BL).

[200] Hunt, 'The Sacrifice', 6–8.

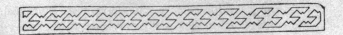

Reliable Quinine

For the treatment of malaria.
Of exceptional purity and alkaloidal value.

TRADE MARK 'TABLOID' BRAND
Quinine Bisulphate

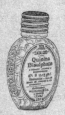

Famed throughout the world for its purity, accuracy, convenience and palatability.

Supplied as follows: gr. 1/2, in bottles of 50 and 100; gr. 1, in bottles of 36 and 100; gr. 2, gr. 3, gr. 4, gr. 5, gr. 10, 0·1 gm., 0·25 gm. and 0·5 gm., in bottles of 25 and 100. Issued *plain* or *sugar-coated*, except gr. 10 and 0·5 gm., which are *plain* only.

TRADE MARK 'WELLCOME' BRAND
Quinine Sulphate

Attains a much higher standard of purity than required by the British Pharmacopœia.

Supplied in "Compact Crystals" and "Large Flake" (the ordinary form), both being identical in composition.

Issued in bottles and tins of convenient sizes.

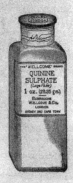

Prices and supplies of all B. W. & Co.'s fine Quinine Products obtainable of Pharmacists in all parts of the world.

BURROUGHS WELLCOME & CO., LONDON
NEW YORK   MONTREAL   SYDNEY   CAPE TOWN
XX 190   MILAN   SHANGHAI   *Copyright*

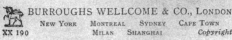

Figure 5.12 Advertisement of 'Wellcome Tabloid Quinine Bisulphate' published in R. Ross, *The Prevention of Malaria* (London: John Murray, 1910). [Credit: Wellcome Library, London]

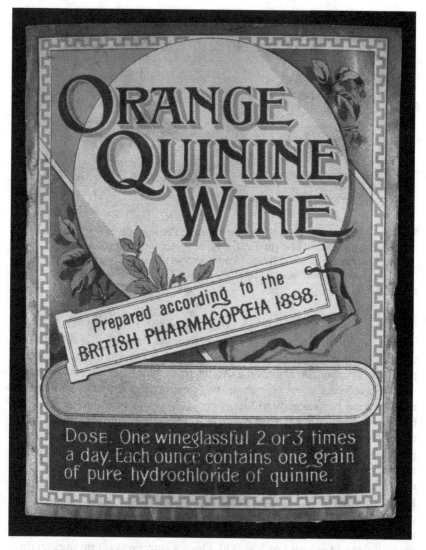

Figure 5.13 Ephemera containing the note 'Orange Quinine Wine, prepared according to the British Pharmacopoeia, 1898'. Credit: Wellcome Library, London.

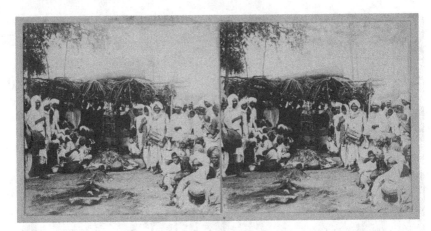

Figure 5.14 © British Library Board. Photograph of 'Buffalo sacrifice, Mettaguda, 1917 (malaria)'. Note: 'View of villagers gathered round sacrificed buffalo head'. Photographer: Edmund Henderson Hunt. [India Office Select Material, British Library]. Shelfmark: MSS Eur F222/11 (2).

'demonstrate to the people' the benefits of the drug and the 'correct way in which to use it'.[201] In every selected area of a district, each camp, consisting of a hospital assistant and a compounder, was supposed to operate for a period ranging from six weeks to two months. At any given period, its operations were expected to remain confined to a population not exceeding 2000 people. Visits to every house were to be occasioned with a prepared 'little lecture', inducing the inhabitants to convince themselves and their neighbours of the merits of consuming prophylactic doses of quinine every night. James had an estimate of the numbers of people who could be reached out through such camps. If a camp remained for two months each in areas inhabited by 2000 people, James speculated, 12,000 people could be 'educated' annually by each camp. If every province consisted of a minimum of thirty districts each with a camp of its own, James reasoned, 'the number of people educated annually' could amount to 360,000. Once a camp was set up in each district of British India, James hoped, about '3 million people per annum would learn thoroughly the benefits to be derived from quinine, where to obtain it and how to use it'. James considered such acts of 'teaching

---

[201] S. P. James, 'Experimental Demonstration Camps', *Proceedings of the Imperial Malaria Conference held at Simla in October 1909* (Simla: Government Central Branch, 1910), 83–85. Home, Sanitary, May 1910, 189–231 A (NAI).

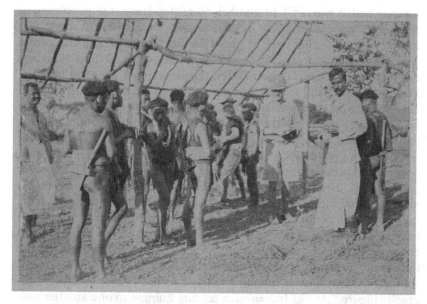

Figure 5.15 © British Library Board. Photograph of 'Sadiya. Captain Robertson and Hospital Assistant giving quinine to Nagas'. Photographer: Frederick Marshman Bailey; 1911–1912 [India Office Select Material, British Library], Photo 1083/34 (162).

the people' more relevant than instructing them 'in the arts of reading and writing'.[202]

Besides, vernacular booklets about malaria were recommended as parts of primary school curriculum. The 'future citizens of the Empire', once exposed to such 'lessons on quinine', were expected to inspire their relatives into consuming the drug.[203] Such pedagogical faith in the relaying of internalised 'lessons' by more diligent pupils of Empire to their closer associates was variously replicated. Apart from binding themselves into consuming 15 grains of quinine per week, the members of the Gurdaspur Quinine Distribution Society, for instance, pledged to induce as many as possible to become members of the society. Branches were set up in various villages, tehsils and districts. Every member had to pay a subscription of 6 annas and join by a contribution of

[202] Ibid.
[203] Comment attributed to Mr Chaudhuri, *Proceedings of the Imperial Malaria Conference held at Simla in October 1909* (Simla: Government Central Branch, 1910), 90 Home, Sanitary, May 1910, 189–231 A (NAI).

1 rupee and 2 annas.[204] In another correspondence, the possibility of organising 'popular lectures by Hindu and Mohamedan leaders' was considered a judicious way of preaching and 'popularising the use of quinine'.[205] Similarly, having described malaria as 'a question of highest national importance', Herbert Risley, the president of the 1909 Imperial Malaria Conference, argued that the people could not help themselves unless they were cooperating with the priorities of the government. 'The people must help us', declared Risley in his concluding comments, 'for only by helping us they can help themselves'. He urged Indian landholders, bankers, professors, merchants, lawyers, schoolmasters, journalists, doctors and influential operators in the subdivisions, to enthuse greater participation in anti-malaria programmes: 'They would be in closest touch with all ranks of people, they could teach, they could persuade, they could do all the things than an official agency would attempt in vain'. If Risley was speaking to whomever he considered 'natural leaders of the people',[206] colloquial official leaflets continued to address the individual, empowering them with immediate access to 'self-treatment' through the medium of quinine.[207] Later in the 1920s, as this photograph (Figure 5.16) of Indian men feeding quinine to one another suggests, the drug was reasserted as a means through which collective well-being and solidarity within local communities could be reinforced.

Thus, the drug quinine and the efforts to enforce its consumption in British India revealed various depths and reaches of the imperial state. However, quinine itself did not figure as a passive, rigid and unchanging object. Its relevance and resilience was recurrently underscored, while it kept changing hands, reconstituting itself considerably in the process.

Conclusion

A colonial consumer field for an overabundant drug was produced by imperial regimes in British India in the late nineteenth and early twentieth centuries. Ironically, this happened at a time when the radical redefinition of the corresponding disease, malaria, was being occasioned by the same imperial world.

Quinine and mosquitoes represented two most visible public faces associated with malaria in British India between the late 1890s and

---

204 C. M. King to the Commissioner Lahore Division, 8 November 1909. Home, Sanitary, May 1910, 232–235 A (NAI).

205 Chaudhuri, *Proceedings*, 90 Home, Sanitary, May 1910, 189–231 A (NAI).

206 H. H. Risley, 'Popular Cooperation in the Prevention of Malaria', *Proceedings*, 96, ibid.

207 W. G. King to the Secretary to the Government of Madras, 30 December 1903, 'Notes'. Home, Medical, April 1904, 46–47 A (NAI).

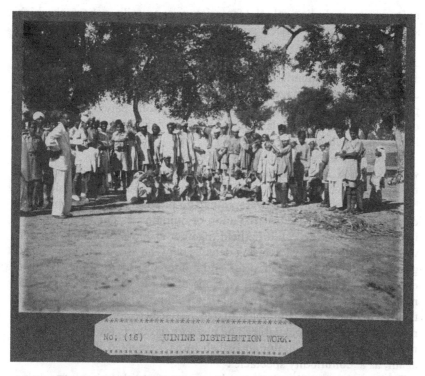

Figure 5.16 © British Library Board. Photograph of 'Quinine distribution work, (Jhelum). Villagers being given doses of quinine'. Photographer: Anonymous, c. 1929. [India Office Select Material, British Library]. Shelfmark: Photo 23/2 (16).

the 1910s. Through my focus on quinine and mosquitoes, I have here emphasised the need for greater acknowledgment of deep historical entanglements of Empire with nonhumans in British India. First, various imperial departments, personnel and provinces shared a commitment for producing perceptions and realities about mosquitoes and quinine. This chapter has refrained from judging whether anopheles mosquitoes indeed transmitted malarial parasites between human bodies or whether quinine indeed cured malaria. It has instead examined the traffic between the imperial worlds of pharmaceutical business, vernacular markets, colonial governance and scientific knowledge in British India through which mosquitoes and quinine could be endowed with such enduring attributes.

Imperial investments were geared towards producing and 'maintaining' the image of quinine as a valuable drug while it circulated through a range of sites including colonial factories, prisons, military barracks, high schools, government offices, post offices, imperial conferences, bazaars, legal codes and primary school curriculums.[208] Efforts to project quinine as compatible with the familiar icons, figures, castes, religions, tastes and languages of intended consumers, I have argued, communalised the drug. Similarly the image of mosquitoes as a potential disease-causing pest was sustained and reinforced by interactions between the worlds of colonial laboratories, plantation economy, field works and vernacular literary production.

At the same time, imperial processes and structures themselves were reshaped and sustained by the constructs, such as quinine and mosquitoes, which they occasioned. Thus, Empire itself could have hardly remained a distant, overarching and imposing entity independent of the script it mobilised. Circulation of quinine was one of many ways in which the Empire could be held together as a profit-making mission veiled by benevolence. Enduring debates between contending provincial governments about the fair price and colour of pure quinine, in turn, exposed several fault lines and tensions of empire. In many ways, quinine seems to have been a metaphor for empire: bitter, expensive and transformative which could be mutated variously to appear as charitable, reasonable and even palatable. The plethora of efforts towards enforcing the consumption of quinine in British India, cemented the Empire, yet again, as a 'commodity spectacle'.[209]

Particularly revealing is to make sense of the location of quinine and mosquitoes in imperial biopolitics. Efforts towards imposing the consumption of quinine in British India, for instance, reinforced various aspects of imperial biopower: utilitarian governance, pedagogical machineries, rule of law and strictures of incarceration. While claiming to produce 'future citizens of the Empire', such facets continued simultaneously to flirt with diverse visions of self-treatment and nationhood. As a tool to nurture regimented and productive subjects in the prisons, high schools, barracks, families, congregations, plantations, public offices, quinine must have informed what Stoler and Cooper call the 'embourgeoisement of imperialism' in the late nineteenth and early twentieth centuries.[210]

---

208 For repair and maintenance See, B. Latour, 'Whose Cosmos, Which Cosmopolitics? Comments on the Peace Terms of Ulrich Beck', *Common Knowledge*, 10, 3 (2004), 459.

209 McClintock, *Imperial Leather*, 56.

210 A. Laura Stoler and F. Cooper, 'Introduction: Between Metropole and Colony: Rethinking a Research Agenda', in A. Laura Stoler and F. Cooper (eds.), *Tensions of*

Empire was shaped as well by what Nicole Shukin calls a 'zoopolitics' involving insects, particularly mosquitoes.[211] Regimes of governing human bodies extended over and were integrally tied with sustained investments in knowing, observing, exchanging, maiming, classifying, delimiting and narrating mosquitoes. Such widespread efforts metamorphosed mosquitoes into subjects of Empire. Engagement with mosquitoes indicated the depth and extent of Empire. In anthropomorphic accounts, mosquitoes symbolised colonial poverty, insanitation, recalcitrance and redundant excesses. Yet, mosquitoes commanded continued attention as an object of imagination, an excuse for intervention and commerce and a mirror against which humanity could be defined. Thus, mosquitoes appeared not only to justify imperial rule, but also figured as its subjects.

It is possible to suggest here that empires, as much as imperial subject/objects like pure quinine and mosquitoes, were cyborgian formations, which were held together by an apparatus of human and nonhuman enmeshes. Interactive networks explored here, for instance, amongst insects, insecticides, tinsmiths, coolies, sweepers, itinerant parasitologists, parasites, vernacular fiction writers, entrepreneurs, bureaucrats, commodities, government factories, post offices, peons, bazaar vendors, policemen, outposts, jailors, inmates, soldiers, sealing bottles, carmine, colouring matter, alkaloids may be said to have constituted not only mosquitoes and quinine, but also an imperial apparatus. I draw upon the anthropologist Viveiros De Castro to define imperial apparatus as an 'inter-subjective field of human and nonhuman relations'.[212] Empire, I argue, could neither precede nor outlive nor be delineated from the discourses about science and nonhumans that it occasioned. The history of how malaria was reassembled in the 1890s and 1900s thus reveals how Empire itself was put together – not as an inflexible institutional apparatus, but as an assemblage in which texts, authorities and materials, and politics, knowledge and nonhumans were, to quote Donna Haraway 'becoming with' one another.[213] Imperial power,

Empire: Colonial Cultures in a Bourgeois World (Berkeley/Los Angeles/London: University of California Press, 1997), 31. On how regimes of governmentality and nonhuman agency enable one another, see P. Joyce, 'What is the Social in Social History?', *Past and Present*, 205 (November 2009), 191–192.

[211] N. Shukin, *Animal Capital: Rendering Life in Biopolitical Times* (Minneapolis and London: University of Minnesota Press, 2009), 9–11.

[212] E. Viveiros De Castro, 'Exchanging Perspectives: The Transformation of Objects into Subjects in Armendian Cosmologies', *Common Knowledge*, 10, 3 (2004), 471.

[213] D. Haraway, *When Species Meet* (Minneapolis and London: University of Minnesota Press, 2008), 2, 23–27.

scientific knowledge, and nonhumans like quinine and mosquitoes were located in a shared and immanent field of co-constitution.[214]

Finally, the history of malaria, quinine and mosquitoes in late-nineteenth and early-twentieth centuries also reveals how distinctions between the human and the nonhuman were constantly invoked, policed and dismantled within the imperial apparatus. The ascription of humanly attributes to nonhumans often coalesced with the relegation of various colonised subjects to the status of less-than-humans. Human-nonhuman binaries were transgressed in various ways: quinine seemed to acquire lifelike relations with people inhabiting the interiors; insects emerged as focus of projects which mobilised a series of labourers and commodities alike; the urban poor and mosquitoes as well as parasites and 'primitives', it was claimed, shared analogous attributes. Simultaneous operation of anthropomorphism and dehumanisation was fundamental rather than incidental to imperial exercise of power.

[214] On the theme of co-constitution: See F. Trentmann, 'Materiality in the Future of History: Things, Practices and Politics', *The Journal of British Studies*, 48, 2 (April 2009), 297, 300; S. Kirsch and D. Mitchell, 'The Nature of Things: Dead Labor, Nonhuman Actors and the Persistence of Marxism', *Antipode*, 36 (2004), 688; A. Pickering, 'The Mangle of Practice: Agency and Emergence in the Sociology of Science', *American Journal of Sociology*, 99, 3 (November 1993), 559, 567, 576.

6   Epilogue

Empire, Medicine and Nonhumans

The British geographer, botanist and ethnographer Clements Robert Markham's memoir detailing the transportation of cinchona seeds and plants from South America to South India, one might recall, was published in 1862. A few years after the Sepoy Mutiny, which marked the transition from East India Company rule to the British Raj, Markham argued that trees planted by rulers were the most enduring legacies of imperial regimes, comparing the recently imported cinchona plants in British India with the melon trees planted by Emperor Babur, the founder of the Mughal dynasty. He envisioned that these cinchona plants, much like Babur's melons, would outlast not only spectacular political events and engineering marvels, but also withstand the rise and fall of empires themselves. These plants, he thought, should be considered an everlasting gift to Her Majesty's Indian subjects from their imperial rulers.[1]

Cinchona plants and their most valuable extract, quinine, continued to remain significant in commerce, public health and global politics in the interwar period[2]. Across South Asia, as the last chapter has shown, the interrelationships amongst cinchona plants, the drug quinine, the tropical disease malaria and anopheles mosquitoes were already widely recognised by the start of World War I. However, the first two decades of the twentieth century also witnessed the beginnings of widespread disillusionment with imperial cinchona plantations and government quinine factories in British India. Insofar as cinchona plantations were concerned, the superiority of Dutch Java was almost entirely established

---

[1] See Chapter 1.

[2] The entanglement of quinine and cinchona with war and commerce continued. See, for example, F. R. Fosberg, 'Cinchona Plantation in the New World', *Economic Botany*, 1, 3 (July–September, 1947), 330–333; W. H. Hodge, 'Wartime Procurement in Latin America', *Economic Botany*, 2, 3 (July–September, 1948), 229–257; W. Popenoe, 'Cinchona Cultivation in Guatemala: A Brief Historical Review up to 1943', *Economic Botany*, 3, 2 (April–June, 1949), 150–157.

by then.[3] Private planters in northeastern India and Ceylon, as I have indicated, began replacing cinchonas from their plantations with other commercial crops. Books published from other parts of the Empire in the 1910s ironically claimed that cinchonas were not only frequently vulnerable to different diseases, but they were also sources of occupational skin diseases amongst those who handled these plants while 'making pharmaceutical preparations'.[4] The effectiveness of quinine itself was questioned amidst allegations of extensive adulteration in the medical markets, poisonous side effects, the emergence of cheaper pharmaceutical alternatives and the suggestion that eradicating mosquitoes was a more efficient way of resisting malaria than quinine prophylaxis.[5] Many of these limitations of quinine were highlighted in debates between colonial medical officials regarding the most effective ways of controlling malaria in the 1900s and 1910s. These debates were conducted in a range of imperial political contexts including colonial public health campaigns, everyday municipal governance, or in spectacular military frontiers during the World War I.[6] The recognition of quinine as an anti-malarial

---

[3] R. Drayton, *Nature's Government: Science, Imperial Britain and the 'Improvement' of the World* (New Haven and London: Yale University Press, 2000), 210, 230–231; A. Goss, 'Building the World's Supply of Quinine: Dutch Colonialism and the Origins of a Global Pharmaceutical Industry', *Endeavour*, 31, 1 (March 2014), 8–18. See also A. R. Hoogte and T. Pieters, 'Science, Industry and the Colonial State: A Shift from the German- to a Dutch-Controlled Cinchona and Quinine Cartel (1880–1920)', *History and Technology*, 31, 1 (2 January, 2015), 2–36; A. R. Hoogte and T. Pieters, 'Science in the Service of Colonial Agro-Industralism: The Case of Cinchona Cultivation in the Dutch and British East Indies, 1852–1900', *Studies in the History and Philosophy of Biological and Biomedical Sciences*, 47, PA (September 2014), 12–22.

[4] M. T. Cook, *The Diseases of Tropical Plants* (London: Macmillan, 1913), 175, 192, 244; R. Prosser White, *Occupational Affections of the Skin; A Brief Account of the Trade Processes and Agents Which Give Rise to Them* (London: H. K. Lewis, 1915) 49.

[5] P. Barton, "Powders, Potions and Tablets: The 'Quinine Fraud' in British India, 1890–1939" in J. H. Mills and P. Barton (eds.), *Drugs and Empire: Essays in Modern Imperialism and Intoxication, c. 1500–1930* (Basingstoke: Palgrave Macmillan, 2007), 144–161; Anonymous, 'Quinine and World War', *BMJ*, 1, 4230 (31 January 1942), 152–153; Anonymous, 'The Quinine Problem', *BMJ*, 1, 3777 (27 May 1933), 923–924; Anonymous, 'Wanted: A Cheap Antimalarial Drug in India', *BMJ*, 1, 4228 (17 January 1942), 78; Anonymous, 'Acute Quinine Poisoning', *BMJ*, 1, 3882 (1 June 1935), 1130; M. Harrison, *Disease and the Dilemmas of Development: A Malaria Strategy for Bombay Presidency, 1902–1942 (Eighth Hasi Majumdar Oration on History and Philosophy of Medicine and Science)* (Calcutta: Estate and Trust Officer, University of Calcutta, 2011); M. Harrison, *The Medical War: British Military Medicine in the First World War* (Oxford: Oxford University Press, 2010), 229–238; M. Harrison, *Public Health in British India: Anglo-Indian Preventive Medicine, 1859–1914* (Cambridge: Cambridge University Press, 1994) 159–161.

[6] P. S. Lelean, *Quinine as a Malarial Prophylactic: A Criticism* (London: John Bale Sons and Danielsson, Ltd., undated) reprinted from *Journal of Royal Army Medical Corps*, November 1911. [Archives and Manuscripts, RAMC/565/10/10. WL]; R. Ross and D. Thomson, *A Case of Malarial Fever, Showing a True Parasitic Relapse, During Vigorous and*

survived these debates, and yet the effectiveness of the drug was subjected to unprecedented scrutiny during these years.

In concluding this book, I want to offer three distinctive analytical
perspectives. The first draws together the threads of the argument in
the preceding chapters, demonstrating that British imperial agency not
only shaped the histories of quinine and malaria, but also occasioned the
interactions between these categories. The second section of the epilogue
reasserts the significance of non-European vernacular public culture in
the history of British imperial medicine. I explore Bengali writings on
malaria, quinine and mosquitoes in some detail to suggest ways to go
beyond the twin tropes of imposition and resistance in the history of
British imperial medicine. The final section will focus on nonhuman
objects and organisms to critique anthropocentrism in standard historiography of British Empire. Taken together these two sections extend
existing conceptions of British imperial agency by focusing on interactive relationships between the British Empire and different components
within imperial history. I will argue that the focus on imperial agency in
this book does not imply the methodological marginalisation of either
vernacular public cultures or nonhumans. Instead, I conclude by suggesting that various vernacular public cultures and nonhumans were not
only co-constituted with British imperial history, but also were integral
to it.

A Cure and Its Disease

Although I began this book with an analysis of the discovery of the alkaloid quinine in 1820, I have focused especially on the period between
Markham's programmatic statements in the early 1860s (marking the
establishment of cinchona plantations in British India) and the beginning
of systematic doubts about the effectiveness of quinine in the late 1900s
and early 1910s. In these intervening decades, British India was one of
most significant parts of the colonial world where quinine was established as the quintessential cure for diseases associated with malaria.

Continuous Quinine Treatment (Liverpool: Liverpool School of Tropical Medicine, 1912)
reprinted from the *Annals of Tropical Medicine and Parasitology*, 5, 4 (February 1912),
539–543 [Shelfmark: WC750 1912R82c. WL]; W. F. Bynum, '"Reasons for Contentment": Malaria in India, 1900–1920', *Parassitologia*, 40 (1998), 25–26; W. F., Bynum,
'An Experiment that Failed: Malaria Control at Mian Mir', *Parassitologia*, 36 (1994),
112, 115–116; Harrison, *Disease and the Dilemmas of Development*, 13, 17, 18; Harrison,
The Medical War, 229–238. See also L. Monnais, 'Rails, Roads and Mosquito Foes: The
State Quinine Service in French Indochina', in R. Peckham and D. M. Pomfret (eds.),
Imperial Contagions: Medicine, Hygiene and Cultures of Planning in Asia (Hong Kong:
Hong Kong University Press, 2013), 198, 199, 203, 208–212.

Rather than proposing a self-contained history of malaria or quinine, I have explored the ways in which the historical trajectories of a disease, a cure, a group of plants and (subsequently) insects intersected. While examining the interconnected histories of quinine and malaria during this period, I have questioned the conventional chronologies of medical knowledge production. Such established chronologies have often assumed a definite pattern according to which: problems inevitably precede a solution, an answer takes shape only after a coherent question has been posed, and preexisting understandings about a disease necessitate knowledge about a cure. Instead, this book has argued that knowledge about a cure and a disease-causing entity, to a considerable extent, shaped one another. In fact, it is not entirely implausible to think about situations in which knowledge about cinchona and quinine preceded, and effected crucial shifts in the history of malaria. Chapters 1 and 2 indicate that the establishment of colonial cinchona plantations in Dutch Java, French Algeria and British India in the mid-nineteenth century converged with the redefinition of malaria from a predominantly European to an almost exclusively colonial concern. While the word malaria certainly had a presence in English language sources in the previous centuries, the discovery of quinine in 1820 was followed by unprecedented circulation of malaria as a diagnostic category and as a matter of governmental preoccupation. Chapter 3 has shown, while commenting on the making of Burdwan fever, that quinine could be invoked to establish the malarial identity of a malady. In many instances during the epidemic, confirmed diagnoses did not lead to the prescription of cure. On the contrary, quinine was employed as a pharmacological agent in quick-fix diagnostic tests. Thus the malarial identity of a malady was ascertained by the response of the ailing body to quinine.

At the same time, the incorruptibility and inflexibility of the pharmaceutical category quinine itself was not necessarily taken for granted by contemporary officials. Therefore, British colonial bureaucrats, who assumed that the Burdwan fever assured the supply of bodies affected with malaria, used the 'opportunity of the epidemic', in turn, to verify the 'purity' of certain drugs circulating extensively as quinine in the medical market. Focusing on attempts to manufacture pure quinine in government factories in British India, Chapter 4 has further explored the irony that despite being employed to establish whether an ailing body was suffering from malaria, quinine itself remained an unstable, malleable as well as elusive entity over many decades. Quinine continued being described as a quintessential remedy in the early 1900s, as has been shown in the previous chapter, even when the corresponding diagnostic category malaria itself was redefined substantially: from an elusive cause of many diseases to the name of a mosquito-borne fever disease. In this decade, prevailing insights about how quinine cured an ailing body were altered to adapt to the newer meanings associated with the category malaria.

I have contributed to attempts within the wider historiography of science to demystify expressions such as experiments, discovery and invention. While narrating the history of quinine manufacture in British India, for example, I have urged that these expressions should not only be read as indicators of the teleological development of pharmaceutical technology, but also as politically contingent, historically produced labels. Similarly, I have indicated that the chemical separation of two newer alkaloids from extracts of cinchona barks was not termed as an exceptional discovery in the world of phytochemistry in 1820 itself. The accomplishment of Pelletier and Caventou was retrospectively glorified as a momentous event in the history of pharmaceutical chemistry because of the recognition quinine eventually received from the market in subsequent decades. Likewise, the mosquito brigades organised in the 1900s were not applications to the 'field' of an already established discovery achieved within the walls of enclosed laboratories. Instead, such elaborate 'expeditions' emerged as occasions for reconfirming tentative laboratory findings, and reasserting them before a global audience. This book, therefore, reinforces persisting efforts to recast the histories of scientific milestones, while at the same time questioning the established chronologies in the relationships between a disease and its cure. In the process, it contradicts the suggestion that modern medicine necessarily represents an objective, teleological and progressive uncovering of scientific reason.

The mutual co-constitution of the drug quinine and the disease malaria was shaped, to a great extent, by the histories of British Empire in the long nineteenth century. In concluding in the late 1900s and early 1910s, I have situated the crystallisation of interrelationships amongst malaria, quinine and mosquitoes within wider trends of the links between natural knowledge and modern imperial rule. As in the case of malaria, other scholars have shown, various developments in the early twentieth century in the fields of natural knowledge and practice, particularly in bacteriology, anthropology and ecology were culminations of processes that had their roots in the imperial history of the nineteenth century.[7] Indeed, the consolidation of natural knowledge about

---

[7] See for example P. Chakrabarti, *Bacteriology in British India: Laboratory Medicine and the Tropics* (Rochester: University of Rochester Press, 2012); G. W. Stocking Jr., 'The Ethnographer's Magic: Fieldwork in British Anthropology from Tylor to Malinowski', in G. W. Stocking Jr. (ed.), *Observers Observed: Essays on Ethnographic Fieldwork* (Madison: University of Wisconsin Press, 1983), 70–120; S. Qureshi, *Peoples on Parade: Exhibitions, Empire and Anthropology in Nineteenth-Century Britain,* (London and Chicago: University of Chicago Press, 2011); P. Anker, *Imperial Ecology: Environmental Order in the British*

cinchonas, malaria, quinine, and mosquitoes, and the establishment of interrelationships between them were not inevitable or accidental, but rather the exigencies and apparatuses of imperial rule shaped them. The British Empire occasioned not only the imbrications of the worlds of medical knowledge, pharmaceutical commerce, colonial governance and (as I will elaborate further in the next section) vernacular public cultures, but also bound South Asian history with events unfolding in distant parts of the world, particularly in South America, the West Indies, German, French and British Africa, and Dutch Java. While analysing the persistence of malaria as a diagnostic category, I have focused on the nineteenth century in its own right. I have refused to treat it as a period characterised by flawed archaic understandings about the disease which would be rectified eventually in course of the next century.

Malaria, of course, continued to remain a significant concern in world history and politics in the interwar period. Many recent books on the history of malaria have focused predominantly on the twentieth century.[8] This book has provided a historical backdrop to the period covered by these existing scholarly works by identifying the ways in which malaria was reconfigured as a major concern for global governance in the imperial context of the long nineteenth century. This context also shaped the interactions between the scholarly disciplines of tropical medicine, parasitology and entomology, and these interactions in turn, resulted in the preponderance of narratives about blood, parasites and mosquitoes in the literature concerning malaria in the early twentieth century.

By focusing on this period, this book reveals how certain nineteenth-century trends in the history of malaria persisted into the next century. Events in the early decades of the twentieth century, particularly the redefinition of malaria as a mosquito-borne, parasite-caused fever disease and the discrediting of quinine did not immediately constitute an incommensurable epistemological break in the history of malaria and its cures. Indeed, as I have indicated in Chapter 5, in various quarters, practices such as the therapeutic prescription of quinine, the use

Empire, 1895–1945 (Cambridge, Mass. and London: Harvard University Press, 2001); D. Haraway, 'Teddy Bear Patriarchy: Taxidermy in the Garden of Eden, New York City, 1908–1936', *Social Text*, 11 (Winter, 1984–1985), 20–64; J. Beattie, *Empire and Environmental Anxiety: Health, Science, Art and Conservation in South Asian and Australasia, 1800–1920* (Basingstoke: Palgrave Macmillan, 2011).

8　F. M. Snowden, *The Conquest of Malaria, Italy 1900–1962* (New Haven: Yale University Press, 2006); S. M. Sufian, *Healing the Land and the Nation: Malaria and the Zionist Project in Palestine, 1920–1947* (Chicago and London: University of Chicago Press, 2007); L. B. Slater, *War and Disease: Biomedical Research on Malaria on the Twentieth Century* (New Brunswick: Rutgers University Press, 2009); M. Cueto, *Cold War, Deadly Fevers: Malaria Eradication in Mexico, 1955–1975* (Baltimore: Johns Hopkins University Press, 2007).

of drugs such as quinine for clinical diagnosis of malaria, and the projection of malaria as a commodious cause of many maladies did not entirely cease.[9] One of the lasting legacies of the nineteenth-century literature about malaria was the continued association of the category predominantly with colonial and postcolonial landscapes. Undoubtedly, malaria reemerged as a prominent concern that afflicted various parts of Europe, extending beyond 'the semicolonial appendage' of southern Italy in the late nineteenth and the early twentieth centuries.[10] However, before long, malariologists celebrated the 'disappearance' of malaria from various parts of the United States and Europe, particularly, England.[11] It was argued that the 'disappearance' of malaria could be attributed to 'civilising social influences' and 'scientific agriculture' that were in vogue in these parts of the world.[12] Published in 1946, *A Malariologist in Many Lands*, a scientific memoir written by Marshall A, Barber, a public health professional associated with the Rockefeller Foundation amongst other organisations, did not devote any of the chapters to Western Europe or even Italy.[13] A reviewer of this account took note of Barber's claim that 'decrease (of malaria) in the United States is almost universal' and that

[9] On the widespread use of quinine as an anti-malarial in twentieth-century South Asia, see Harrison, *Disease and the Dilemmas of Development*. On the continued use of quinine in clinical diagnosis of malaria, see P. Manson, 'The Diagnosis of Malaria from the Standpoint of the Practitioner in England', *Lancet*, 159, 4107 (17 May 1902), 1378. On the persistence of malaria as a perceived commodious cause of many diseases, see Anonymous, 'The Diagnosis of Latent Malaria', *Lancet*, 186, 4805 (2 October 1915), 768; Anonymous, 'Latent Malaria', *Lancet*, 170, 4376 (13 July 1907), 100. On the 'plasticity of disease concepts' and on 'the shifting boundaries of what constitutes as adequate model of disease' in relation to malaria as late as the 1940s, see Slater, *War and Disease*, 8.

[10] Snowden, *The Conquest of Malaria*, 3; P. Zylberman, 'A Transatlantic Dispute: The Etiology of Malaria and the Redesign of the Mediterranean Landscape', in S. G. Solomon, L. Murard, and P. Zylberman (eds.), *Shifting Boundaries of Public Health: Europe in the Twentieth Century* (Rochester: University of Rochester Press, 2008), 269–297; D. H. Stapleton, 'Internationalism and Nationalism: The Rockefeller Foundation, Public Health and Malaria in Italy, 1923–1951', *Parassitologia*, 42, 1–2 (June, 2000), 127–134; H. Evans, 'European Malaria Policy in the 1920s and 1930s: The Epidemiology of Minutiae', *Isis*, 80, 1 (March 1989), 40–59; S. P. James, 'The Disappearance of Malaria from England', *Proceedings of the Royal Society of Medicine*, 23, 1 (November, 1929), 71–87.

[11] James, 'The Disappearance of Malaria from England'; L. W. Hackett, 'The Disappearance of Malaria in the United States and Europe', *Rivista di Parassitologia*, 13, 1 (January, 1952), 43–56.

[12] James, 'The Disappearance of Malaria from England', 83; Hackett quoted in G. Majori, 'Short History of Malaria and its Eradication in Italy with Short Notes on the Fight Against the Infection in the Mediterranean Basin', *Mediterranean Journal of Hematology and Infectious Diseases*, 4, 1 (2012), www.ncbi.nlm.nih.gov/pmc/articles/PMC3340992/ [Retrieved on 6 June 2016.]

[13] M. A. Barber, *A Malariologist in Many Lands* (Lawerence, Kansas: University of Kansas Press, 1946).

'an analogous decrease in malaria has occurred in northern and central Europe'.[14] Instead, the memoir focused predominantly on various corners of the colonial and postcolonial world such as parts of Central America, the West Indies, the Philippine Islands, Malaya and the Fiji islands, Equatorial Africa, Egypt, India and Brazil. A twentieth-century poster (Figure 6.1) which was released in London by Her Majesty's Stationary Office as an instruction for travellers identified the vast expanses of the colonial and postcolonial world including 'Africa, Tropical America, India and the Far East' as the 'danger areas' for acquiring malaria, and recommended everyday use of quinine and mosquito nets in these 'areas'.[15]

More recent scholarly assessments have described malaria as a 'leading cause of...underdevelopment in the world today...a major contributor to the inequalities between (the Global) North and (the Global) South, and of the dependency of the Third World'.[16] Many historians who have written about early and mid-twentieth-century South Asia, Africa, Egypt, Palestine, Philippines, Indochina or postwar Mexico, have examined the significance of concerns about malaria in shaping the late imperial and postcolonial world. These scholars have shown that malaria in the twentieth century was not only a recurrent issue in imperial governance and geopolitics; but the disease was also entangled within local aspirations of development and ethnic nationalism.[17]

In reemphasising the significance of European empires in the making of modern medical knowledge, I have drawn upon the extant historiography linking science, medicine and empires. I have also been inspired by

---

[14] S. Jarcho, 'Review of M. A. Barber, *A Malariologist in Many Lands*', *Journal of History of Medicine and Allied Sciences*, 2, 2 (Spring, 1947), 268–270.

[15] R. Mount, 'The Malaria Mosquito under a Spotlight, with Scenes Showing How to Avoid Catching Malaria. Colour Lithograph after a Design Attributed to Reginald Mount' (London: HM Stationary Office, c. 1943–c. 1953). [Credit: Wellcome Library, London. Photo number L0024907.]

[16] F. M. Snowden and R. Bucala, 'Introduction', in F. M. Snowden and R. Bucala (eds.), *The Global Challenge of Malaria: Past Lessons and Future Prospects* (Singapore: World Scientific Publishing, 2014), vii.

[17] Harrison, *Disease and the Dilemmas of Development*; S. Watts, 'British Development Policies and Malaria in India 1897–c. 1929', *Past & Present* 165 (November 1999), 141–181; R. Packard, 'Malaria Blocks Development Revisited: The Role of Disease in the History of Agricultural Development in the Eastern and Northern Transvaal Lowveld, 1890–1960', *Journal of Southern African Studies*, 27, 3 (2001), 591–612; T. Mitchell, *Rule of Experts: Egypt, Techno-politics, Modernity* (Los Angeles: University of California Press) 2002, 19–53; S. M. Sufian, *Healing the Land and the Nation*; W. Anderson, *Colonial Pathologies: American Tropical Medicine, Race and Hygiene in the Philippines* (Durham: Duke University Press, 2006), 207–225; Monnais, 'Rails, Roads and Mosquito Foes', 215–225; M. Cueto, *Cold War, Deadly Fevers*.

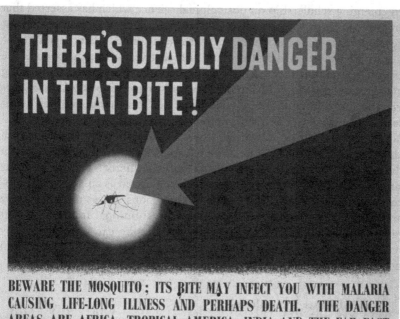

THERE'S DEADLY DANGER IN THAT BITE!

BEWARE THE MOSQUITO ; ITS BITE MAY INFECT YOU WITH MALARIA CAUSING LIFE-LONG ILLNESS AND PERHAPS DEATH. THE DANGER AREAS ARE AFRICA, TROPICAL AMERICA, INDIA AND THE FAR EAST

DEFEAT THE MOSQUITO IN THESE WAYS

Go ashore as little as possible in the danger zones. If you do go ashore return to your ship before sundown. The mosquito usually attacks by night.

Take a dose of quinine the day before your ship arrives at a danger zone. Take a dose daily as long as you remain and for four weeks after you leave. Quinine won't hurt you, but it will kill malaria germs in your blood.

Make your quarters mosquito proof. Keep them clean and see that there are no pools of stagnant water (for example in the boats) where mosquitoes may breed. Sleep under a mosquito net.

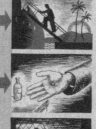

QUININE EVERY DAY KEEPS MALARIA AWAY

Figure 6.1 Colour lithograph attributed to R. Mount, 'The malaria mosquito under a spotlight, with scenes showing how to avoid catching malaria.' (London: HM Stationary Office, c. 1943–c.1953.) [Credit: Wellcome Library, London. Photo number L0024907.]

an emerging scholarship on postcolonial science which has asserted that empire can be a crucial analytical frame in understanding more recent developments in the sciences.[18] At the same time, I have been attentive to the ways in which historians in recent years have questioned the exclusive attention accorded to imperial agency in analysing the making of the modern world.[19] Inspired by these diverse positions, *Malarial Subjects* has contributed to recent conceptual literature about empires themselves. The history of British Empire in the long nineteenth century cannot be reduced to the activities of the colonial state alone. Instead, each chapter describes the Empire as an occasion for the interaction between the worlds of governance, knowledge and commerce. The Empire was simultaneously an overarching causal agent, as well as an immanent process that was itself sustained by these interactions. It was not necessarily an inflexible, top-down and preordained institutional framework. But rather, the long and violent life of British Empire can be explained by its ability to shape and in turn be reconstituted by various human and nonhuman histories.

'Morbus Bengalensis'

Non-European colonised groups have featured in different ways in the recent historiography of British imperial science and medicine. One of the most enduring strands of this historiography has acknowledged that science and medicine were crucial means through which imperial rule and violence were inflicted on colonised groups.[20] Other scholars have argued that the colonial state-endorsed science and medicine were not shaped by the activities of Europeans alone, but rather such forms of knowledge were also built upon the physical and intellectual labour of indigenous groups in the colonised locales.[21] While extending these insights, postcolonial scholars have further revealed that colonised vernacular groups were not passive recipients of the dictates of imperial

---

[18] W. Anderson, 'From Subjugated Knowledge to Conjugated Subjects: Science and Globalisation, or Postcolonial Studies of Science', *Postcolonial Studies*, 12, 4 (2009), 389–400; A. Prasad, 'Science in Motion: What Postcolonial Science Studies Can Offer', *Electronic Journal of Communication Information & Innovation in Health (RECIIS)* 2, 2 (July–December 2008), 35–47.

[19] See R. Deb Roy, 'Nonhuman Empires', *Comparative Studies of South Asia, Africa and the Middle East*, 35, 1 (May 2015), 72.

[20] See for example P. Chakrabarti, *Materials and Medicine: Trade, Conquest and Therapeutics in the Eighteenth Century* (Manchester: Manchester University Press, 2010).

[21] See especially K. Raj, *Relocating Modern Science: Circulation and the Construction of Scientific Knowledge in South Asia and Europe, 1650–1900* (Houndmills and New York: Palgrave Macmillan, 2007).

science and medicine. These scholars have shown how the contents of the colonial state-informed science and medicine were eventually translated, displaced, reinterpreted and appropriated by the colonised people to suit their own agendas.[22] Inspired by these different scholarly positions, this section comments on Bengali publications on malaria, quinine and mosquitoes in the late nineteenth and early twentieth centuries. I have focused on a specific South Asian language for the sake of in-depth analysis, apart from my own interests in the region. Besides, Bengal had one of the most enduring exposures to imperial rule in the modern world. It was home to a thriving vernacular print market, as well as one of the earliest cinchona plantations and quinine factories to be set up in the colonial world. Yet it retained the notoriety of being considered as one of the most malarial provinces of the British Empire until decolonisation. This section argues that resisting, translating and reappropriating insights about quinine, malaria and mosquitoes in the Bengali public sphere should not necessarily be regarded as extraneous to the history of imperial medicine. Rather, along with details unfolding in bureaucratic files, commercial private papers, or colonial medical journals, these processes need to be acknowledged as episodes within the history of empire and imperial medicine. I suggest that the history of imperial medicine was shaped through interactions between the more peripatetic concerns of colonial bureaucrats, medical officials, and Europeans pharmaceutical businessmen, on the one hand, and vernacular public cultures, on the other.[23] This section ends by hinting that in the final decades of British imperial rule, Bengali (often anti-imperial) writings on mosquitoes reflected the various concerns of British colonial officials, multinational charitable organisations, the US military and other dominant players in global governance in the interwar period.

British Indian subjects were not necessarily docile bodies who were inescapably colonised into consuming quinine. Colonised subjects often rejected or criticised medicines prescribed to them by the colonial state, and this constituted an integral aspect of the history of imperial medicine. Indeed, the elaborate disciplinary as well as punitive measures

---

[22] P. B. Mukharji, *Nationalizing the Body: The Medical Market, Print and Daktari Medicine* (London and New York: Anthem Press, 2009); I. Pande, *Medicine, Race and Liberalism: Symptoms of Empire*, (Abingdon and New York: Routledge, 2010).

[23] This is not to deny that some of these processes associated with vernacular public sphere were eventually appropriated within the emerging anti-imperial nationalist projects. These suggest overlaps and continuities between imperial medicine, on the one hand, and emergent anti-imperial nationalist medicine, on the other. For details see Mukharji, *Nationalizing the Body*.

adopted by the British Indian government to enforce the consumption of quinine amongst the colonial subjects indicate the hesitation with which the drug must have been initially received. Indigenous rejection of quinine took various forms. Female tea plantation labourers in North Bengal often refused their daily dosage of quinine by spitting the drug out.[24] More patrician critics of quinine claimed that the drug was a symbol of moral decadence and excessive reliance upon Western ways of living. An article published in the 1870s in the homoeopathic *Calcutta Journal of Medicine*, as discussed in Chapter 3, sarcastically renamed Burdwan fever as a 'cinchona disease'. The article argued that Burdwan fever was a side effect of excessive consumption of quinine in colonial Bengal. Similarly, Bengali medical journals like *Chikitsa Sammilani* published editorials titled 'Quinine is malaria', and in the process refused to distinguish between the cause and cure of disease. These kinds of statements did not merely express doubts about the efficacy of quinine as a therapeutic substance. By equating the quintessential cure with malaria, these critics were simultaneously calling into question the validity of the diagnostic category malaria itself.[25] Echoing these thoughts, an early twentieth-century Bengali article entitled 'Malaria Rahasya' or the 'Malaria Mystery' rejected quinine by labelling it as a poison. It also described malaria as an 'airy-fairy word', and an 'imaginary unfounded idea'.[26]

Most Bengali commentators, however, underscored the significance of malaria as an experiential reality, even when they continued to suspect the efficaciousness of quinine.[27] In a paper read out to the Calcutta Medical Society in the early 1880s on the theme 'Use and Abuse of Quinine in Fever', Rakhal Chandra Ghose, a Bengali trained in one of the medical colleges set up by the colonial government, argued that the 'old sufferers living in the endemic districts of Bengal and constantly imbibing the malarial poison' were victims of a peculiar form of malarial fever. He called this malarial malady which was unique to Bengal, 'Morbus Bengalensis'. He asserted that quinine was 'literally useless' in curing 'Morbus Bengalensis'.[28] These doubts were expressed in the context of the proliferation of various indigenous substitutes of

[24] Anonymous, 'The Indian Tea Industry. The Labour Question. Malaria as a Factor. VI-The application of Principles of Protection', Cutting from *The Statesman*, 1 January 1909. Home, Sanitary, May 1910, 189–231 A (NAI).

[25] Anonymous, 'Quinine i Malaria', *Chikitsa Sammilani*, 9, 10 (1893), 402–405.

[26] N. Majumdar, 'Malaria Rahasya', *Hahnemann*, 9, 11 (c. 1910), 577, 578, 583, 584.

[27] J. Basu, 'Quinine', *Chikitsa Sammilani*, 4, 1 (April–May 1887), 16–18; Anonymous, 'Quininer Opobebohar' (Abuse of Quinine), *Chikitsa Sammilani*, 6, 10/11/12 (Mid-January to Mid-April 1890), 388–391; Anonymous, 'Quinine', *Chikitsak*, 1, 1 (January/February, 1890), 93–100.

[28] R. C. Ghose, 'Use and Abuse of Quinine in Fever', *IMG* (1 May 1882), 138–142.

quinine in the Bengali vernacular medical marketplace. Many locally produced pills and tonics were advertised as superior alternatives to quinine in contemporary Bengali almanacs, manuals and pamphlets. These drugs included *Atyashcharya Batika* (The most wonderful pill), *Dasyadi Pachan*, Sarkar's tonic, *Chaitanya batika* (Chaitanya pills), *Bijoy batika* (Victory pills) amongst others.[29] All commodities associated with curing malaria, however, were not to be orally consumed. Certain advertisements recommended ritually sanctioned lockets which were supposedly endowed with divine powers that could stave off malaria and its effects.[30] A range of advertisements claimed that these local commodities were more suited than quinine to combat malaria in Bengal.

Nonetheless, the colonial state and its vernacular subjects did not always adopt completely opposite positions on quinine. The image of a unanimous medical bureaucracy imposing quinine on a reluctant Bengali people did not necessarily hold. A section of English bureaucrats themselves criticised the widespread distribution of quinine amongst 'Indian patients'. Drawing on various physiological surveys conducted in India in the early 1900s, this group of officials emphasised the differences in the 'composition of the blood of non–flesh-eating natives of India from that of the blood of the flesh-eating Europeans'. They argued that the red blood corpuscles of local inhabitants in India were characterised by a relative deficiency of haemoglobin, and this rendered the consumption of significant doses of quinine 'deleterious'.[31] On the other hand, apart from selling indigenous substitutes of quinine, Bengali shopkeepers and medics in the vernacular marketplaces also innovated their own versions of quinine. While many of them were sceptical about the effectiveness of an imported drug, others were increasingly aware of the credibility the label quinine carried with it, because of its enduring

[29] Anonymous, 'N. C. Pul & Co.'s Most Wonderful Pills', *Anubikshan*, 1, 5 (November/December, 1875), 5; Anonymous, 'D. Gupta and Company's Antiperiodic Pill', in *Nutan Panjika* (Calcutta: Benimadhab De and Company, 1887–1888), 2 [Box 1 File 7 CSSSC]; Anonymous, 'Nalhati Pharmacy: Sarkar's Tonic', *Bharat-Suhrid*, 1,10 (March–April, 1903), in M. Mamun (ed.), *Unish Satakey Bangladeser Sangbad Samayik patra Volume 7*, 363–364 [Box 5 CSSSC]; Anonymous, 'Noakhali Haldar and Company's famous Chaitanya Pills', *Asha*, 1, 7–8, (October–December, 1902), in Mamun (ed.), *Unish Satakey*, 289 [Box 5 CSSSC]; Anonymous, 'Bijoy Batika', *B. Basu and Company's Salsa* (B. Basu and Company: Calcutta, c. 1900), 2 [Author's collection]; G. Nandi, 'Malaria Jvarey Dasyadi Pachan' ('Dasyadi Pachan in Malaria Fever'), *Chikitsak*, 1,1 (1889), 70–72.

[30] Anonymous, 'Desh Bides Bikshyato' ('World Famous'), *Benimadhab De and Company's Panjika*, (1896–97), [Box 1, File7, CSSSC].

[31] S. P. James, 'Problems Relating to the Use of Quinine', and C. Donovan, 'The Most Useful Salt of Quinine for Distribution in Malarial Tracts', *Proceedings of the Imperial Malaria Conference held at Simla in October 1909* (Simla: Government Central Branch Press, 1910), 69 and 75. Home, Sanitary, May 1910, 189–231 A (NAI).

association with the colonial government. As the case of Shashi Bhu-
san Dutta detailed in the previous chapter suggests, various operators in
the vernacular marketplace appropriated the label of quinine to describe
their disparate medical products. By the 1890s, the colonial state had
installed a network of mechanisms to detect and punish these acts. Contemporary Bengali novelists, as well, shared the governmental perception
that the original purity of quinine was being tampered with by Indian
rural shopkeepers.[32]

The interactions between state medicine and vernacular medical markets in Bengal were enabled by the increasing participation of Bengalis
such as Jodunath Mukhopadhyay as subordinate members in the colonial
medical apparatus. Mukhopadhyay pursued multiple careers, and inhabited different cultural worlds. He was educated in the colonial medical
institutions, authored various medical manuals in Bengali, and traded
in indigenous alternatives to quinine.[33] Many Bengali medical manuals
written by Mukhopadhyay emphasised the virtues of quinine as a remedy
for diseases associated with malaria.[34] At the same time, an advertisement published in March 1888 claimed that he had himself started manufacturing a more effective remedy for malarial fever which he called *Sarvajvarankusha*, which meant 'The cure of all fevers'.[35] This suggests that
Bengalis who advertised the virtues of quinine and those who traded in
its indigenous alternatives did not necessarily constitute mutually exclusive worlds. In fact, many spokesmen in favour of anti-malarial patent
medicine or indigenous alternatives of quinine in Bengal were employed
in the colonial medical department.[36] Therefore, it is not unlikely that
directly or indirectly they were also associated with the colonial state's
project of popularising quinine amongst the Indians. Bengali advocates
of quinine and its indigenous substitutes were often drawn from the same
cultural world, and used similar expressions in praise of these competing
drugs. For example, appealing to the sensibilities of a Hindu readership, Bengali articles and advertisements referred to both quinine and
anti-malarial patent medicines in Bengal as 'Brahmastra', an invincible

[32] S. Chattopadhyay, 'Ramer Sumati', in S. Chattopadhyay, *Sarat Sahitya Samagra* (Calcutta: Ananda Publishers, 1986/1913), 1572–1588.
[33] The category indigenous itself is historically constructed. See P. B. Mukharji, 'Symptoms of Dis-Ease: New Trends in Histories of "Indigenous" South Asian Medicines',
History Compass, 9, 12 (2011), 887–899.
[34] J. Mukhopadhyay, *Quinine* (Calcutta, 1893); J. Mukhopadhyay, *Bishamjvare Quinine
Proyog-pronali* (Chinsurah: Chikitsaprokash Press, 1879).
[35] K. Mukhopadhyay, 'Sarvajvarankusha', *Education Gazette and Saptahik Vartabaha* (9
March 1888), 733 [UJPL, 6/7, CSSSC].
[36] Anonymous, 'Noakhali Haldar and Company's famous Chaitanya Pills'; Anonymous,
'Sudhanidhi', *Bharat Suhrid*, 1, 10 (March/April, 1903), in Mamun, *Unish Satakey*, 363
[Box 5, CSSSC].

weapon described in Hindu mythology. Bengali medical publications did not pursue the single-minded agenda of contesting the curative properties ascribed on quinine. These were also sites in which the relevance of quinine was reasserted before a Bengali-reading audience.[37]

Those who wrote about malaria, quinine and its indigenous substitutes in Bengali medical journals, books, newspapers, magazines and almanacs (and who were cited in the advertisements of various anti-malarial medicines in the late nineteenth century) mostly belonged to a class of bilingual Bengali men, who were trained in the emerging medical colleges in and around Calcutta. A majority of these Bengali authors, such as Mukhopadhyay, held 'a license for medicine and surgery' (LMS). Others possessed more respectable degrees such as Doctor of Medicine (MD) or a baccalaureate degree in medicine (MB).[38] These qualifications, which were recognised by the colonial government, enabled these authors to seek employment in a hierarchy of positions within the colonial medical establishment ranging from assistant surgeons to resident medical officers in government hospitals.[39] Bengali writings on malaria and its cures were authored not only from Calcutta, but also from other parts of Bengal including Chandannagore, Chinsurah, Murshidabad and Bolpur.[40] As already noted, apart from doubting the efficacy of quinine, some of these authors questioned the existence of malaria itself.[41] Others attributed malarial epidemics in Bengal to flaws in government policies.[42] However, most of these texts echoed the dominant concerns of the colonial government, and circulated significant contemporary medical theories about malaria and its cures.[43]

---

[37] Bengali texts that described quinine as 'Brahmastra' included Anonymous, 'Quininer Opobebohar', 388; Mukhopadhyay, *Quinine*, 58; J. Mukhopadhyay, *Saral Jvar Chikitsa Prothom Bhag* (Calcutta: Nityananda Ghosh, 1880), 15. Bengali texts that described patent medicines as 'Brahmastra' included Mukhopadhyay, 'Sarvajvarankusha'; Anonymous, 'Sudhanidhi'; Anonymous, 'Bijoy Batika'.

[38] See Mukharji, *Nationalizing*, 4–7. Basu, 'Quinine', 18; P. Sanyal, 'Remittent Fever e Quinine', *Chikitsa Sammilani*, 4, 1 (April/May, 1887), 245; Mukhopadhyay, *Bishamjvare Quinine*.

[39] D. K. Ghosh, *Malaria* (Sultangachi, Hooghly: Doyal Kishen Ghosh, 1878); A. Bhattacharya, *Jvar Chikitsa* (Calcutta: Valmiki Press, 1878).

[40] Nandi, 'Dasyadi Pachan'; Mukhopadhyay, *Bishamjvare Quinine*; Majumdar, 'Malaria Rahasya'; A. Pal, *Malaria* (Bolpur, 1927).

[41] Anonymous, 'Quinine i Malaria'; Majumdar, 'Malaria Rahasya'; Anonymous, 'Burdwan fever', *Calcutta Journal of Medicine*, 6, 6 (June 1873), 198.

[42] D. Mitter, *The Epidemic Fever in Bengal* (Calcutta: Hindu Patriot Press, 1873); Ghosh, *Malaria*, 50.

[43] Sanyal, 'Remittent Fever e Quinine'; R. Mitra, 'Quinine', *Chikitsa Sammilani*, 3, 1 (April/May 1886), 131–136; H. Sengupta, 'Quinine O Ihar Bebohar', *Bhishak Darpan*, 6, 11(May 1897), 447–450; Anonymous, 'Malaria', *Swasthya*, 4, 9 (December/January, 1900/1901), 257–287; K. Sen, 'Malaria o Moshok', *Bhisak Darpan*, 10, 4 (April, 1900),

While claiming to translate and disseminate knowledge about malaria and quinine in the Bengali language, these texts were highly creative and original works in themselves.[44] They displayed their authors' ability to blend wisdom acquired from superiors in the colonial medical service, college lecturers and English textbooks, on the one hand, with experiential references to more intimate landscapes, places, vegetation, cultural icons and events encountered in Bengal, on the other.[45] These were cosmopolitan texts in which references to ancient Ayurvedic verses and nineteenth-century British medical commentators (such as John Mac-Culloch) were intimately interspersed; some of these Bengali texts contained quotations in Latin, Sanskrit and English.[46] In his book-length treatise on malaria published in 1878, assistant surgeon Doyal Krishen Ghosh indicated that malaria was not only an enigmatic medical problem, but also a moral problem that was caused by laziness, inadequate sleep, excessive sexual activity and undisciplined diet.[47] Ghosh, therefore, combined insights from English medical journals with lessons prescribed in Bengali medico-moral manuals, which were widely in circulation in the print market.[48]

These texts did not represent a distortion of preordained imperial medical knowledge. But rather, along with English medical journals and colonial bureaucratic correspondence analysed in Chapters 2 and 3, these Bengali texts were also integral sites where imperial insights about malaria were reshaped and consolidated. As liminal go-betweens, their authors played an important role in shaping the vocabulary in which literate Bengalis, who were crucial agents in the imperial world, addressed the disease. Their mediation enabled the enmeshing of European medical categories with Bengali cultural repertoires, which paved the way for various literary liberties. If quinine was referred to as a 'brahmastra', malaria was described as a 'rakshashi' (female demon); a 'jujuburi' (witch); 'jamopam rakshash' ('a demon comparable to Lord Yama, the mythical God of Death'; and a 'dabanol' ('forest fire').[49] When he mentioned malarial fever as 'maloyarir jvar' in his well-known novel

---

143–154; Anonymous, 'Malariar Prokop', *Swasthya*, 3, 7 (October–November, 1899), 215–218.

[44] For more on this claim see Mukharji, *Nationalizing the Body*.

[45] Ghosh, *Malaria*, 1–26; Bhattacharya, *Jvar Chikitsa*, see especially the title page, preface and 1–18.

[46] Majumdar, 'Malaria Rahasya', 575–585; Bhattacharya, *Jvar Chikitsa*, 'The title page'.

[47] Ghosh, *Malaria*, 10–18.

[48] On Bengali medical manuals, see R. Deb Roy, 'Debility, Diet, Desire: Food in Nineteenth- and Early Twentieth-Century Bengali Manuals,' in S. Chaudhuri and R. B. Chatterjee (eds.), *The Writer's Feast: Food and the Cultures of Representation* (New Delhi: Orient Blackswan, March 2011), 179–205.

[49] K. Basu, *Malaria Nibaraner Upay o Onyanyo Prabandho* (Calcutta: Swasthya Dharma Sangha, 1924), 11; Majumdar, 'Malaria Rahasya', 577; S. Lahiri, 'Ayurbedey Malaria',

Arakshaniya (*The Unmarriageable*), the iconic Bengali writer Sarat Chandra Chattopadhyay hinted at the way in which the word malaria may have been slightly tweaked in its everyday colloquial usage in certain parts of contemporary Bengal.[50] In the same novel, Chattopadhyay suggests how young women ostensibly suffering from malaria in poverty-stricken, rural, patriarchal Bengal were perceived as ugly and unmarriageable. *Arakshaniya* represents malaria not as a distant governmental jargon, but as an everyday reality that shaped, by the 1910s, experiences of intimacy and romance in Bengal.[51]

Bengali writers on malaria shaped attitudes not only of the manual and novel reading public in Bengal, but of the colonial state also. Despite punishing fraud and adulteration, the colonial state itself drew upon various local cultural symbols to popularise government quinine amongst the Indian subjects. These state-initiated innovations also shaped the interactions between local cultural icons and apparently secular medical items. As discussed in the previous chapter, the imperial postal department distributed a signboard in the 1890s that described quinine as a remedy gifted by the Hindu deity Lord Shiva to the ailing peasants of rural Bengal.[52] The colonial state also initiated the translation of advertisements of government quinine from English into a range of South Asian languages, including Bengali. The publicity for government quinine in Indian regional languages and the use of religious icons like Lord Shiva in quinine posters must have been made easier by the increasing presence of South Asians, including Bengalis, in different levels of colonial medical governance. Bengalis, whether in their capacity as medics trained in the colonial medical colleges in India, or as employees in the colonial bureaucracy drafted unpublished routine correspondence in English, contributed to English medical journals and wrote book-length treatises in English. Their opinions may not necessarily have formed the backbone of imperial malaria policy. However, the fact that their writings made it into journals such as the *Indian Medical Gazette* indicates that their insights about the locality were given cognizance by the colonial medical establishment.[53] In Chapter 3, I have suggested that some

---

Bhisak Darpan, 21, 12(December, 1911), 462; Anonymous, 'Swasthyaprosongo', *Swasthya*, 3, 8 (November/December, 1899), 226.

[50] S. Chattopadhyay, 'Arakshaniya', in S. Chattopadhyay, *Sarat Sahitya Samagra* (Calcutta: Ananda Publishers, 1986/1916), 251–252.

[51] Ibid., 244–267.

[52] It is worthy of note that in an undated advertisement even an anti-malarial patent medicine in Bengal was projected as an outcome of the blessings of Lord Shiva. Advertisement of 'Bisswesswar Ross Pills' (Calcutta: Febrona Limited) [Image number DP0003, CSSSC].

[53] K. D. Ghose, 'A Plea for Malaria', *IMG* 17 (1 June 1882), 150–154; Ghose, 'Use and Abuse of Quinine'; Anonymous, 'Tincture of Iodine and Burnt Alum in Intermittent Fever', *IMG*, 17 (2 October 1882), 279.

Bengali members in the British Indian administration, such as Sunjeeb Chunder Chatterjee and Gopaul Chandra Roy, played significant roles in shaping colonial discourse about Burdwan fever. In a letter addressed to the Secretary of the Government of Bengal in 1863, Chatterjee, who was one of the first Bengali members in the colonial bureaucracy and also the elder brother of the pioneering Bengali novelist Bankim Chandra Chattopadhyay, recommended intense anti-malarial administrative intervention by the colonial state in the interiors of Bengal. That this letter was cited again seven years later in official correspondence suggests that his recommendations were taken seriously.[54] Roy, who studied medicine in Glasgow and London, was employed as inspecting medical officer of dispensaries in Burdwan, and in the 1870s wrote a book on Burdwan fever. That the book was published simultaneously by different English firms in London and Calcutta, and went into multiple editions suggests that Roy's work attracted a considerable audience.[55] Such widespread interest in how the members of the colonised society defined malaria and its solutions was not exceptional. One might recall that the Viceroy Lord Northbrook declared in 1872 a prize of Rs. 1000 for the best essay written by a 'native' sub-assistant surgeon on the causes and prevention of Burdwan fever.[56] It can be argued that regional expertise asserted by Bengalis writing on malaria in English was appropriated by the imperial project of pathologising colonised lands, landscapes and people. By sharing intimate information about plants, places and landscapes in Bengal, these writers added greater depth, texture and local flavour to imperial medical narratives about malaria.

The interchange between South Asian colonised voices and the colonial state manifested in other ways. The Bengali medical journal *Bhishak Darpan* published an article in 1911 entitled 'Ayurbedey Malaria' ('Malaria in the Ayurveda') by a physician Saracchandra Lahiri, who asserted that the authors of key texts of Ayurveda in ancient India already knew the aetiology and cures of malaria.[57] In a speech delivered as the

[54] S. C. Chatterjee, Cantalpara, to A. Eden, Secretary to the Government of Bengal, dated 1 May 1863. Home, Public, 7 May 1870, 65–71 A (NAI).

[55] G. C Roy, *The Causes, Symptoms and Treatment of Burdwan Fever, or the Epidemic Fever of Lower Bengal* (London: J and A Churchill; Calcutta: Thacker, Spink and Co. New Edition, Revised and Improved, 1876). For more see Chapter 3.

[56] General, Medical, 147–148 B, August 1872 (WBSA).

[57] Lahiri, 'Ayurbedey Malaria', 461–467. Various other contemporary texts authored by Bengalis made similar claims. K. Vidyabhushan, *What is Malaria and the Germ Theory* (Calcutta: Narendranath Vidyanidhi, 1914); Majumdar, 'Malaria Rahasya', 575–585. The *Bhishak Darpan* also published two articles subsequently that added nuance to Lahiri's assertions. P. Bhattacharya, 'Ayurbedey Malaria', *Bhishak Darpan*, 21, 12 (December, 1911), 443–461; M. Kabyatirtha, 'Ayurbedey Malaria Probondher Samalochona', *Bhisak Darpan*, 22, 6 (June 1912), 209–216.

President of the Imperial Malaria Conference held in Shimla in 1909, H.H. Risley almost anticipated Lahiri's opinions when he argued that the authors of Atharvaveda knew about malaria and its cures.[58] Therefore, Bengali revivalist ideologues in the immediate aftermath of the Swadeshi movement in the 1900s appropriated colonial medical categories such as malaria to assert the relevance of Ayurveda in modern India. In turn, senior colonial officials such as Risley invoked ancient Indian wisdom to assert the enduring historical roots of colonial medical categories such as malaria in the subcontinent.

Therefore, notions about malaria and quinine were not unilaterally imposed on Bengal by the colonial state. Imperial notions of malaria and quinine were reshaped and sustained by Bengali idioms, icons, words and politics. As evident from these examples, these interactions informed the intellectual and material meanings of malaria and quinine in Bengal. These interactions also influenced the routes and networks through which the government organised the circulation of quinine in the province. Well before the government embarked in the 1890s and 1900s on a policy of aggressively enforcing the consumption of quinine in the interiors of South Asia, there thrived in Bengal a vernacular medical market in which various medical products, indigenous as well as imported (such as quinine), circulated.[59] Advertisements published in Bengali newspapers, almanacs and medical manuals in the 1870s and 1880s indicate that Bengali operators in local medical marketplaces already devised networks through which to circulate their products into the interiors of districts, subdivisions, 'outposts', police stations, and 'small, remote, and cluttered villages'.[60] They sold their medical products in the various corners of the province through many sites closely associated with the colonial state: merchants' offices, tea plantations, government medical stores, veterinary dispensaries, district boards, municipalities, port commission offices, railway stores, collieries and dispensaries.[61] They also recruited various ostensibly credible figures in rural Bengal such as teachers, pundits, postmasters, sub-inspectors, head-constables, the rural gentry, 'native doctors' and kavirajas to sell anti-malarial drugs

---

[58] H. Risley, 'Popular Cooperation in the Prevention of Malaria', *Proceedings of the Imperial Malaria Conference held at Simla in October 1909* (Simla: Government Central Branch Press, 1910), 95. Home, Sanitary, May 1910, 189–231 A (NAI).

[59] Anonymous, 'D. Gupta and Company's Antiperiodic Pill'; Anonymous, 'Wanted', *Sadharani* (28 December 1879) [Box 1, File 7, CSSSC].

[60] Mukhopadhyay, 'Sarvajvarankusha'.

[61] Anonymous, 'Batakrishna Pal and Company Chemists and Druggists', in *Nutan Panjika,* (Calcutta: Benimadhab De and Company, 1904–1905), [Box 5, NL, 20c, CSSSC].

in lieu of a commission.[62] These advertisements instructed prospective consumers to request for medicines from Calcutta-based firms directly through the post, and to make payments through various postal innovations like money order and bearer's post.[63] As I have elaborated in the previous chapter, many of these strategies would in subsequent decades form the backbone of aggressive quinine distribution efforts initiated under the watch of the government.

Similarly, regarding attitudes towards mosquitoes, the views of the colonised people and of the imperial medical entomologists often coalesced. It may be pointed out as a digression that in his address on the occasion of awarding the Nobel Prize in medicine to Ronald Ross, the rector of the Caroline Institute reportedly claimed that Ross's discovery was anticipated by East African tradition. He explained his point by suggesting that 'negroes in East Africa use the same name for the mosquito and malaria'.[64] While both the politics and content of the rector's statement deserve greater scrutiny, it is undeniable that in the imperial world of the late nineteenth and early twentieth centuries, many groups of people, besides imperial medical entomologists were concerned about mosquitoes. I have shown in Chapter 5 how prejudices against insects more generally and mosquitoes in particular were shared between the worlds of colonial plantation economy, late Victorian advertisements, sanitary governance, entomological laboratory and Bengali literature.

In British India, the government continued to organise mosquito-killing initiatives into the interwar period.[65] Cleansing the environment of mosquitoes was seen to be part of a wider sanitising project through which the colonial state asserted itself as the custodian of medical well-being in the colony.[66] In the early twentieth century, the British Empire in India, however, was not the only global power which prioritised protection from or annihilation of mosquitoes as a governmental agenda. These concerns were shared by fledgling multinational philanthropic organisations such as the Rockefeller Foundation, which started interacting closely with regional caretakers of development and health across

[62] Anonymous, 'Wanted'.
[63] Anonymous, 'D. Gupta and Company' in *Nutan Panjika* (Calcutta: Benimadhab De and Company, 1887–1888), 1 [Box 1, File 7, CSSSC].
[64] Anonymous, 'The Nobel Prize for Medicine, 1902', *Lancet*, 161, 4141 (10 January 1903), 122.
[65] Harrison, *Disease and the Dilemmas of Development*, 26–42.
[66] On the wider political context in which medicalisation of insects was carried out, see H. Raffles, 'Jews, Lice and History', *Public Culture*, 19, 3 (Fall, 2007), 521–566; N. Rogers, 'Germs with Legs: Flies, Disease and the New Public Health', *Bulletin of the History of Medicine*, 63 (Winter, 1989), 599–617.

the world in Italy, Egypt and Brazil.[67] Mosquitoes also featured prominently in the military predicaments of the United States. This was manifested not just in manuals that instructed soldiers engaged in overseas military expeditions about the most effective means to protect themselves from malaria and mosquitoes.[68] I have indicated that mosquitoes even emerged as a symbol of legitimate US military aggression in the early 1950s when a squadron of the US air force during the Korean War was named after mosquitoes. Photographs taken during this period from Malaysia, Mauritius, Trinidad and Ghana, and currently held at the archives of the Royal Commonwealth Society in Cambridge, suggest that the obsession to seek protection from malarial mosquitoes dictated patterns of entomological research, urban planning, architectural design and housewifery curriculum across the colonial world.[69] These concerns even made their way into children's comic literature. Herge's 1930 work *Tintin in Congo* warns readers about the perils of venturing into the interiors of Belgian Congo without a mosquito net![70]

In this wider context, as I have indicated in the last chapter, mosquitoes also attracted considerable attention in Bengali publications across a range of literary genres including fantasies, social treatises, educational pamphlets, crime fiction, comic short stories, poems, medical manuals and popular magazines. Of course, these literary works represented disparate aesthetic, satirical and political projects, and most of them did not directly promote the medicalisation of mosquitoes. However, it is significant that over the same period both imperial medical entomology and these Bengali literary texts contributed to the metamorphosis of mosquitoes into objects of enduring public spectacle. Even when Bengali humorous pamphlets and short stories caricatured these entomological projects, they were reminiscent of the global reality that

[67] Stapleton, 'Internationalism and Nationalism'; Mitchell, *Rule of Experts*, 26–51; R. M. Packard and P Gadehla, 'A Land Filled with Mosquitoes: Fred L. Soper, the Rockefeller Foundation, and the Anopheles Gambiae Invasion of Brazil', *Medical Anthropology: Cross-Cultural Studies in Health and Illness*, 17, 3 (1997), 215–238.

[68] A. Wells, 'Mosquitoes: American soldiers in World War II can encourage them to breed them by leaving ruts in roads and unfilled earth holes, causing mosquito-borne diseases', (Washington, DC: US Government Printing Office, 1944) [Credit: Wellcome Library, London, Photo Number: L74413].

[69] These photographs are held at the Royal Commonwealth Society Collections at the Cambridge University Library. Anonymous, 'Institute of Medical Research, Antimalarial Work, Kuala Lumpur' (c. 1940s–1950s) [RCS-Y3011R-7]; Anonymous, 'Mauritius: Map Showing the Location of Mosquitoes' (Sir Henry Hesketh Bell Collection, 1922) [RCS-RCMS-36/5/4]; Anonymous, 'Mosquito-Proof House, Pitch Lake, Brighton' (Fisher Photograph Collection, August 1912) [RCS/Fisher/Y3075C/3]; Anonymous, 'Housewifery at Achimota College' (c. 1945) [RCS/Y3011U/211].

[70] Herge, *Tintin in the Congo* (London: Egmont, 1930/2005), 10–11.

public health officials were indeed engaged in a 'war with mosquitoes'.[71] Some of these texts echoed medical entomology, overtly or symbolically, to suggest that mosquitoes were villainous enemies of humans, and therefore, should be exterminated.[72]

In the 1920s, many Bengali books about public health and medicine identified malaria as one of the severest problems that plagued the 'desh' – the country. Although written at the height of anti-imperial nationalist movements in South Asia, these books rarely invoked the vision of an overarching Indian nation. Instead, words like 'desh', 'bangla', 'bangadesh', 'bangladesh' were frequently used to conjure up the image of a Bengali homeland.[73] Mosquitoes, as vectors of malaria, were described as inimical to the 'desh' – the Bengali homeland.[74] The villages – 'Gram' or 'palligram' – were projected as particularly vulnerable.[75] These texts appealed to the colonial municipal governments for devising mechanisms to protect rural Bengal from the virulence of malarial mosquitoes.

Yet, the purging of mosquitoes from the homeland, and the reconstruction of rural Bengal, it was argued, could not be the exclusive prerogative of the municipalities. It was recommended that these projects could only be emboldened through collective action involving the participation of Bengali society more generally.[76] To that end, authors of these books instructed their readers to establish associations such as 'Pallisamiti' ('Village association'), 'Malaria Nibaroni Samiti' (Society for the prevention of malaria') and 'Swasthya-raksha samiti' ('Society for the preservation of health').[77] These organisations were supposed to undertake various steps to protect the 'desh' of the Bengalis, and particularly

---

[71] K. Bhattacharya, *Moshar Juddha (War of Mosquitoes)* (Calcutta: Kulja Sahitya Mandir, 1922); P. Mitra, 'Mosha' ('Mosquito'), in S. Dasgupta (ed.), *Ghanada Samagra 1* (Kolkata: Ananda Publishers), 21–30.

[72] R. Thakur, 'Samavaye Malaria Nibaran' ('Malaria Eradication Through Cooperatives: Text of a lecture delivered on 29 August 1923'), in *Rabindra Rachanabali*, Volume 13 (Calcutta: West Bengal Government, November 1990), 795–798; D. Ray, *Moshar Hul (The Sting of Mosquitoes)*, (Meherpur: Manasi Press, 1922).

[73] U. Chakrabarti, *Malaria* (Kolkata: Souredrakumar Chakrabarti, 1923/24), 77–81; K. Basu, *Malaria Nibaraner Upay O Onyanyo Prabandho (How to Prevent Malaria and Other Essays)*, (Calcutta: Swasthya Dharma Sangha, 1924/25), 10; G. K. Mitra, *Malaria o Bongodesh-Sulabh Onyanyo Jvarer Protikar Samasyar Porikalpana (Scheme for Preventing Malaria and Other Fevers Prevalent in Bengal)*, (Calcutta: Public Health Department, Bengal Government, c. 1924), 14; A. Pal, *Malaria* (Bolpur: Publisher not mentioned, 1927/1928), 'Preface'.

[74] Basu, *Malaria Nibaraner Upay*, 10–11; Mitra, *Malaria o Bongodesh*, 4–14; Pal, *Malaria*, 6–14, 191–218.

[75] Chakrabarti, *Malaria*, 77–89; Basu, *Malaria Nibaraner Upay*, 10; Mitra, *Malaria o Bongodesh*, 1–7.

[76] Chakrabarti, *Malaria*, 90; Basu, *Malaria Nibaraner Upay*, 10; Mitra, *Malaria o Bongodesh*, 14.

[77] Chakrabarti, *Malaria*, 87; Basu, *Malaria Nibaraner Upay*, 10–11.

the villages of Bengal from mosquitoes. These steps included not just the
mobilisation of resources from within the localities for the destruction of
the habitats of mosquitoes by sanitising puddles; putting kerosene into
pits of stagnant water;[78] improving rural drainage networks;[79] replacing
old decaying vegetation with newly planted trees;[80] and informing villagers about the means to protecting themselves from mosquitoes.[81]

These authors also pointed out that the goal of minimising the threat
of malarial mosquitoes necessitated that these organisations set up free
primary schools and schemes to reduce poverty; encourage agriculture and the weaving industry; revive a culture of athletics and physical training; establish rural courts to adjudicate local disputes; and
put together plebeian Hindu gatherings, such as 'dharmasabha' and
'harisabha'.[82] According to these texts, the control of malaria and its vectors in Bengal was connected to the restoration of social cohesion, harmony, prosperity and religious values within rural communities. At the
same time, it was argued that protection of the 'desh' from mosquitoes
could not be ensured through activities in the public sphere alone. The
shared project of resisting mosquitoes required, it was claimed, the sub-
mission of individual householders to specific codes of morality and
everyday routine. These included the obligation to keep the household
clean and tidy; to cover the body with clothes at all times; to fumigate
the home in the evening with flames of incense sticks and camphor;[83] to
remain inside a mosquito net and within the secure marital confines of
one's home in the evenings and at night.[84]

Some of these instructions to the householders were particularly
meticulous in their detail. A book published in 1927, for example, argued
that anopheles mosquitoes were especially attracted to certain colours
(such as navy blue, dark red, brown and scarlet), and that householders should avoid sleeping in mosquito nets, which bore such colours.[85]
The same book began by suggesting that countries, which had effectively
eradicated malaria and its insect vectors, were relatively more 'cultured
and politically free' than Bengal.[86] It claimed that widespread malaria
in Bengal was a reflection of a deeper cultural crisis; a crisis resulting from the inability of the Bengalis to retain their indigenous culture

---

[78] Chakrabarti, *Malaria*, 22; Basu, Ibid; Mitra, *Malaria o Bongodesh*, 9–10.
[79] Chakrabarti, *Malaria*, 77; Mitra, *Malaria o Bongodesh*, 10.
[80] Chakrabarti, *Malaria*, 88; Mitra, Ibid., 11.
[81] Basu, *Malaria Nibaraner Upay*, 10; Mitra, Ibid., 9, 11, 13.
[82] Chakrabarti, *Malaria*, 80–89.   [83] Basu, *Malaria Nibaraner Upay*, 11.
[84] Chakrabarti, *Malaria*, 22; Basu, Ibid.; Mitra, *Malaria o Bongodesh*, 10–11.
[85] Pal, *Malaria*, 13.
[86] Ibid., 'Preface', 1–2. He uses the Bengali word 'sabhya' which could have been translated as 'civilised'. However, in page 201 he himself translates 'sabhya' as 'culture'.

during colonial rule as well as their failure to embrace 'western culture' conclusively.[87] In this phase of cultural flux, continued the author, the Bengalis had given in to excessive consumption, material pleasures and 'fashion'.[88] To resist the onslaught of malarial mosquitoes, he urged the Bengalis to observe restraint and self-discipline in their everyday life.[89] Therefore, the challenge of protecting the 'desh' from mosquitoes opened up the need for greater sanitary governance, as well as social and moral discipline in rural Bengal.

The perception that mosquitoes were a threat to Bengali health, household and homeland was reflected in the world of radio broadcasts, literature and advertisements of the time. *Betar Jagat*, a widely circulated magazine associated with the radio-broadcasting agency, published articles in consecutive issues in the 1930s, alerting the Bengali householders of the crucial role they could play in restraining mosquitoes.[90] Sarat Chandra Chattopadhyay's novel *Palli Samaj* (*Village Society*), published earlier in the 1910s, hints at how collective social projects against malaria and its vectors were appropriated within contemporary programmes of rural reconstruction.[91] In tune with the wider trends of the period, the need to protect the 'desh' from malarial mosquitoes was also articulated in military vocabulary. An advertisement of an anti-malarial drug (Figure 6.2), Baikol, published during World War II in 1942, compared the threat of mosquitoes to the fear of 'raids' carried out by Japanese fighter aeroplanes during those years in Bengal. The advertisement carries the caption 'The enemy attacks Bengal', and depicts a gigantic mosquito followed by waves of smaller mosquitoes hovering over the map of Bengal.[92]

Similarly, in a lecture delivered to the 'Anti-malaria Society' earlier in August 1923, Rabindranath Tagore, already a Nobel laureate in literature, described mosquitoes as one of the 'greatest enemies of Bangladesh' which needed to be 'evicted' from the homeland. In a speech replete with words such as 'war', 'weapon' and 'killing', Tagore asserted that the shared project of destroying mosquitoes could strengthen solidarity amongst the Bengalis much more effectively than

---

[87] Ibid., 201–202.   [88] Ibid., 188, 201, 202.   [89] Ibid., 188.

[90] S. N. Sur, 'Mosha Nibaroney Grihaster Kartabya' (Duties of Householders in Resisting Mosquitoes), *Betar Jagat*, 4, 16 (5 May 1933), 540–544; S. N. Sur, 'Malaria', *Betar Jagat*, 4, 15 (21 April 1933), 505–508.

[91] S. Chattopadhyay, 'Palli Samaj', in S. Chattopadhyay. *Sarat Sahitya Samagra* (Calcutta: Ananda Publishers, 1986/1916), 167–169.

[92] Advertisement of 'Baikol', *Ananda Bazar Patrika Saradiya* (1942), 172 [AS 46, BSP 32. Credit: The Archive of the CSSSC].

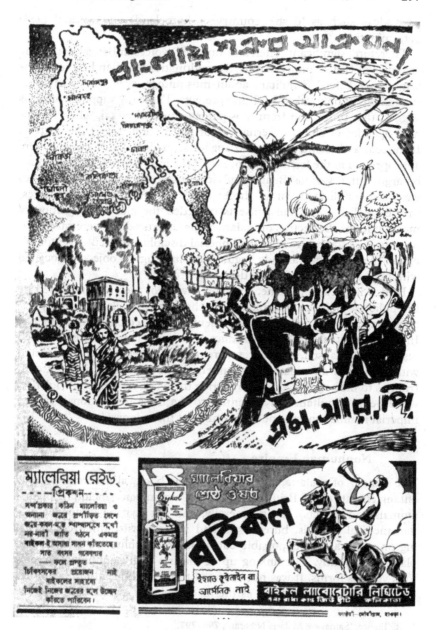

Figure 6.2 Advertisement of 'Baikol', *Ananda Bazar Patrika Saradiya*, (1942), p. 172. [AS 46, BSP 32. Credit: The Archive of the CSSSC.]

lofty ideas such as 'desh' (country or homeland) and 'swaraj' (self-determination).[93]

·Therefore, significant (often anti-imperial) voices in Bengal shared the anxieties of British imperial officials, multinational philanthropic organisations, and the US military about mosquitoes, even when they pursued different political and cultural projects. These overlapping concerns suggest that protection from mosquitoes emerged as one of the dominant agendas of global governance during the first half of the century. If indeed, as Warwick Anderson suggests, medicine and hygiene were appropriated in the 'civilising process' of the interwar period, then it can be argued that various Bengali publications about malarial mosquitoes were also implicated within those processes.[94] A few sources suggest that Bengali biases against insects preceded the global recognition of mosquitoes as the vectors of malaria. These texts which were published prior to the establishment of the imperial discipline of medical entomology in the 1890s had already begun featuring bugs or objects associated with bugs as symbols of moral decadence.[95]

British imperial medicine, therefore, was not merely constituted by the policies, violence, disciplinary mechanisms and classificatory practices shaped by senior British representatives of colonial governments. Imperial medicine was also a product of the ways in which the colonised resisted, internalised, reinterpreted, reinforced, interacted and competed with, and even anticipated governmental impositions. This book contributes to the ongoing efforts to narrate the history of imperial violence, while being simultaneously attentive to the close interactions between imperial regimes and the public cultures of the colonised.

Nonhuman Empire

The history of malaria, as detailed in this book, also reveals various entanglements of the British Empire with nonhumans (including plants, animals and objects), more generally, and not just mosquitoes. Colonial medical officials, bureaucrats and industrialists, while commenting on malaria and its possible cures, invoked nonhuman animals and plants recurrently. The linking up of malaria with nonhuman animals took various forms. It was not confined to the identification of anopheles mosquitoes in the 1900s as the insect vector for malarial parasites.

---

[93] R. Tagore, 'Samavaye Malaria Nibaran', 796–797.
[94] Anderson, *Colonial Pathologies*, 1.
[95] J. Mukhopadhyay, *Korakey kit ba Somaj Chitra* (*Worm in a flower bud*), (Calcutta: Bamacharan Dutta, 1877); S. Saphari, *Moshari Rahasya* (*Mystery of the mosquito curtain*), (Calcutta: Chandi Charan Basu, 1887).

Monsters, for example, were depicted as a symbol of malaria in a late-nineteenth-century advertisement for anti-malarial pills.[96] Architectural designs of houses within tea plantations in Assam in British India in the 1940s were shaped by the ostensible purpose of protecting the planters simultaneously from malaria and wild animals.[97] These trends have survived in postcolonial India. Recent journalistic reports have suggested that the combined threats from snakes and malaria shape military confrontations in the forests of Central India between Maoists, on the one hand, and the state-sponsored militia, on the other.[98] I have noted how the history of malaria in British India reveals a hierarchy of plants in the imperial imagination. Plants appropriated within the cosmopolitan colonial plantation economy such as cinchonas, eucalyptus or sunflower were celebrated for their therapeutic properties. Various other plants, which were described as 'wild' 'undergrowths', even when they were intimately associated with the life-worlds of various groups of people in colonial India, as Chapters 1 and 3 have shown, ran the risk of being labelled as unwanted excesses and pathological sources of malaria.

Historians have exposed, in different ways, the importance of nonhumans (particularly animals) in imperial medicine.[99] Building on these existing works, this book has carried out the methodological challenge of narrating the significance of nonhumans in imperial history, while retaining a critique of scientific determinism. In order to simultaneously resist tendencies of anthropocentrism and scientism in the history of the British Empire, it has explored the ways in which British Empire and medical knowledge about nonhumans were co-constituted. Indeed, the Empire was deeply invested in the production of medical knowledge about nonhuman animals, plants and objects. I have argued that the medical properties attributed to cinchona plants, objects described

---

[96] M. Mayer and Ottoman, Advertisement of 'Mason and Pollard's Anti-Malaria Pills', (Name of publisher and place of publication not mentioned, 1890) [Author's collection].

[97] See the photograph taken by P. Bose entitled, 'The Manager's bungalow, Panitola Tea Estate [Upper Assam]' (c. 1950). Shelfmark: Photo 451/1(4) [BL].

[98] P. K. Maitra, 'Mosquitoes, Snakes Rattle Naxal Leaders', *Hindustan Times* (20 April 2008, Gadchiroli), www.hindustantimes.com/india/mosquitoes-snakes-rattle-naxal-leaders/story-YFcLUrFnfjUo6QwMYxVxzN.html [Retrieved on 20 June 2016]; S. S. Bose, 'No Water, Food or Medicines. Now, Go Fight "Biggest Threat"', *Times of India* (9 April 2010, Dornapal), http://timesofindia.indiatimes.com/india/No-water-food-or-medicines-Now-go-fight-biggest-threat/articleshow/5775869.cms [Retrieved on 20 June 2016].

[99] For recent works on this theme in relation to South Asian history, see, for example, P. Chakrabarti, 'Beasts of Burden: Animals and Laboratory Research in Colonial India', *History of Science*, 48, 2 (June 2010), 125–152; S. Mishra, 'Beasts, Murrains and the British Raj: Reassessing Colonial Medicine in India from the Veterinary Perspective, 1860–1900', *Bulletin of the History of Medicine*, 85, 2 (2011), 587–619.

as malarial, the drug quinine and anopheles mosquitoes did not unfold in a historical and political vacuum. Instead, the exigencies and apparatuses of British imperial rule, to a considerable extent, informed them. At the same time, these nonhumans were not passive constructs, but rather they were integral to the structural, ideological, commercial, prejudicial, biopolitical and physical foundations of the British Empire itself.

Constructs such as cinchonas, quinine, malaria and mosquitoes were amongst the many historical adhesives which bound up disparate groups and distant regions as components of a wider imperial world. As this book demonstrates, they deepened 'connections', 'tensions' and 'fractures' between the imperial realms of British India, Dutch Java, French Algeria, German and British Africa, Mauritius, Burma and the West Indies, while holding together disparate groups claiming to represent scientific and medical knowledge, pharmaceutical commerce, colonial governance and vernacular cultures.[100] The drug quinine and its source cinchona plants reinforced the ideological self-image of the British Empire as a simultaneously benevolent and profit-making enterprise. And yet, the history of the production and maintenance of objects and organisms described here reflects also the prejudices about race, colour, indentured labourers and primitives which were intrinsic to liberal empires of the nineteenth century.[101]

This book has shown that nonhumans were entangled in histories of imperial biopower at least in three different ways. First, nonhumans such as cinchonas, objects described as malarial, quinine and mosquitoes featured as instruments of imperial biopolitics.[102] Discourses and practices relating to them reinforced control over lands, landscapes and people which explain the revealing overlaps amongst geographies of plantations, disease and empire.[103] Imperial discourses about malaria and

---

[100] On connections and tensions see A. Stoler and F. Cooper, 'Between Metropole and Colony: Rethinking a Research Agenda', in A. Stoler and F. Cooper (eds.), *Tensions of Empire: Colonial Cultures in a Bourgeois World* (London and Los Angeles: University of California Press, 1997), 1–27. See also S. Bhattacharya, M. Harrison and M. Worboys, *Fractured States: Small Pox, Public Health and Vaccination Policy in British India, 1800–1947* (New Delhi: Orient Longman, 2005).

[101] For a pioneering work on the liberal justifications of Empire, see U. S. Mehta, *Liberalism and Empire: A Study in Nineteenth-Century British Liberal Thought* (Chicago and London: University of Chicago Press, 1999).

[102] For the overlaps between empire, biopower and race, see especially, A. Stoler, *Race and the Education of Desire: Foucault's History of Sexuality and the Colonial Order of Things* (Durham and London: Duke University Press, 1995), 80–136. See also, Pande, *Medicine, Race and Liberalism.*

[103] For foundational works on the question of biopower and colonial medicine, see M. Vaughan, *Curing Their Ills: Colonial Power and African Illness* (Stanford: Stanford University Press, 1991); D. Arnold, *Colonizing the Body: State Medicine and Epidemic Disease in Nineteenth-Century India* (Los Angeles and London: University of California Press, 1993).

its cures constructed colonial subjects not only as potential labourers, who required remaining healthy and productive, but also shaped them as potential consumers, who needed to be disciplined to consume various curatives. Secondly, our understandings about subjects of imperial biopower need to be extended beyond the human to include insects, plants and inanimate objects.[104] Much like the colonised Indians, cinchona plants, the drug quinine, objects designated as malarial as well as mosquitoes were subjected to imperial regimes of classification, surveillance and knowledge-production. Thirdly, distinctions between humans and nonhumans, considered by many commentators as fundamental to biopower, were asserted as well as blurred in the history of imperial medicine in British India.[105] This was particularly because of the simultaneous operation of the twin processes of anthropomorphism and dehumanisation in British imperial history.[106] The feminisation of cinchona plants imported from South America as 'fairest of Peruvian maids' and as 'delicate, beautiful and tender', as evident in Chapter 1, happened at the precise moment in which colonised 'natives' and 'aborigines' supposedly immune from malaria were being projected to inhabit 'the state of nature'. In different parts of the book I have shown how imperial medical commentators claimed that the lower animals and colonised aboriginal

[104] N. Shukin, *Animal Capital: Rendering Life in Biopolitical Times* (Minneapolis and London: University of Minnesota Press, 2009), 1–45; D. Haraway, *Primate Visions: Gender, Race, and Nature in the World of Modern Science* (Verso: London and New York, 1989), 26–58, 244–275. For a critique of the absence of the category of nonhumans in recent reconceptualisation of 'Empire' and 'multitude' by Michael Hardt and Antonio Negri, see T. E. Lewis, 'Swarm Intelligence: Rethinking Swarm Intelligence from within the Transversal Commons', *Culture, Theory and Critique*, 51, 3 (2010), 223–238.

[105] G. Agamben, *The Open: Man and Animal* (Stanford: Stanford University Press, 2004), 12–27, 80; For a sympathetic critique of Agamben, see D. LaCapra, *History and Its Limits: Human, Animal and Violence* (Ithaca and London: Cornell University Press, 2009), 149–189.

[106] H. Raffles, 'Jews, Lice and History', *Public Culture*, 19.3, 53 (Fall, 2007), 521–566. On dehumanization, see the historiography on 'primitives', for example, K. Ghosh, 'A Market for Aboriginality: Primitivism and Race Classification in the Indentured Labour Market of Colonial India', in G. Bhadra, G. Prakash and S. Tharu (eds.), *Subaltern Studies X: Writings on South Asian History and Society* (New Delhi: Oxford University Press, 1999), 8–48; J. Fabian, *Time and the Other: How Anthropology Makes its Object* (New York: Columbia University Press, 1983); P. Banerjee, *The Politics of Time: 'Primitives' and History Writing in a Colonial Society* (New Delhi: Oxford University Press, 2006). See also S. Muthu, *Enlightenment Against Empire* (New Jersey: Princeton University Press, 2003), 11–71. On anthropomorphism, see S. Sivasundaram, 'Trading Knowledge: The East India Company's Elephants in India and Britain', *The Historical Journal*, 48, 1 (2005), 27–63. For a broader perspective, see L. Daston and G. Mitman, *Thinking with Animals: New Perspectives on Anthropomorphism* (New York: Columbia University Press, 2005). This point about the dual move of anthropomorphising and dehumanising in relation to enlightenment Europe has been made eloquently by Simon Schaffer in 'Enlightened Automata', in W. Clark, J. Golinski and S. Schaffer (eds.), *The Sciences in Enlightened Europe* (Chicago and London: University of Chicago Press, 1999), 126–165.

groups (in Chapter 2), indigenous quacks and locusts (in Chapter 3), parasites and primitives, urban labourers and mosquitoes (in Chapter 5) shared analogous properties. Quinine, as I have explored in Chapter 4, appears to have personified various racial hierarchies of colour. In colonial factory discourses, whiteness symbolised one of the most consistent indicators of quinine's purity, while brownness and yellowness featured amongst the most obvious markers of the impurities that had corrupted the drug.

Finally, I have claimed that nonhumans such as cinchonas, objects described as malarial, quinine and mosquitoes, apart from being shaped by the histories of the British Empire, were also amongst its integral physical constituents. Both the Empire and its co-constituents can also be understood as 'localised'[107] socio-material networks. I have explored networks constituted, for example, of Wardian cases, steamers, small pots, herbariums, plantations, royal gardens, planters, bureaucrats, economic-botanists, geographers (in Chapter 1); of decaying vegetation, friable granite rocks, water casks, mouldy bed sheets, stale mushrooms, geologists, meteorologists, chemists, colonial administrators (in Chapter 2); of sunflower, paddy, bamboo, jute, 'undergrowths', physicians, landed proprietors, local officials, vernacular tradesmen (in Chapter 3); of cinchona barks, alkaloids, colouring matter, labelled bottles, sealing wax, carmine, European pharmaceutical families, office of the Secretary of State for India, chemical examiners, managers of colonial factories (Chapter 4); and of insecticides, parasites, fishes, hyacinths, tinsmiths, coolies, planters, parasitologists, sanitary commissioners and Bengali fiction writers (in Chapter 5). These social-material amalgamations shaped and sustained not only cinchonas, malaria, Burdwan fever, quinine and mosquitoes, respectively, but also constituted various moments and structures of the British Empire as well.

The British Empire was an extensive technopolitical, material-discursive and natural-cultural formation.[108] Humans alone did not constitute the British Empire. Similarly, cinchonas, malarial objects, quinine and mosquitoes did not represent a self-contained domain of nonhumans. I have argued that the Empire as well as these nonhuman co-constituents can be deconstructed into heterogeneous associations of

---

[107] E. C. Spary, 'Of Nutmegs and Botanists: The Colonial Cultivation of Botanical Identity', in L. Schiebinger and C. Swan (eds.), *Colonial Botany: Science, Commerce and Politics in the Early Modern World* (Philadelphia: University of Pennsylvania Press, 2005), 203.

[108] On technopolitical see Mitchell, *Rule of Experts*, 42–43; on material-discursive see H. Raffles, 'Towards a Critical Natural History', *Antipode* 37, 2 (2005), 377; on natural-cultural see D. Haraway, *When Species Meet* (Minneapolis and London: University of Minnesota Press, 2008), 25, 47, 62.

humans and nonhumans, subjects and objects. Invoking actor-network theory, perspectivist anthropology, sociology of sciences and post-Marxist feminism, I claim that the British imperial apparatus[109] as well as its co-constituents detailed in this book may be described variously as 'mangles',[110] 'inter-subjective fields of human and nonhuman relations',[111] 'cyborgs'[112] and 'collectives' which traversed the domains of 'object-discourse-nature-society'.[113] Therefore, I have refused to prescribe other-than-humans (particularly nonhuman animals, interspecies assemblages, or cyborgs) as definite agents of transgression and resistance.[114] This is because such figures themselves were often implicated within imperial structures. Thus this book has reinforced efforts to go beyond dominant anthropocentric conceptions of Empire, while claiming that nonhumans themselves did not necessarily inhabit a preordained or self-contained realm. It has also reasserted the extraordinary significance and violence of empires in the making of modern medicine, while contesting the assumption that imperial agency can be critiqued comprehensively by examining the activities of Europeans alone.

[109] The use of the word 'apparatus' here is informed by G. Agamben, *What is an Apparatus? And Other Essays* (Stanford: Stanford University Press, 2009), 2–14. Agamben proposes a 'massive partitioning' between 'apparatuses' and 'living beings (or substances)', and defines 'a subject as that which results from the relation . . . and the relentless fight between them'. See 13–14. The interpenetrating histories of empire and malaria reveal how imperial apparatuses, substances and subjects were inseparably intertwined.

[110] A. Pickering, 'The Mangle of Practice: Agency and Emergence in the Sociology of Science', *American Journal of Sociology*, 99, 3 (November, 1993), 559, 567, 576.

[111] E. V. de Castro, 'Exchanging Perspectives: The Transformation of Objects into Subjects in Amerindian Ontologies', *Common Knowledge*, 10, 3 (2004), 471.

[112] My anachronistic invocation of the late-twentieth-century evocative figure of cyborgs, as conceived by Haraway, to understand nineteenth-century imperial actors and artefacts is deliberate. See D. J. Haraway, *Simians, Cyborgs and Women: The Reinvention of Nature* (New York: Routledge, 1991), 149–176.

[113] B. Latour, *We Have Never Been Modern* (Cambridge, Mass.: Harvard University Press, 1993), 144. For 'collectives', see, for instance, B. Latour, 'A Collective of Humans and Nonhumans', in *Pandora's Hope: Essays in the Reality of Science Studies* (Cambridge, Mass.: Harvard University Press, 1999), 174–193. We should note that Latour also uses 'associations' and 'assemblages' as almost interchangeable with 'collectives'. For another dense conceptualisation of 'assemblage', see G. Deleuze and F. Guattari, 'Rhizome', in *A Thousand Plateaus: Capitalism and Schizophrenia* (Minneapolis and London: University of Minnesota Press, 1987), 3–25.

[114] For other opinions on this question, see Haraway, *Simians, Cyborgs and Women*, 149–176; Lewis, 'Swarm Intelligence'.

Bibliography

PRIMARY SOURCES

UNPUBLISHED OFFICIAL SOURCES

National Archives of India
Home Department, Medical Board, 1858
Home Department, Public Branch, 1860–1890
Home Department, Medical Branch, 1874–1911
Home Department, Port Blair Branch, 1880
Home Department, Sanitary Branch, 1882–1910
Home Department, Patents Branch, 1888
Home Department, Jails Branch, 1910
Revenue and Agriculture Department, Agriculture Branch, 1891–1912
Revenue and Agriculture Department, Economic Products Branch, 1896–1904
Revenue and Agriculture Department, Forests Branch, 1901
Revenue and Agriculture Department, Famine Branch, 1903

West Bengal State Archive
General Department, General Branch, 1862–1868
General Department, Medical Branch, 1869–1877
General Department, Sanitation Branch, 1870
General Department, Industry and Science Branch, 1872
General Department, Miscellaneous Branch, 1872
Municipal Department, Sanitation Branch, 1868–1873
Municipal Department, Medical Branch, 1871–1898
Political Department, Medical Branch, 1870
Finance Department, Miscellaneous Branch, 1888–1898

Asia, Pacific and Africa Collections, British Library, London
IOR/V/23/131 (1873)
IOR/L/SUR/2/7/f.193, September 1868
IOR/L/PJ/6/42, File 929 June–July 1881

PRIVATE PAPERS

Wellcome Library
Fayrer, J., 'Malaria', Text of the paper read before the Epidemiological Society of London on 1 February 1882 (S4403 N.s. v. 1 1881/82)
Peretti, P. Pharmacist, Rome (MS.6074)

London Metropolitan Archives
Howard Private Papers (ACC-1037)
Whiffen Papers (B/WHF)

British Library
Hunt, E. H., 'Buffalo Sacrifice', Mettaguda, 1917 (malaria) (MSS Eur. F222/11, India Office Select Material)

PUBLISHED REPORTS

Army Medical Department Report for the Year 1866, Volume viii (London, 1868).
Bryson, A., (ed.), *Statistical Report of Health Navy 1857* (London: House of Commons, 1859).
East India, Chinchona Cultivation (Copy of All Correspondence Between the Secretary of State for India and the Governor General, and the Governors of Madras and Bombay, Relating to the Cultivation of Chinchona Plants from April 1866 to April 1870) (London: House of Commons, 1870).
Elliot, J., *Report on Epidemic Remittent and Intermittent Fever Occurring in Parts of Burdwan and Nuddea Divisions* (Calcutta: Bengal Secretariat Office, 1863).
French, J. H., *Endemic Fever in Lower Bengal, Commonly called Burdwan Fever* (Calcutta: Thacker, Spink 1875).
Meldrum, C., *Weather, Health and Forests: A Report on the Inequalities of the Mortality from Malarial Fever and Other Diseases in Mauritius* (Port Louis: Mercantile Record Co. Printing Establishment, 1881).
Proceedings of the Third Meeting of the General Malaria Committee at Madras November 1912 (Simla: Government Central Branch Press, 1913).
Stephens, J. W., and S. R. Christophers, *Report to the Malarial Committee of the Royal Society*, Seventh Series (London: Harrison and Sons, 1902).
Thompson, R., *Report on Insects Destructive to Woods and Forests* (Allahabad: Government Press, 1868).
Volprignano, P. T., *The Future of the Port of London. A Provision Against the Malaria of the Metropolis, the Pollution of the Thames, the Collisions on the River Being The Outline of a Scheme for an Uninterrupted Navigation to and from the Port of London* (London: H Horne and Sons, 1890).

PUBLICATIONS IN ENGLISH

Barber, M. A., *A Malariologist in Many Lands* (Lawrence, Kans.: University of Kansas Press, 1946).
Barker, T. H., *On Malaria and Miasmata* (London: John W. Davies, 1859).
Bird, G. G., *Observations on Civic Malaria and the Health of Towns* (London: William Wood, 1848).
Bontius, J., *An Account of the Diseases, Natural History, and Medicines of the East Indies, Translated from the Latin of James Bontius, Physician to the Dutch Settlement at Batavia* (London: T. Noteman, 1769).
Caldwell, C., *Essays on Malaria and Temperament* (Lexington, Ky.: N. L. Finnel and J. F. Herndon, 1831).

Chevers, N., *A Manual of Medical Jurisprudence for India* (Calcutta: Thacker, Spink and Co, 1870).

Cook, M. T., *The Diseases of Tropical Plants* (London: Macmillan, 1913).

de Vrij, J. E., *On the Cultivation of Quinine in Java and British India* (London: G. E. Eyre & W. Spottiswoode, 1865).

Dempster, T. E., *The Prevalence of the Organic Disease of the Spleen as a Test for Detecting Malarious Localities in Hot Climates* (Calcutta: Office of the Superintendent of Government Printing, 1868).

Drake, D., *A Systematic Treatise, Historical, Etiological and Practical, On the Principal Diseases of the Interior of North America as They Appear in the Caucasian, African, Indian and Esquimax Varieties of Its Population* (Cincinnati: Winthrop B. Smith & Co., 1850).

Edwards, J., *Malaria: What It Means and How Avoided* (Philadelphia: P. Blakiston, 1881).

Hanbury, D., *Science Papers: Chiefly Pharmacological and Botanical* (London: Macmillan and Co., 1876).

Herge, *Tintin in the Congo* (London: Egmont, 2005/1930).

Holt, V. M., *Why Not Eat Insects?* (London: Field and Tuer, 1885).

Hooker, W. D., *Inaugural Dissertation upon the Cinchonas, Their History, Uses and Effects* (Glasgow: Edward Khull, Dunlop Street, 1839).

Horsfield, T., and F. Moore, *A Catalogue of the Lepidopterous Insects in the Museum of the Hon. East India Company* (London: W. H. Allen, 1857).

Howard, J. E., *Illustrations of Neuva Quinologia of Pavon* (London: Lovell Reeve and Co, 1862).

The Quinology of the East Indian Plantations (London: Lovell Reeve and Co. 1869).

Johnson, J., *The Influence of Tropical Climates on European Constitutions* (London: Thomas and George Underwood, 1827).

Jones, W. H. S., *Malaria, a Neglected Factor in the History of Greece and Rome* (Cambridge: Macmillan & Bowes, 1907).

Jordan, L. J., *Specification of Lewis Jacob Jordan: Tonic* (London: Great Seal Printing Office, 1861).

Kentish, R., *Experiments and observations on a new species of bark, showing its great efficacy in very small doses, also a comparative view of the powers of the red and quilled bark; being an attempt towards a general analysis and compendious history of the valuable genus of Cinchona, or the Peruvian bark* (London: J. Johnson, 1784).

King, G., *A Manual of Cinchona Plantation in India* (Calcutta: Office of the Superintendent of Government Print, 1880).

La Roche, R., *Pneumonia: Its Supposed Connection, Pathological and Etiological, with Autumnal Fevers; Including an Inquiry into the Existence and Morbid Agency of Malaria* (Philadelphia: Blanchard and Lee, 1854).

Lelean, P. S., *Quinine as a Malarial Prophylactic: A Criticism* (London: John Bale Sons and Danielsson, 1911).

Lind, J., *An Essay on Diseases Incidental to Europeans in Hot Climates with the Method of Preventing their Fatal Consequences* (London: T. Beckett and A. De Hondt, 1768).

MacCulloch, J., *An Essay on the Remittent and Intermittent Diseases, including Generically Marsh Fever and Neuralgia* (London: Longman, Rees, Orme, Brown and Green, 1828).

Malaria: An Essay on the Production and Propagation of this Poison; and On The Nature and Localities of The Places by Which it is Produced, with An Enumeration of the Diseases Caused by it and the Means of Preventing or Diminishing Them, Both at Home and in the Naval and Military Service (London: Longman, Rees, Orme, Brown and Green, 1827).

Macgowan, A. T., *Malaria, The Common Cause of Cholera, Intermittent Fever and Its Allies* (London: John Churchill and Sons, 1866).

Macpherson, J., *On Bengal Dysentery and Its Statistics* (Calcutta: Thacker, 1850).

Quinine and Antiperiodics in Therapeutic Relations Including an Abstract of Briquet's Work on Cinchona and a Notice of Indian Febrifuges (Calcutta: R. C. Lepage, 1856).

Magendie, F., *Formulary for the Preparation and Mode of Employing Several New Remedies: Namely, Morphine, Iodine, Quinine* (London: Thomas and George Underwood, 1824).

Mannons, M. A. F., *Specification of Marc Antoine Francois Mannons: Elixir* (London: Great Seal Patent Office 1862).

Markham, C. R., *Travels in Peru and India* (London: John Murray, 1862).

Markham, C. R., *A Memoir of the Lady Ana de Osorio, Countess of Cinchon and Vice Queen of Peru (a.d. 1629–1639) with a Plea for the Correct Spelling of the Cinchona Genus* (London: Trübner & Co., 1874).

McIvor, W. G., *Notes on the Propagation and Cultivation of the Medicinal Cinchonas, or Peruvian Bark Trees* (Madras: Graves, Coodson, 1863).

Mitter, D., *The Epidemic Fever in Bengal* (Calcutta: Hindu Patriot Press, 1873).

Oldham, C. F., *What is Malaria? And Why Is It Most Intense In Hot Climates?* (London: H. K. Lewis, 1871).

Planchon, G., *Peruvian Barks* (London: George E. Eyre and William Spottsiwoode, 1866).

Prosser White, R., *Occupational Affections of the Skin; A Brief Account of the Trade Processes and Agents Which Give Rise to Them* (London: H. K. Lewis, 1915).

Purvis, W., *Specification of William Purvis: Medicinal Biscuit* (London: Great Seal Printing Office, 1871).

Relph, J., *An Inquiry into the Medical Efficacy of a New Species of Peruvian Bark, Lately Imported into this Country Under the Name of Yellow Bark Including Practical Observations Respecting the Choice of Bark in General* (London: James Phillips, 1794).

Ross, R., and D. Thomson, *A Case of Malarial Fever, Showing a True Parasitic Relapse, During Vigorous and Continuous Quinine Treatment* (Liverpool: Liverpool School of Tropical Medicine, 1912).

Ross, R., *Mosquito Brigades and How to Organise Them?* (London: Longmans, Green, 1902).

The Best Antimalarial Organization for the Tropics (Leipzig: Johann Ambrosius Barth, 1909).

Roy, G. C., *The Causes, Symptoms and Treatment of Burdwan Fever. Or the Epidemic Fever of Lower Bengal* (Calcutta: Thacker, Spink and Co., 1876).

Russell, E. G., *Malaria: Cause and Effects, Malaria and the Spleen: An Analysis of Thirty-nine Cases* (Calcutta: Thacker, Spink, 1880).

Salisbury, J. H., *Malaria* (New York: W. A. Kellogg, 1885).

Sanders, W., *Observations on the Superior Efficacy of the Red Peruvian Bark, in the Cure of Fevers*, (London: J. Johnson 1782).

Shaw, G. E., *Quinine Manufacture in India* (London: Institute of Chemistry of Great Britain and Ireland, 1935).

Sternberg, G. M., *Malaria and Malarial Diseases* (New York: Wood, 1884).

Vidyabhushan, K., *What is Malaria and the Germ Theory* (Calcutta: Narendranath Vidyanidhi, 1914).

Wilson, T., *An Enquiry into the Origin and Intimate Nature of Malaria* (London: Renshaw, 1858).

PERIODICALS IN ENGLISH

British Medical Journal (1857–1942)
Bulletin of Miscellaneous Information (Royal Gardens, Kew) (1888–1932)
Calcutta Journal of Medicine (1873)
Economic Botany (1947–1949)
Edinburgh Medical Journal (1856/57–1887/88)
Hindu Patriot (1873)
Hindustan Times (2008)
Indian Annals of Medical Science (1866–1877)
Indian Medical Gazette (1870–1897)
Journal of the Asiatic Society of Bengal (1837–1904)
Journal of the Royal African Society (1903–1907)
Medical Records (1874)
Medical Times and Gazette of London (1854–1885)
Philosophical Transactions of the Royal Society of London (1871)
Proceedings of the Royal Society of Medicine (1929)
Rivista di Parassitologia (1952)
Science (1900–1906)
The American Economic Review (1912)
The American Journal of Nursing (1901)
The Brisbane Courier (1868)
The Lancet (1848–1915)
The Practitioner (1874–1875)
The Straits Times (1870)
Times of India (2010)
Transactions of the Epidemiological Society of London (1889–1890)
Transactions of the Medical and Physical Society of Calcutta (1831)
Wellington Independent (1868)

PUBLICATIONS IN BENGALI

Basu, K., *Malaria Nibaraner Upay o Anyanyo Prabandho* (Calcutta: Swasthya Dharma Sangha, 1924).

Bhattacharya, A., *Jvar Chikitsa* (Calcutta: Valmiki Press, 1878).

Bhattacharya, K., *Moshar Juddha* (Calcutta: Kulja Sahitya Mandir, 1922).

Chakrabarti, U., *Malaria* (Calcutta: Souredrakumar Chakrabarti, 1923/1924).

Chattopadhyay, B., 'Sanjibchandra Chattopadhyayer Jiboni', in J. C. Bagal (ed.), *Bankim Rachanabali Volume 2* (Calcutta: Sahitya Samsad, 1954/1890), 790–795.

Chattopadhyay, K. C., *Bibidha Mahaushadh* (Calcutta: Iswar Chandra Basu and Company, 1876).

Chattopadhyay, S., *Sarat Sahitya Samagra* (Calcutta: Ananda Publishers, 1986).

Devi, M., *Mungpoote Rabindranath* (Calcutta: Prima Publications, 1943).

Ghosh, D. K., *Malaria* (Sultangachi, Hooghly: Doyal Krishen Ghosh, 1878).

Mitra, G. K., *Malaria o Bangadesh-Sulabh Anyanyo Jvarer Pratikar Samasyar Parikalpana* (Calcutta: Public Health Department, Bengal Government, c. 1924).

Mitra, P., 'Mosha', in Surajit Dasgupta (ed.), *Ghanada Samagra 1* (Kolkata: Ananda Publishers, 2000/1945), 21–30.

Mukhopadhyay, J., *Bishamjvare Quinine Proyog-pronali* (Chinsurah: Chikitsaprokash Press, 1879).

Korakey kit ba Somaj Chitra (Calcutta: Bamacharan Dutta, 1877).

Quinine (Calcutta: publisher unknown, 1893).

Saral Jvar Chikitsa Prothom Bhag (Calcutta: Nityananda Ghosh, 1880).

Mukhopadhyay, T., *Kankabati* (Calcutta: Kebalram Chattapadhyay, 1892).

Pal, A., *Malaria,* (Bolpur: publisher unknown, 1927).

Ray, A. S., 'Kaduni', in B. Basu (ed.), *Adhunik Bangla Kabita* (Calcutta: M. C. Sarkar and Sons Private Limited, 1973/1940), 148–150.

Ray, D., *Moshar Hul* (Meherpur: Manasi Press, 1922).

Saphari, S., *Moshari Rahasya* (Calcutta: Chandi Charan Basu, 1887).

Thakur, R., 'Likhi Kichu Saddho Ki', *Rabindra Rachanabali*, Volume 12 (Kolkata: Vishwabharati, 1995/1941), 55.

'Moshak Mangal Gitika', *Rabindra Rachanabali*, Volume 12 (Kolkata: Vishwabharati, 1995/1940), 55–56.

'Samavaye Malaria Nibaran' (Text of lecture delivered on 29 August 1923), in *Rabindra Rachanabali*, Volume 13 (Calcutta: West Bengal Government, November 1990), 795–798.

BENGALI PERIODICALS

Anubikshan (1875)
Asha (1902)
Benimadhab De and Company Panjika (1896/1897)
Betar Jagat (1933)
Bharat Suhrid (1903)
Bhisak Darpan (1897–1912)
Chikitsa Sammilani (1885–1893)
Chikitsak (1889–1890)
Education Gazette and Saptahik Vartabaha (1888)
Hahnemann (c. 1910)

Nutan Panjika (1887–1905)
Sadharani (1879)
Sambad Purna Chandroday (1862)
Somprakash (1867)
Swasthya (1896–1901)

SECONDARY SOURCES

Ackerknecht, E., 'The Development of Our Knowledge of Malaria', *Ciba Symposia*, 7, 3/4 (1945–1946), 38–50.
Ackerknecht, E. H., *Malaria in the Upper Mississippi Valley, 1760–1900* (Baltimore: The Johns Hopkins Press, 1945).
Agamben, G., *The Open: Man and Animal* (Stanford: Stanford University Press, 2004).
   What is an Apparatus? And Other Essays (Stanford: Stanford University Press, 2009).
Alavi, S., *Islam and Healing: Loss and Recovery of an Indo-Muslim Medical Tradition, 1600–1900* (Basingstoke: Palgrave Macmillan, 2008).
Anderson, W., *Colonial Pathologies: American Tropical Medicine, Race and Hygiene in the Philippines* (Durham: Duke University Press, 2006).
   'From Subjugated Knowledge to Conjugated Subjects: Science and Globalisation, or Postcolonial Studies of Science', *Postcolonial Studies*, 12, 4 (2009), 389–400.
   'Postcolonial Histories of Medicine', in F. Huisman and J. H. Warner (eds.), *Locating Medical History: The Stories and Their Meanings* (Baltimore: Johns Hopkins University Press, 2004), 285–306.
   The Cultivation of Whiteness: Science, Health and Racial Destiny in Australia (Durham: Duke University Press, 2006).
Anker, P., *Imperial Ecology: Environmental Order in the British Empire, 1895–1945* (Cambridge, Mass.: Harvard University Press, 2001).
Appadurai, A., 'Introduction: Commodities and the Politics of Value', in A. Appadurai (ed.), *The Social Life of Things: Commodities in Cultural Perspective* (Cambridge: Cambridge University Press, 1986), 3–60.
   'Number in the Colonial Imagination', in C. Breckenridge and P. Van der Veer, (eds.), *Orientalism and the Postcolonial Predicament: Perspectives from South Asia* (Philadelphia: University of Pennsylvania Press, 1993), 314–339.
Arnold, D., '"An ancient race outworn": Malaria and Race in Colonial India, 1860–1930', in W. Ernst and B. Harris (eds.), *Race, Science, Medicine, 1700–1960* (London: Routledge, 1999), 122–143.
   'Disease, Medicine and Empire' in D. Arnold (ed.), *Imperial Medicine and Indigenous Societies* (Manchester: Manchester University Press, 1988), 1–26.
   Colonizing the Body: State Medicine and Epidemic Disease in Nineteenth-Century India (Los Angeles: University of California Press, 1993).
   Everyday Technology: Machines and the Making of India's Modernity (Chicago: University of Chicago Press, 2013).

Science, Technology and Medicine in Colonial India (Cambridge: Cambridge University Press, 2000).

The Tropics and the Travelling Gaze: India, Landscape and Science, 1800–1856 (Seattle: University of Washington Press, 2006).

'Touching the Body: Perspectives on the Indian Plague' in R. Guha and G. Spivak (eds.), *Selected Subaltern Studies* (New York: Oxford University Press, 1988), 391–426.

Attewell, G. *Refiguring Yunani Tibb: Plural Healing in Late Colonial India* (Hyderabad: Orient Blackswan, 2007).

Bailkin, J., 'The Boot and the Spleen: When Was Murder Possible in British India?', *Comparative Studies in Society and History*, 48, 2 (April, 2006), 462–493.

Banerjee, P., *The Politics of Time: 'Primitives' and History Writing in a Colonial Society* (New Delhi: Oxford University Press, 2006).

Barton, P., 'Powders, Potions and Tablets: The "Quinine Fraud" in British India, 1890–1939' in J. H. Mills and P. Barton (eds.), *Drugs and Empire: Essays in Modern Imperialism and Intoxication, c. 1500–1930* (Basingstoke: Palgrave Macmillan 2007), 144–161.

Basalla, G., 'The Spread of Western Science', *Science*, 156(May 1967), 611–622.

Bashford, A., *Global Population: History, Geopolitics, and Life on Earth* (New York: Columbia University Press, 2014).

Beattie, J., *Empire and Environmental Anxiety: Health, Science, Art and Conservation in South Asian and Australasia, 1800–1920* (Basingstoke: Palgrave Macmillan, 2011).

Beinart, W., and L. Worshela, *Prickly Pear: Social History of a Plant in the Eastern Cape* (Johannesburg: Wits University Press, 2013).

Bennett, J., *Vibrant Matter: A Political Ecology of Things* (Durham: Duke University Press, 2010).

Bennett T., and P. Joyce (eds.), *Material Powers: Cultural Studies, History and the Material Turn* (London: Routledge, 2010).

Berger, R., *Making Ayurveda Modern: Political Histories of Indigenous Medicine in North India, 1900–1955* (Basingstoke: Palgrave Macmillan, 2013).

Bewell, A., *Romanticism and Colonial Disease* (Baltimore: Johns Hopkins University Press, 1999).

Bhattacharya, N., 'The Logic of Location: Malaria Research in Colonial India, Darjeeling and Duars, 1900–1930', *Medical History*, 55, 2 (April 2011), 183–202.

Bhattacharya, S., M. Harrison and M. Worboys, *Fractured States: Small Pox, Public Health and Vaccination Policy in British India, 1800–1947* (New Delhi: Orient Longman, 2005).

Bleichmar, D., 'Atlantic Competitions: Botanical Trajectories in the Eighteenth-Century Spanish Empire', in J. Delbourgo and N. Dew (eds.), *Science and Empire in the Atlantic World* (Abingdon: Routledge, 2007), 225–252.

Bloor, D., *Wittgenstein: A Social Theory of Knowledge* (New York: Columbia University Press, 1983).

Braun B., and S. J. Whatmore (eds.), *Political Matter: Technoscience, Democracy and Public Life* (Minneapolis: University of Minnesota Press, 2010).

Bravo, M. T., 'Mission Gardens: Natural History and Global Expansion, 1720–1820', in L. Schiebinger and C. Swan (eds.), *Colonial Botany: Science, Commerce and Politics in the Early Modern World* (Philadelphia: University of Pennsylvania Press, 2005), 49–65.

Brockway, L. H., *Science and Colonial Expansion: The Role of the British Royal Botanic Gardens* (New Haven: Yale University Press, 2002).

Bruce-Chwatt, L. J., 'John Macculloch (1773–1835): The Precursor of the Discipline of Malariology', *Medical History*, 21 (1977), 156–165.

Burke, T., *Lifebuoy Men, Lux Women: Commodification, Consumption and Cleanliness in Modern Zimbabwe* (Durham: Duke University Press, 1996).

Bynum, W. F., 'An Experiment That Failed: Malaria Control at Mian Mir', *Parassitologia*, 36 (1994), 107–120.

'"Reasons for Contentment": Malaria in India, 1900–1920', *Parassitologia*, 40 (1998), 19–27.

Chakrabarti, P., 'Beasts of Burden: Animals and Laboratory Research in Colonial India', *History of Science*, 48, 2 (June 2010), 125–152.

Bacteriology in British India: Laboratory Medicine and the Tropics (Rochester: University of Rochester Press, 2012).

'Empire and Alternatives: Swietenia Febrifuga and Cinchona Substitutes', *Medical History*, 54 (2010), 75–94.

Materials and Medicine: Trade, Conquest and Therapeutics in the Eighteenth Century (Manchester: Manchester University Press, 2010).

Medicine and Empire, 1600–1960 (Basingstoke: Palgrave Macmillan, 2014).

Chakrabarty, D., 'Postcolonial Studies and the Challenge of Climate Change', *New Literary History*, 43, 1 (Winter, 2012), 1–18.

'Postcoloniality and the Artifice of History: Who Speaks for "Indian" Pasts'?, in R. Guha (ed.), *A Subaltern Studies Reader:1986–1995* (New Delhi: Oxford University Press, 1997), 263–293.

Provincializing Europe: Postcolonial Thought and Historical Difference (New Jersey: Princeton University Press, 2000).

Chatterjee, P., *Black Hole of Empire: History of a Global Practice of Power* (New Jersey: Princeton University Press, 2012).

'The Constitution of Indian Nationalist Discourse', in P. Chatterjee, *Empire and Nation: Selected Essays* (New York: Columbia University Press, 2010/1987), 37–58.

'The Disciplines in Colonial Bengal', in P. Chatterjee (ed.), *Texts of Power: Emerging Disciplines in Colonial Bengal* (Minneapolis: University of Minnesota Press, 1995), 1–29.

Chatterjee, P., T. Guha-Thakurta and B. Kar (eds.), *New Cultural Histories of India: Materiality and Practices* (New Delhi: Oxford University Press, 2014).

Cipolla, C. M., *Miasma and Disease: Public Health and the Environment in the Pre-Industrial Age* (New Haven: Yale University Press, 1992).

Cohen, W. B., 'Malaria and French Imperialism', *Journal of African History*, 24 (1983), 23–36.

Cook, H. J., *Matters of Exchange: Commerce, Medicine and Science in the Dutch Golden Age* (New Haven: Yale University Press, 2007).

Coronil, F., *The Magical State: Nature, Money and Modernity in Venezuela* (Chicago: University of Chicago Press, 1997).

Crawford, M. J., *Empire's Experts: The Politics of Knowledge in Spain's Royal Monopoly of Quina, 1751–1808* (unpublished doctoral dissertation, University of California, San Diego, 2009).

Cueto, M., *Cold War, Deadly Fevers: Malaria Eradication in Mexico, 1955–1975* (Baltimore: Johns Hopkins University Press, 2007).

Cumming, D. A., 'John Macculloch at Addiscombe: The Lectureships on Chemistry and Geology', *Notes and Records of the Royal Society of London*, 34, 2 (February 1980), 155–183.

'MacCulloch, John (1773–1835)', *Oxford Dictionary of National Biography* (Oxford: Oxford University Press, 2004).

Dasgupta, R., 'Justice in a Landscape of Trees', http://humanitiesunderground .wordpress.com/2012/08/05/justice-in-a-landscape-of-trees/ [retrieved on 29 April 2013].

Daston, L., 'Historical Epistemology', in J. Chandler, A. I. Davidson and H. Harootunian (eds.), *Questions of Evidence: Proof, Practice and Persuasion Across the Disciplines* (Chicago: University of Chicago Press, 1994), 282–289.

'Science Studies and the History of Science', *Critical Inquiry*, 35, 4 (Summer 2009), 798–813.

Daston, L., and G. Mitman, *Thinking with Animals: New Perspectives on Anthropomorphism* (New York: Columbia University Press, 2005).

de Castro, E. V., 'Exchanging Perspectives: The Transformation of Objects into Subjects in Armendian Cosmologies', *Common Knowledge*, 10, 3 (2004), 463–484.

de Certeau, M., *The Practice of Everyday Life* (Los Angeles: University of California Press, 1984).

Dean, W., *Brazil and the Struggle for Rubber: A Study in Environmental History* (Cambridge: Cambridge University Press, 1987).

Deb Roy, R., 'Debility, Diet, Desire: Food in Nineteenth- and Early Twentieth-Century Bengali Manuals,' in S. Chaudhuri and R. B. Chatterjee (eds.), *The Writer's Feast: Food and the Cultures of Representation* (New Delhi: Orient Blackswan, 2011), 179–205.

'Mal-areas of Health: Dispersed Histories of a Diagnostic Category', *Economic and Political Weekly*, 42, 2 (January13–19, 2007), 122–129.

'Nonhuman Empires', *Comparative Studies of South Asia, Africa and the Middle East*, 35, 1 (May 2015), 66–75.

'Quinine, Mosquitoes and Empire: Reassembling Malaria in British India, 1890–1910', *South Asian History and Culture*, 4, 1 (January 2013), 65–86.

'Science, Medicine and New Imperial Histories', *British Journal for the History of Science*, 45, 3 (September 2012), 443–450.

Deleuze, G., 'Postscript on the Societies of Control', *October*, 59 (Winter, 1992), 3–7.

Deleuze, G., and F. Guattari, 'Rhizome', in *A Thousand Plateaus: Capitalism and Schizophrenia* (Minneapolis: University of Minnesota Press), 3–25.

Dobson, M., '"Marsh Fever": The Geography of Malaria in England', *Journal of Historical Geography*, 6, 4 (1980), 357–380.

Drayton, R., 'Maritime Networks and the Making of Knowledge', in D. Cannadine (ed.), *Empire, the Sea and Global History* (Basingstoke: Palgrave Macmillan, 2007), 72–82.

  Nature's Government: Science, Imperial Britain and the 'Improvement' of the World (New Haven: Yale University Press, 2000).

  'Science, Medicine and the British Empire', in R. W. Winks (ed.), *The Oxford History of the British Empire*, vol. 5, *Historiography* (Oxford: Oxford University Press, 1999), 264–275.

Dube, S., 'Terms that Bind: Colony, Nation, Modernity', in S. Dube (ed.), *Postcolonial Passages: Contemporary History-writing on India* (New Delhi: Oxford University Press, 2004), 1–37.

Elshakry, M., *Reading Darwin in Arabic: 1860–1950* (Chicago: University of Chicago Press, 2014).

Endersby, J., *Imperial Nature: Joseph Hooker and the Practices of Victorian Science* (Chicago: University of Chicago Press, 2008).

Evans, H., 'European Malaria Policy in the 1920s and 1930s: The Epidemiology of Minutiae', *Isis*, 80, 1 (March 1989), 40–59.

Fabian, J., *Time and the Other: How Anthropology Makes its Object* (New York: Columbia University Press, 1983).

Fan, F., 'The Global Turn in the History of Science,' *East Asian Science, Technology, and Society*, 6(2012), 249–258.

Farley, J., 'Parasites and the Germ Theory of Disease', in C. E. Rosenberg and J. Golden (eds.), *Framing Disease: Studies in Cultural History* (New Jersey: Rutgers University Press, 1992), 33–49.

  'The Spontaneous Generation Controversy (1700–1860): The Origin of Parasitic Worms', *Journal of the History of Biology*, 5, 1 (Spring, 1972), 95–125.

Foster, W. D., *A History of Parasitology* (Edinburgh: E&S Livingstone Ltd., 1965).

Ghosh, A., *The Calcutta Chromosome: A Novel of Fevers, Delirium and Discovery* (New Delhi: Ravi Dayal Publishers, 1996).

Ghosh, K., 'A Market for Aboriginality: Primitivism and Race Classification in the Indentured Labour Market of Colonial India', in G. Bhadra. G. Prakash and S. Tharu (eds.), *Subaltern Studies X: Writings on South Asian History and Society* (New Delhi: Oxford University Press, 1999), 8–48.

Gibson, S., *Animal, Vegetable, Mineral? How Eighteenth-Century Science Disrupted the Natural Order* (Oxford: Oxford University Press, 2015).

Golinsky, J., *Making Natural Knowledge: Constructivism and the History of Science* (Chicago: University of Chicago Press, 2005).

Goss, A., 'Building the World's Supply of Quinine: Dutch Colonialism and the Origins of a Global Pharmaceutical Industry', *Endeavour*, 31, 1 (March 2014), 8–18.

Goswami, M., 'From Swadeshi to Swaraj: Nation, Economy, Territory in Colonial South Asia', *Comparative Studies in Society and History*, 40, 4 (October, 1998), 609–636.

Goswami, M., *Producing India: From Colonial Economy to National Space* (Chicago: University of Chicago Press, 2004).

Grove, R. H., *Green Imperialism: Colonial Expansion, Tropical Island Edens and the Origins of Environmentalism, 1600–1860* (Cambridge: Cambridge University Press, 1996).

Guha-Thakurta, T., *Monuments, Objects, Histories: Institutions of Art in Colonial and Postcolonial India*, (New York: Columbia University Press, 2004).

Haas, L. F., 'Pierre Joseph Pelletier (1788–1842) and Jean Bienaime Caventou (1795–1887)', *Journal of Neurology, Neurosurgery and Psychiatry*, 57(1997), 1333.

Hacking, I., *Social Construction of What?* (Cambridge, Mass.: Harvard University Press, 1999).

Haraway, D., *Primate Visions: Gender, Race, and Nature in the World of Modern Science* (New York: Verso, 1989).

'Situated Knowledges: The Science Question in Feminism and the Privilege of Partial Perspective', in M. Biagioli (ed.), *Science Studies Reader* (London: Routledge, 1999), 172–188.

'Teddy Bear Patriarchy: Taxidermy in the Garden of Eden, New York City, 1908–1936', *Social Text*, 11 (Winter, 1984–1985), 20–64.

When Species Meet (Minneapolis: University of Minnesota Press, 2008).

Haraway, D. J., *Simians, Cyborgs and Women: The Reinvention of Nature* (New York: Routledge, 1991).

Harrison, M., *Climates and Constitutions: Health, Race, Environment and British Imperialism in India, 1600–1850* (New Delhi: Oxford University Press, 1999).

Disease and the Dilemmas of Development: A Malaria Strategy for Bombay Presidency, 1902–1942 (Calcutta: Estate and Trust Officer, University of Calcutta, 2011).

'"Hot Beds of Disease': Malaria and Civilisation in Nineteenth-Century British India", *Parassitologia*, 40 (1998), 11–18.

Medicine in an Age of Commerce and Empire: Britain and its Tropical Colonies, 1660– 1830 (Oxford: Oxford University Press, 2010).

Public Health in British India: Anglo-Indian Preventive Medicine, 1859–1914 (Cambridge: Cambridge University Press, 1994).

'Science and the British Empire', *Isis* 96(2005), 56–63.

The Medical War: British Military Medicine in the First World War (Oxford: Oxford University Press, 2010).

Hazareesingh, S., 'Cotton, Climate and Colonialism in Dharwar, Western India, 1840–1880', *Journal of Historical Geography*, 38, 1 (2012), 1–17.

Headrick, D., *The Tools of Empire: Technology and European Imperialism in the Nineteenth Century* (Oxford: Oxford University Press, 1981).

Hobhouse, H., *Seeds of Change: Five Plants that Transformed Mankind* (New York: Harper Collins, 1987).

Hodges, S., 'Governmentality, Population and the Reproductive Family in Modern India', *Economic and Political Weekly*, 39, 11 (13–19 March 2004), 1157–1163.

'The Global Menace', *Social History of Medicine*, 25, 3 (2012), 719–728.

Hoffman, M. A., *Malaria, Mosquitoes and Maps: Practices and Articulations of Malaria Control in British India and WWII* (Unpublished doctoral dissertation, University of California, San Diego, 2016).

Holger Maehle, A., *Drugs on Trial: Experimental Pharmacology and Therapeutic Innovation in the Eighteenth Century* (Amsterdam: Rodopi, 1999).

Honigsbaum, M., *The Fever Trail: The Hunt for the Cure for Malaria* (London: Macmillan, 2001).

Hoogte, A. R., and T. Pieters, 'Science in the Service of Colonial Agro-Industralism: The Case of Cinchona Cultivation in the Dutch and British East Indies, 1852–1900', *Studies in the History and Philosophy of Biological and Biomedical Sciences*, 47, PA (September 2014), 12–22.

'Science, Industry and the Colonial State: A Shift from the German- to a Dutch-controlled Cinchona and Quinine Cartel (1880–1920)', *History and Technology*, 31, 1 (2 January 2015), 2–36.

Hoskins, J., *Biographical Objects: How Things Tell the Stories of People's Lives* (New York: Routledge, 1998).

Hughes, J. E., *Animal Kingdoms: Hunting, the Environment and Power in the Indian Princely States* (Cambridge, Mass.: Harvard University Press, 2013).

Humphreys, M., *Malaria: Poverty, Race and Public Health in the United States* (Baltimore: Johns Hopkins University Press, 2001).

Jansen, S., 'An American Insect in Imperial Germany: Visibility and Control in the Making of the Phylloxera in Germany, 1870–1914', *Science in Context*, 13, 1 (2000), 31–70.

Jarcho, S., *Quinine's Predecessor: Francesco Torti and the Early History of Cinchona* (Baltimore: Johns Hopkins University Press, 1993).

'Review of M. A. Barber, *A Malariologist in Many Lands*', *Journal of History of Medicine and Allied Sciences*, 2, 2 (Spring, 1947), 268–270.

Jones, R., *Mosquito* (London: Reaktion Books, 2012).

Joyce, P., 'What is the Social in Social History?', *Past and Present*, 205 (November, 2009), 175–210.

Kar, B., 'Historia Elastica: A Note on the Rubber Hunt in the North-Eastern Frontier of British India', *Indian Historical Review*, 36, 1 (2009), 131–150.

Kaviraj, S., 'The Imaginary Institution of India', in P. Chatterjee and G. Pandey (eds.), *Subaltern Studies VII* (Delhi: Oxford University Press, 1992), 1–39.

Keevak, M., *Becoming Yellow: A Short History of Racial Thinking* (New Jersey: Princeton University Press, 2011).

Kirkwood, J. H., and C. H. Lloyd, *John Eliot Howard: A Budget of Papers on His Life and Work* (Oxford: Lloyd, 1995).

Kirsch S., and D. Mitchell, 'The Nature of Things: Dead Labor, Nonhuman Actors, and the Persistence of Marxism', *Antipode*, 36 (2004), 687–705.

Klein, I., 'Malaria and Mortality in Bengal, 1840–1921', *Indian Economic and Social History Review*, 9 (1972), 132–160.

Kowal, E., J. Radin and J. Reardon, 'Indigenous Body Parts, Mutating Tempo-ralities, and the Half-lives of Postcolonial Technoscience', *Social Studies of Science*, 43, 4 (2013), 465–483.

Kumar, P., *Indigo Plantations and Science in Colonial India* (Cambridge: Cambridge University Press, 2013).

LaCapra, D., *History and its Limits: Human, Animal and Violence* (Ithaca: Cornell University Press, 2009).

Latour, B., 'On the Partial Existence of Existing and Nonexisting Objects,' in L. Daston (ed.), *Biographies of Scientific Objects* (Chicago: University of Chicago Press, 1999), 247–269.

Pandora's Hope: Essays in the Reality of Science Studies (Cambridge, Mass.: Harvard University Press, 1999).

Reassembling the Social: An Introduction to Actor-Network Theory (Oxford: Oxford University Press, 2005).

Science in Action: How to Follow Scientists and Engineers through Society (Cambridge, Mass.: Harvard University Press, 1987).

'The Promises of Constructivism' in D. Ihde and E. Selinger (eds.), *Chasing Technoscience: Matrix of Materiality* (Bloomington: Indiana University Press, 2003), 27–46.

We Have Never Been Modern (Cambridge Mass.: Harvard University Press, 1993).

'Whose Cosmos, Which Cosmopolitics? Comments on the Peace Terms of Ulrich Beck', *Common Knowledge* 10, 3 (2004), 450–462.

Law, R. S., *The End of a Chapter: The Story of Whiffen and Sons Limited, Fine Chemical Manufacturers* (London: Fisons, 1973).

LaWall, C. H., 'The History of Quinine', *Medical Life*, 38, 4 (April 1931), 195–216.

Lewis, T. E., 'Swarm Intelligence: Rethinking Swarm Intelligence from within the Transversal Commons', *Culture, Theory and Critique*, 51, 3 (2010), 223–238.

Li, S., 'Natural History of Parasitic Disease: Patrick Manson's Philosophical Method', *Isis*, 93 (2002), 206–228.

Livingstone, D. N., 'Tropical Climate and Moral Hygiene: The Anatomy of a Victorian Debate', *The British Journal for the History of Science*, 32, 1 (March 1999), 93–110.

Mackinnon, A. S., 'Of Oxford Bags and Twirling Canes: The State, Popular Responses, and Zulu Antimalaria Assistants in the Early-Twentieth Century Zululand Malaria Campaigns', *Radical History Review*, 80 (Spring, 2001), 76–100.

Macleod, R., (ed.), *Nature and Empire: Science and the Colonial Enterprise, Osiris*, 15 (Chicago: University of Chicago Press, 2000).

Majori, G., 'Short History of Malaria and its Eradication in Italy with Short Notes on the Fight Against the Infection in the Mediterranean Basin', *Mediterranean Journal of Hematology and Infectious Diseases*, 4, 1 (2012), www.ncbi.nlm.nih.gov/pmc/articles/PMC3340992/ [retrieved on 6 June 2016].

Marks, S., 'What is Colonial about Colonial Medicine? And What Has Happened to Imperialism and Health', *Social History of Medicine*, 10 (1997), 205–219.

McClintock, A. *Imperial Leather: Race, Gender and Sexuality in the Colonial Context* (New York: Routledge, 1995).

McNeill, J. R., *Mosquito Empires: Ecology and War in the Greater Caribbean* (Cambridge: Cambridge University Press, 2010).

Mehta, U. S., *Liberalism and Empire: A Study in Nineteenth-Century British Liberal Thought* (Chicago: University of Chicago Press, 1999).

Miller, D. P., and P. H. Reill (eds.), *Visions of Empire: Voyages, Botany and Representations of Nature* (Cambridge and New York: Cambridge University Press, 1996).

Mintz, S., *Sweetness and Power: The Place of Sugar in Modern History* (New York: Penguin Group, 1985).

Mishra, S., 'Beasts, Murrains and the British Raj: Reassessing Colonial Medicine in India from the Veterinary Perspective, 1860–1900', *Bulletin of the History of Medicine*, 85, 2 (2011), 587–619.

Mitchell, T., *Carbon Democracy: Political Power in the Age of Oil* (New York: Verso, 2011).

Rule of Experts: Egypt, Techno-politics, Modernity (Los Angeles: University of California Press, 2002).

'Society, Economy and the State Effect', in G. Steinmetz (ed.), *State/Culture: State Formation After the Cultural Turn* (Ithaca: Cornell University Press, 1999), 76–97.

Mitman, G., 'In Search of Health: Landscape and Disease in American Environmental History', *Environmental History*, 10, 2 (April 2005), 184–210.

Moll, J. M. H., 'William Saunders, 1743–1817', *Journal of Medical Biography*, 1(November 1993), 235.

Monnais, L., 'Rails, Roads and Mosquito Foes: The State Quinine Service in French Indochina', in R. Peckham and D. M. Pomfret (eds.), *Imperial Contagions: Medicine, Hygiene and Cultures of Planning in Asia* (Hong Kong: Hong Kong University Press, 2013), 195–213.

Mukharji, P. B., *Nationalizing the Body: The Medical Market, Print and Daktari Medicine* (London: Anthem Press, 2009).

'Symptoms of Dis-Ease: New Trends in Histories of "Indigenous" South Asian Medicines', *History Compass*, 9, 12 (2011), 887–899.

'The "Cholera Cloud" in the Nineteenth-Century "British World": History of an Object-Without-an-essence', *Bulletin of the History of Medicine*, 86 (Fall, 2012), 303–332.

Mukherjee, A., 'The Peruvian Bark Revisited: A Critique of British Cinchona Policy in Colonial India', *Bengal Past and Present*, 117 (1998), 81–102.

Mukhopadhyay, B., *Sanjibchandra: Jibon o Sahitya (Sanjibchandra: His Life and Works)* (Calcutta: Pustak Biponi, 1988).

Murray Fallis, A., 'Malaria in the Eighteenth and Nineteenth Centuries in Ontario', *Bulletin of the Canadian History of Medicine*, 1, 2 (1984), 25–38.

Muthu, S., *Enlightenment Against Empire* (New Jersey: Princeton University Press, 2003).

Nappi, C., *The Monkey and the Inkpot: Natural History and its Transformations in Early Modern China* (Cambridge Mass.: Harvard University Press, 2009).

Naraindas, H., 'Poisons, Putrescence and the Weather: A Genealogy of the Advent of Tropical Medicine', *Contributions to Indian Sociology*, 30, 1 (1996), 1–35.

Osborne, M. A., and R. A. Fogarty, 'Medical Climatology in France: The Persistence of Neo-Hippocratic Ideas in the First Half of the Twentieth Century', *Bulletin of the History of Medicine*, 86, 4 (Winter 2012), 543–563.

Packard, R. M. and P. Gadehla, 'A Land Filled with Mosquitoes: Fred L. Soper, the Rockefeller Foundation, and the Anopheles Gambiae Invasion of Brazil', *Medical Anthropology: Cross-Cultural Studies in Health and Illness*, 17, 3 (1997), 215–238.

Packard, R. M., 'Maize, Cattle and Mosquitoes: The Political Economy of Malaria Epidemics in Colonial Swaziland', *The Journal of African History*, 25, 2 (1984), 189–212.

'Malaria Blocks Development Revisited: The Role of Disease in the History of Agricultural Development in the Eastern and Northern Transvaal Lowveld, 1890–1960', *Journal of Southern African Studies*, 27, 3 (2001), 591–612.

The Making of a Tropical Disease: A Short History of Malaria (Baltimore: Johns Hopkins University Press, 2007).

Palmero, J. R., and A. R. Vega, 'Spanish Agriculture and Malaria in the Eighteenth Century', *History and Philosophy of Life Science*, 10 (1998), 343–362.

Pande, I., *Medicine, Race and Liberalism: Symptoms of Empire* (New York: Routledge, 2010).

Pearse, D. E., 'Author', in F. Lentricchia and T. McLaughlin (eds.), *Critical Terms for Literary Study* (Chicago: University of Chicago Press, 1990), 105–117.

Perez, C., *Quinine and Caudillos: Manual Isidoro Belzu and the Cinchona Bark Trade in Bolivia, 1848–1855* (unpublished doctoral dissertation, University of California at Los Angeles, 1998).

Philip, K., *Civilising Natures: Race, Resources and Modernity in South Asia* (Hyderabad: Orient Longman, 2004).

Pickering, A., 'The Mangle of Practice: Agency and Emergence in the Sociology of Science', *American Journal of Sociology*, 99, 3 (November, 1993), 559–589.

Prasad, A., 'Science in Motion: What Postcolonial Science Studies Can Offer', *Electronic Journal of Communication Information & Innovation in Health (RECIIS)* 2, 2 (July–December 2008), 35–47.

Qureshi, S., *Peoples on Parade: Exhibitions, Empire and Anthropology in Nineteenth-Century Britain* (Chicago: University of Chicago Press, 2011).

Raffles, H., 'Jews, Lice and History,' *Public Culture*, 19, 3 (Fall, 2007), 521–566.

'Towards a Critical Natural History', *Antipode* 37, 2 (2005), 374–378.

Raj, K., 'Beyond Postcolonialism . . . and Postpositivism: Circulation and the Global History of Science', *Isis*, 104, 2 (June 2013), 337–347.

Relocating Modern Science: Circulation and the Construction of Scientific Knowledge in South Asia and Europe, 1650–1900 (Palgrave Macmillan: New York, 2007).

Ramaswamy, S., 'Catastrophic Cartographies: Mapping the Lost Continent of Lemuria', *Representations*, 67 (Summer, 1999), 92–129.

Ramesh, A., 'Scientific Commodities, Imperial Dreams', *Studies in the History and Philosophy of Biological and Biomedical Sciences*, (2016), http://dx.doi.org/10.1016/j.shpsc.2016.04.006 [retrieved on 10 July 2016].

Rangarajan, M., 'The Raj and the Natural World: The War Against Dangerous Beasts in Colonial India', *Studies in History*, 14, 2 (1998), 265–299.

Ravi, S., 'Indian Police fighting Maoists "dying of malaria"', *BBC* (Tuesday, 23 February 2010), http://news.bbc.co.uk/1/hi/world/south_asia/8529615.stm [retrieved on 24 March 2014].

Rocco, F., *Quinine: Malaria and the Quest for a Cure that Changed the World* (London: Harper Collins, 2003).

Rogers, N., 'Germs with Legs: Flies, Disease and the New Public Health', *Bulletin of the History of Medicine*, 63 (Winter, 1989), 599–617.

Roy, A., *The God of Small Things* (London: Flamingo, 1997).

Rupke, N. A. (ed.), *Medical Geography in Historical Perspective, Medical History, Supplement No. 20* (London: Wellcome Trust Centre for the History of Medicine at UCL, 2000).

Russell III, E. P., '"Speaking of Annihilation", Mobilizing for War against Human and Insect Enemies, 1914–1945', *The Journal of American History*, 82, 4 (March 1996), 1505–1529.

Saha, J., 'A Mockery of Justice: Colonial Law, the Everyday State and Village Politics in the Burma Delta, c. 1890–1910', *Past and Present*, 217, 1 (2012), 187–212.

Said, E. W., 'Invention, Memory, and Place', *Critical Inquiry*, 26, 2 (Winter, 2000), 175–192.

Sallares, R., *Malaria and Rome: A History of Malaria in Ancient Italy* (Oxford: Oxford University Press, 2002).

Samanta, A., *Malarial Fever in Colonial Bengal, 1820–1939: Social History of an Epidemic* (Kolkata: Firma KLM, 2002).

Samyn, J., 'Cruel Consciousness: Louis Figuier, John Ruskin and the Value of Insects', *Nineteenth-Century Literature*, 71, 1 (2016), 89–114.

Sarma, S., *The Ecology and the Epidemic: A Study on the Nineteenth-Century Controversy* (Calcutta: India Book Exchange, 1999).

Schaffer, S., 'Enlightened Automata', in W. Clark, J. Golinski and S. Schaffer (eds.), *The Sciences in Enlightened Europe* (Chicago: University of Chicago Press, 1999), 126–165.

'Self Evidence', in J. Chandler, A. I. Davidson and H. Harootunian (eds.), *Questions of Evidence: Proof, Practice and Persuasion Across the Disciplines* (Chicago: University of Chicago Press, 1994), 56–91.

Schiebinger, L., and C. Swan, 'Introduction' in Schiebinger and Swan (eds.), *Colonial Botany: Science, Commerce and Politics in the Early Modern World* (Philadelphia: University of Pennsylvania Press, 2005), 1–18.

Schiebinger, L., *Plants and Empire: Colonial Bioprospecting in the Atlantic World* (Cambridge, Mass.: Harvard University Press, 2004).

Secord, J. A., 'John MacCulloch: Geology and the Appreciation of Landscape', [Unpublished manuscript].

'King of Siluria: Roderick Murchison and the Imperial Theme in Nineteenth-Century British Geology', *Victorian Studies*, 25, 4 (Summer 1982), 413–442.

Shapin, S. and S. Schaffer, *Leviathan and Air Pump: Hobbes, Boyle and the Experimental Life* (New Jersey: Princeton University Press, 1985).

Shukin, N., *Animal Capital: Rendering Life in Biopolitical Times* (Minneapolis: University of Minnesota Press, 2009).

Sismondo, S., 'Some Social Constructions', *Social Studies of Science*, 23, 3 (August 1993), 515–553.

Sivaramakrishnan, K., *Modern Forests: Statemaking and Environmental Change in Colonial Eastern India* (Stanford: Stanford University Press, 1999).

Old Potions, New Bottles: Recasting Indigenous Medicine in Colonial Punjab (New Delhi: Orient Longman, 2006).

Sivasundaram, S., *Nature and the Godly Empire: Science and the Evangelical Mission in the Pacific* (Cambridge: Cambridge University Press, 2005).

'Sciences and the Global: On Methods, Questions and Theory', *Isis*, 101 (2010), 146–158.

'Trading Knowledge: The East India Company's Elephants in India and Britain', *The Historical Journal*, 48, 1 (2005), 27–63.

Skaria, A., *Hybrid Histories: Forests, Frontiers and Wildness in Western India* (New Delhi: Oxford University Press, 1999).

Slater, L. B., *War and Disease: Biomedical Research on Malaria on the Twentieth Century* (New Brunswick: Rutgers University Press, 2009).

Snowden, F. M. and R. Bucala (eds.), *The Global Challenge of Malaria: Past Lessons and Future Prospects* (Singapore: World Scientific Publishing, 2014).

Snowden, F. M., *The Conquest of Malaria, Italy 1900–1962* (New Haven: Yale University Press, 2006).

Soren, D., 'Can Archaeologists Excavate Evidence of Malaria?', *World Archaeology*, 35, 2 (October 2003), 193–209.

Spary, E. C., 'Of Nutmegs and Botanists: The Colonial Cultivation of Botanical Identity', in L. Schiebinger and C. Swan (eds.), *Colonial Botany: Science, Commerce and Politics in the Early Modern World* (Philadelphia: University of Pennsylvania Press, 2005), 187–203.

Special Correspondent, 'Maoist Link to Malaria', *The Telegraph* (Thursday, 29 October 2009), www.telegraphindia.com/1091029/jsp/frontpage/story_11672759.jsp [retrieved on 24 March 2014].

Srivastava, M. (ed.), *Branding New: Advertising Through the Times of India* (Faridabad: Thomson, India, 1989).

Stapleton, D. H., 'Internationalism and Nationalism: The Rockefeller Foundation, Public Health and Malaria in Italy, 1923–1951', *Parassitologia*, 42, 1–2 (June, 2000), 127–134.

Stocking Jr., G. W., (ed.), *Observers Observed: Essays on Ethnographic Fieldwork* (Madison: University of Wisconsin Press, 1983).

Stoler, A. L., *Race and the Education of Desire: Foucault's History of Sexuality and the Colonial Order of Things* (Durham: Duke University Press, 1995).

Stoler, A. L. and F. Cooper, 'Between Metropole and Colony: Rethinking a Research Agenda', in A. L. Stoler and F. Cooper (eds.), *Tensions of Empire:*

Colonial Cultures in a Bourgeois World (Los Angeles: University of California Press, 1997), 1–46.

Strickland, W. A., 'Quinine Pills: Manufactured on the Missouri Frontier (1832–1862)', *Pharmacy in History*, 25, 2 (1983), 61–68.

Sufian, S. M., *Healing the Land and the Nation: Malaria and the Zionist Project in Palestine, 1920–1947* (Chicago: University of Chicago Press, 2007).

Swellengrebel, N. H., 'How the Malaria Service in Indonesia Came into Being, 1898–1948', *The Journal of Hygiene*, 48, 2 (June 1950), 146–157.

Tomic, S., 'Chemical Analysis of Plants: The Case of Cinchona', *Annals of Science*, 58, 3 (2001), 287–309.

Totelin, L., 'Botanizing Rulers and their Herbal Subjects: Plants and Political Power in Greek and Roman Literature', *Phoenix*, 66, 1–2 (2012), 122–144.

Trease, G. E., 'Pierre-Joseph Pelletier (1788–1842): The Discoverer of Quinine', *British Journal of Pharmaceutical Practice*, 2, 7 (1980), 32–33.

Trentmann, F., "Materiality in the Future of History: Things, Practices and Politics', *The Journal of British Studies*, 48, 2 (April 2009), 283–307.

Tresch, J., *The Romantic Machine: Utopian Science and Technology after Napoleon* (Chicago: University of Chicago Press, 2012).

Unwin, T., 'A Waste of Space? Towards a Critique of the Social Production of Space', *Transactions of the Institute of British Geographers*, New Series, 25, 1 (2000), 11–29.

van Binsbergen, W., 'Commodification: Things, Agency, and Identities', in W. van Binsbergen and P. Geschiere (eds.), *Commodification: Things, Agency and Identities: The Social Life of Things Revisited* (Berlin/Muenster/Vienna/London: LIT, 2005), 9–51.

Vaughan, M., *Curing their Ills: Colonial Power and African Illness* (Stanford: Stanford University Press, 1991).

Veale, L., *A Historical Geography of the Nilgiri Cinchona Plantations, 1860–1900* (unpublished doctoral dissertation, University of Nottingham, 2010).

Watts, S., 'British Development Policies and Malaria in India 1897–c. 1929', *Past & Present* 165, (November 1999), 141–181.

Webb Jr, J. L. A., *Humanity's Burden: A Global History of Malaria* (Cambridge: Cambridge University Press, 2008).
    The Long Struggle Against Malaria in Tropical Africa (Cambridge: Cambridge University Press, 2014).

Western, J., and S. Frenkel, 'Pretext or Prophylaxis? Racial Segregation and Malarial Mosquitoes in a British Tropical Colony: Sierra Leone', *Annals of the Association of American Geographers*, 78, 2 (June 1988), 211–228.

Whitcombe, E., 'The Environmental Costs of Irrigation in British India: Waterlogging, Salinity, Malaria', in D. Arnold and R. Guha (eds.), *Nature, Culture and Imperialism: Essays on the Environmentalist History of South Asia* (New Delhi: Oxford University Press, 1996), 237–257.

White, L., 'Tsetse Visions: Narratives of Blood and Bugs in Colonial Northern Rhodesia, 1931–1939', *Journal of African History*, 36 (1995), 219–245.

Wickramasinghe, N., *Metallic Modern: Everyday Machines in Colonial Sri Lanka* (New York and Oxford: Berghahn Press, 2014).

Williams, D., 'Clements Roberts Markham and the Introduction of the Cinchona Trees into British India, 1861,' *The Geographical Journal*, 128, 4 (December 1962), 431–442.

Wilson, J., *The Domination of Strangers: Modern Governance in Eastern India, 1780–1835* (Basingstoke: Palgrave Macmillan, 2008).

Winther, P., *Anglo-European Science and the Rhetoric of Empire: Malaria, Opium and British Rule in India, 1756–1895* (Oxford: Lexington Books, 2005).

Worboys, M., 'From Miasmas to Germs: Malaria 1850–1879', *Parassitologia*, 36 (1994), 61–68.

'Germs, Malaria and the Invention of Mansonian Tropical Medicine', in D. Arnold (ed.) *Warm Climates and Western Medicine: The Emergence of Tropical Medicine, 1500–1900* (Amsterdam-Atlanta: Rodopi, 1996), 181–207.

Spreading Germs: Disease Theories and Medical Practice in Britain, 1865–1900 (Cambridge: Cambridge University Press, 2000).

Wrigley, R., and G. Revill (eds.), *Pathologies of Travel* (Amsterdam: Rodopi, 2000).

Yip K., (ed.), *Disease, Colonialism and the State: Malaria in Modern East Asian History* (Hong Kong: Hong Kong University Press, 2009).

Zurbrigg, S., 'Hunger and Epidemic Malaria in Punjab, 1868–1940', *Economic and Political Weekly*, 27, 4 (25 January 1992), 2–26.

Zwierlein, A., 'Unmapped Countries: Biology, Literature and Culture in the Nineteenth Century' in A. Zwierlein (ed.), *Unmapped Countries: Biological Visions in Nineteenth-Century Literature and Culture* (London: Anthem Press, 2005), 1–14.

Zylberman, P., 'A Transatlantic Dispute: The Etiology of Malaria and the Redesign of the Mediterranean Landscape', in S. G. Solomon, L. Murard and P. Zylberman (eds.), *Shifting Boundaries of Public Health: Europe in the Twentieth Century* (Rochester: University of Rochester Press, 2008), 269–297.

Index

Printed in the United States
By Bookmasters

Printed in the United States
By Bookmasters